CHILDBIRTH AND THE DISPLAY OF
AUTHORITY IN EARLY MODERN FRANCE

Women and Gender in the Early Modern World

Series Editors: Allyson Poska and Abby Zanger

In the past decade, the study of women and gender has offered some of the most vital and innovative challenges to scholarship on the early modern period. Ashgate's new series of interdisciplinary and comparative studies, *Women and Gender in the Early Modern World*, takes up this challenge, reaching beyond geographical limitations to explore the experiences of early modern women and the nature of gender in Europe, the Americas, Asia, and Africa. Submissions of single-author studies and edited collections will be considered.

Titles in the series include:

Midwiving Subjects in Shakespeare's England
Caroline Bicks

Widowhood and Visual Culture in Early Modern Europe
Edited by Allison Levy

Women and the Book Trade in Sixteenth-Century France
Susan Broomhall

Publishing Women's Life Stories in France, 1647–1720
From Voice to Print
Elizabeth C. Goldsmith

The Power and Patronage of Marguerite de Navarre
Barbara Stephenson

Architecture and the Politics of Gender in Early Modern Europe
Edited by Helen Hills

Women, Art and the Politics of Identity in Eighteenth-Century Europe
Edited by Melissa Hyde and Jennifer Milam

Childbirth and the Display of Authority in Early Modern France

LIANNE MCTAVISH
University of New Brunswick, Canada

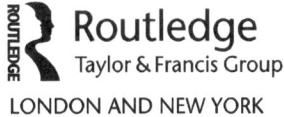

Routledge
Taylor & Francis Group

LONDON AND NEW YORK

First published 2005 by Ashgate Publishing

Published 2016 by Routledge
2 Park Square, Milton Park, Abingdon, Oxon OX14 4RN
711 Third Avenue, New York, NY 10017, USA

Routledge is an imprint of the Taylor & Francis Group, an informa business

British Library Cataloguing in Publication Data
McTavish, Lianne
  Childbirth and the display of authority in early modern
  France. – (Women and gender in the early modern world)
  1. Midwives – France – History – 16th century 2. Midwives –
  France – History – 17th century 3. Midwives –
  History – 18th century 4. Midwifery – France – History –
  16th century 5. Midwifery – France – History – 17th century
  6. Midwifery – France – History – 18th century 7. Childbirth
  – France – History 8. Midwives in art 9. Childbirth in art
  10. Obstetrics – France – History
  I. Title
  618.2'00944'0903

Library of Congress Cataloging-in-Publication Data
McTavish, Lianne, 1967–
    Childbirth and the display of authority in early modern France / Lianne McTavish.
      p. cm. — (Women and gender in the early modern world)
    Includes bibliographical references and index.
    ISBN 0-7546-3619-4 (alk. paper)
    1. Childbirth—France—History. 2. Pregnancy—France—History. 3. Obstetrics—
France—History. I. Title. II. Series.

  RG652.M385 2004
  618.2'00944—dc22

                                                                    2004008774

ISBN 13: 978-0-7546-3619-9 (hbk)

For Lee

Contents

List of Figures

Acknowledgements

My interest in early modern midwifery was sparked during a period of intense anti-abortion activity in upper New York state. When the pro-life group Operation Rescue attempted to blockade clinics in Buffalo during the Spring of 1992, I joined hundreds of other pro-choice volunteers to defend access to abortion. Standing side by side with arms linked, we shielded the clinic entrances with our bodies, keeping the handful of ostensible rescuers at bay. Overhearing a great deal of abortion rhetoric on the front lines, I desired to learn more about the history of women's reproduction. I could not launch into a new research project, however, before completing my doctoral dissertation in the University of Rochester's Program of Visual and Cultural Studies. Training to become an art historian steeped in critical theory, my thesis was on representations of the Académie royale de peinture et de sculpture [Royal Academy of Painting and Sculpture] in Paris, an initially small association of artists founded in 1648. Nevertheless, while undertaking research in Paris in 1994, I started ferreting out early modern sources related to pregnancy and childbirth. Captivated by the engravings of unborn figures and author portraits in French obstetrical treatises, I resolved to study their social, cultural, and medical significance. This book is the result.

My interdisciplinary interpretation of obstetrical treatises incurred substantial scholarly debts. Generous funding was provided by the Social Sciences and Humanities Research Council of Canada (1997–2000), and Associated Medical Services/Hannah Institute for the History of Medicine (2001). These grants allowed me to travel to European and North American libraries and archives. I thank the helpful staff at the Archives nationales, Bibliothèque nationale, Cabinet des estampes, Archives de l'assistance publique, Musée du Louvre, Bibliothèque interuniversitaire de médecine, Musée d'histoire de la médecine, Bibliothèque de l'Académie nationale de médecine, and Bibliothèque Sainte-Geneviève in Paris; British Library and Wellcome Library in London; National Library of Medicine in Bethesda, MD; Edward G. Miner Library, University of Rochester Medical Center, in Rochester, NY; and libraries of the University of Rochester, University of Western Ontario, University of Toronto, and University of New Brunswick.

I could not have completed this project without the warm welcome of historians of medicine Hilary Marland, Helen King, and David Harley. Adrianna Bakos, Lisa Cartwright, Elizabeth Harvey, Ludmilla Jordanova, and Gerhild Williams encouraged me to give papers at conferences. My colleagues in the Department of

History at the University of New Brunswick provided a stimulating learning environment; Steven Turner and Beverly Lemire deserve special mention for responding to portions of the manuscript in progress, while Linda Kealey commented on a more polished draft. Gillian Thompson, Wladyslaw Cichocki, and Nathalie Comeau checked some of my French translations. When quoting directly from the early modern texts, I have retained original spelling and accent use. Colleagues at other universities, including Susan Broomhall and Lisa Forman Cody, read the manuscript before it was published, providing feedback and criticism. Professors Cristelle Baskins, Jeffrey Ravel, Holly Tucker, and graduate student Heather Molyneaux also supplied important assistance.

Thanks are due to the anonymous referees of the manuscript as well as to my editors at Ashgate, Erika Gaffney, Allyson Poska, and Abby Zanger.

Parts of Chapters 3 and 4 were previously published in the *Journal of the Social History of Medicine*, and its editors have kindly granted permission to reprint that material here.

Friends and family supporting me over the years include Chris Black, Hart Caplan, Janice Wright Cheney, Lorrie McTavish Egerter, Hannah Lane, Dale McTavish, Maja Padrov, Jill Ruby, Laura Soskin, the Spence family, Vlad Tasic, and Alice Taylor. Although they may not know it, fellow members of Pro-Choice New Brunswick provided constant motivation, especially while escorting in frigid weather outside the Morgentaler clinic in Fredericton. Finally, I owe a debt of gratitude to Lee Spence, for showing me there is much more to life than work. This book is dedicated to him.

Introduction

Interpreting Obstetrical Treatises

Throughout the early modern period in France, *chirurgiens accoucheurs* [surgeon men-midwives] were predominantly associated with both sexual impropriety and physical danger. Female midwives governed the birthing chamber, inviting men to assist at deliveries after days of unsuccessful labour, when the child was likely dead and the life of the mother in peril.[1] These men attempted to turn the child in the womb manually, or used instruments, such as *crochets* [hooks], to perform craniotomies, a procedure that entailed crushing the infant's head and extracting its body piece by piece. Not surprisingly, the appearance of the surgeon man-midwife was identified with death, and he was regularly likened to both a butcher and a hangman.[2] French surgeons slowly managed, however, to change their image, attending even the uncomplicated deliveries of wealthy, urban clients by the late eighteenth century.

The transitional period heralding the rise of male birth assistants has attracted attention from scholars determined to discover the complex medical, social, and cultural factors that encouraged the increased role of men in childbirth.[3] Like these academics, I am interested in how men-midwives began to appear at deliveries. Unlike accounts that emphasize the development of male medical knowledge and use of instruments, however, my primary concern is with how surgeon men-midwives were recognized as experts embodying obstetrical authority, instead of threatening intruders. How did men ever appear to be skilled, trustworthy birth assistants at a time when women – equipped with an intimate experience of pregnancy and labour – were 'naturally' associated with childbirth?

In order to answer this question, I analyse a range of sources, focusing on 24 obstetrical treatises produced in France between 1550 and 1730.[4] Primarily written by surgeon men-midwives, the lengthy treatises cover all aspects of childbirth, from theories of conception to signs of pregnancy, labour, and postpartum complaints. Male practitioners described in detail the emergency situations to which they had been called. Their writing is accompanied by vivid images representing unborn figures floating in large oval wombs, surgical tools classified according to use, and portraits of authors. Obstetrical treatises enjoyed numerous editions as well as translations into multiple languages, addressing a diverse audience that consisted of male medical practitioners, female midwives, pregnant women, lay people, and even readers in search of a sex manual.

Scholars have long recognized obstetrical treatises as influential sources contributing to the acceptance of male attendance at births.[5] For the most part, the treatises are identified with the transmission of male medical theory and denigration of female midwives: the medicalization of childbirth that severed the 'natural' link between maternal knowledge and the female body. My study offers a different point of view. I argue that obstetrical treatises were sites for both the production and contestation of what anthropologist Brigitte Jordan calls authoritative knowledge in childbirth.[6] Jordan asserts that while numerous knowledge systems exist in any given domain, one tends to dominate, being perceived as obvious rather than a result of negotiation and struggle. During the early modern period, the belief that childbirth was best left to women was challenged, but the technocratic model of birth now commonplace in Canada, the United States, and much of Western Europe – with its lack of respect for women's bodily knowledge – was far from established; it became dominant in the twentieth century.[7] There was no single kind of authoritative obstetrical knowledge in early modern France, but rather various articulations of knowledge vying for that status. I consider how claims about authority in childbirth were organized and displayed, advanced and defended in obstetrical treatises.

I argue the treatises neither merely delivered male medical knowledge nor disparaged maternal experience. Surgeon men-midwives formulated male obstetrical authority both in relation to and distinction from representations of female midwives and the maternal body. Though these authors championed men's anatomical knowledge, they also appreciated the firsthand, bodily experience of maternity traditionally associated with women. Exploring the contradictory images of male and female midwives in obstetrical treatises, my study reveals early modern masculinity as precarious, not hegemonic. Representations of femininity are equally unstable, especially in publications written by women such as Louise Bourgeois, royal midwife to Queen Marie de Médicis from 1601 to 1609. My interpretations undermine characterizations of the practice of childbirth in early modern Europe as a gender war which men ultimately won, an inaccurate description already criticized by historians Hilary Marland and Adrian Wilson.[8]

Emphasizing the display of obstetrical authority leads me to pay special attention to the images in the treatises, fascinating woodcuts and engravings that have never before been studied. I investigate, for example, the author portraits that regularly acted as frontispieces to treatises, noting how they present visual arguments about status, gender, and the sources of expertise in midwifery. My approach is in dialogue with the scholarship of Ludmilla Jordanova, an art historian who argues that portraiture was central to the individual and collective identities of eighteenth- and nineteenth-century British medical practitioners.[9] Drawing on my knowledge of art history, cultural studies, and the history of medicine, I insist that the plates in obstetrical treatises are crucial to a fuller understanding of both the publications themselves and the claims made about birthing practices in early modern Europe.

Obstetrical treatises portray social and visual relations that are otherwise difficult to grasp. They discuss royal births, medical rivalries, and appropriate behaviour in the lying-in chamber. A host of characters appear in the publications, including surgeon men-midwives, physicians, female midwives, unborn children, and women in labour. The significance of this material extends far beyond the birthing chamber. My study addresses important instances of the construction of identity, performance of gender, definition of the body, and negotiation of social roles in early modern France. It considers the history and representation of gestures, looking, status, authority, and print culture. A wide range of scholars, consisting of art historians, literary critics, practitioners of women's studies, and political as well as cultural historians, should therefore find relevant information in the pages that follow.

Thinking Visually

The images in early modern French obstetrical treatises are worthy of careful visual analysis. Many art historians specializing in seventeenth-century France concentrate on the work of canonized artists such as Nicolas Poussin.[10] Their neglect of medical imagery results, in part, from the longstanding privileging of painting at the expense of printmaking in the history of French visual culture. Ranked beneath painting and sculpture by the Académie royale de peinture et de sculpture in Paris, engraving continues to be awarded a lower status notwithstanding the substantial role of reproducible plates in the production of knowledge during the early modern period. In contrast, historians generally rely on written records more than visual ones, in keeping with traditional hierarchies linking writing with intellectual activity, and images with material artifice. Art historian Barbara Maria Stafford argues that even as optical demonstration is considered crucial to enlightenment, images are linked with misleading illusion.[11] According to her, collaboration between art historians and other scholars is hindered by the enduring presumption that visual images are unreliable unless explicated by written texts.

Though historians of childbirth favour written documents, they examine an impressive range of them, including midwifery licenses, personal letters, unpublished record books, and published medical treatises.[12] Visual sources are not entirely overlooked; for example, Jordanova performs sophisticated analyses of British images related to childbirth. In a fascinating study of Allan Ramsay's painted portrait of the famous eighteenth-century man-midwife William Hunter, made around 1764, she notes the strategic omission of reference to the sitter's still controversial practice of midwifery.[13] Turning to a consideration of Hunter's obstetrical atlas of 1774, *The Anatomy of the Human Gravid Uterus*, Jordanova argues that the way in which Hunter's fetuses confidently inhabit their mothers' bodies should be associated with the cultural shift toward beliefs in maternal bonding and the imbrication of children's rights with those of their mothers.[14]

Less research has been undertaken on comparable images produced in other parts of Europe. There is at least one scholar in addition to me working on French images of childbirth. Pierre Bertrand studies the iconography of early modern French childbirth, outlining the visual conventions of scenes of lying-in and breast feeding.[15] Though these representations are often engraved, they do not usually appear in the obstetrical treatises that interest me. As an art historian, Bertrand is especially adept at applying his knowledge of the rituals of childbirth to paintings, shedding new light on their contents. For example, he argues that the anonymously painted *Portrait of Gabrielle d'Estrées at her Bath* from around 1599 is a celebration of the fecundity of King Henri IV's newly-delivered mistress, not a political satire of her immorality as was previously thought.[16]

Bertrand's work confirms that the practice of art history can be enriched by interdisciplinary exchanges with the history of medicine; the history of medicine also benefits from the intrusion of 'outsiders.' To date, such interdisciplinary encounters have usually converged on anatomical rather than obstetrical knowledge. Literary critic Jonathan Sawday, for example, argues that Renaissance dissections produced a new image of the interior of the body, transforming understandings of identity and influencing the work of artists and poets.[17] Using a different approach, art historian Bette Talvacchia foregrounds issues of gender in a study of the anatomical plates in Charles Estienne's sixteenth-century French treatise.[18] She contends these images were influenced by contemporary erotic imagery, especially scenes from the sexually explicit Italian publication, *I Modi*.

Perhaps because of such studies, historians of medicine are becoming more receptive to examinations of the visual realm. This interest conforms to broader developments in the discipline of history, sometimes characterized as a pictorial turn.[19] A recent publication by Roy Porter is a case in point: after a prolific career in which he studied written documents relating to early modern English medicine, Porter turned to the contemplation of visual images concerned with the same subject. He argues they are 'embodiments, in form and content alike, of discursive practices and aesthetic expectations, governed by moral tropes and comic conventions, to be approached hermeneutically.'[20] Porter's aim is to contextualize a range of images, showing how they conveyed anxieties about the body and medical ethics, often by ridiculing physicians and other medical practitioners.

When Porter applies his extensive knowledge of medicine to images, he continues to favour writing. The author describes early modern medical engravings with reference to their captions as well as literary texts. For the most part he recounts the complicated narratives portrayed in the images, identifying key characters and themes. In part, the written inscriptions beneath, and textual character of, eighteenth-century English prints encourage this approach. Nevertheless, Porter portrays images as extensions of writing instead of attending to their visual nature. He also assumes the images were relevant primarily to the highly literate viewer, without considering how different understandings of the visual material might have been gleaned by less educated audiences.[21]

Distinguishing his work from art history, Porter claims to leave the interpretation of artistic practice to those experts.[22] Yet many art historians no longer subscribe to a narrow interest in artists, their working methods, and developing styles. They undertake detailed visual analyses of images, considering them in relation to other representations to study how visual conventions both endure and change. Approaching visual images as productive sites of meaning, art historians scrutinize the ways in which knowledge is shaped and reshaped in them. These scholars are concerned with the specificity of visual images, exploring them as signifying systems that are imbricated in – even as they offer challenges to – written texts.

In the chapters that follow, I consider how visual elements such as framing, composition, and the spatial relationships between represented objects contribute to the hermeneutics of images in early modern French obstetrical treatises. Instead of producing a chronological survey of the plates, I analyse them within a nexus of associated images, examining how visual conventions are reworked over time. It will be clear from my references to visual images as signifying systems that my overall approach is in the spirit of semiotics, the study of signs developed by Swiss linguist Ferdinand de Saussure, who argued that the relationship between signifiers (a spoken or written word) and signifieds (things in the world) is arbitrary and not fixed. His claim that language is a conventional rather than a natural system has been taken up by art historians and applied to the visual realm to undermine the commonsense notion that visual images reflect the world. Understanding that 'human culture is made up of signs, each of which stands for something other than itself,' art historians analyse the conventional codes of visual representation.[23]

Many art historians turn to the work of American semiotician Charles Sanders Peirce because he emphasizes the specific operation of visual signs instead of exclusively focusing on linguistic ones. Arguing that there are different kinds of relationships between signs and their (signified) objects, Peirce examines how a range of visual signs convey meaning. Peirce's system is both more precise and more flexible than those based on Saussure, stressing how meanings change, with signs typically alluding to other signs rather than to a stable signified.[24] While Peirce's theories inform my overall approach to interpreting images, they will be more implicit than explicit for my purposes – which after all concern the analysis of the images and texts comprising obstetrical treatises, rather than a reconceptualization of semiotic methods. Peirce's influence will nevertheless be evident in my contention that the early modern images usually have multiple potential meanings. The impact of Peirce is most clearly defined in Chapter 6, where I evaluate engravings of the unborn. Drawing on Peirce's distinctions between iconic, symbolic, and indexical signs, I challenge the notion that these images reflect what people in the past thought about the 'fetus.'

My approach foregrounds the images themselves, instead of prioritizing the artists who made them. In a discussion of different methods of analysing visual material, cultural critic Gillian Rose argues there are three crucial sites at which the meaning of an image is made – production, the image itself, and its interactivity with audiences.[25] According to Rose, distinctions between methodologies can be explained in terms of which site theorists prioritize in their analyses. Rose claims that methods emphasizing the site of production attend to the technologies determining what is visually possible during specific historical periods, as well as the agents involved in making images.[26] Despite specializing in the artistic production of seventeenth-century France, I decided that concentrating on it would not provide a reliable basis for my analyses of obstetrical plates. Like most art historians, I realize that visual texts do not have a single, discernible intention located in individual artists.[27]

In any case, a preoccupation with artists might reinforce a modern approach to images that construes artists as independent, creative beings. For many early modern audiences, the identity of artists was not a primary consideration when regarding images; they were often more interested in the quality of the representation, its materials, and how the details conveyed meaning.[28] Nor were artists autonomous, as important decisions about images were made by patrons. Images in obstetrical treatises were commissioned by the books' publishers and authors, who specified their subject matter and perhaps even such formal matters as composition. In that sense, the subject positions of the authors of obstetrical treatises were more important than those of artists, and I devoted proportionate research time to them. Though there is some biographical information about early modern French surgeon men-midwives, it does not provide a stable foundation for interpreting the obstetrical images. For the most part, what we think we know about these authors is produced in and through the texts they wrote. But as I hope to make clear, obstetrical treatises conform to a genre and do not mirror the thoughts of their authors in any straightforward way.

Although my analyses stress the form and content of images, I also consider issues of reception. In some ways, close readings of images reveal modes of reception because ideal viewing positions are encoded in the representations. Yet as scholars such as cultural theorist Stuart Hall have argued, spectators do not always adopt dominant viewing positions.[29] Drawing on their own knowledge and experiences, viewers can actively produce mediated or oppositional understandings of visual texts. Recognizing the diversity of potential interpretations, practitioners of cultural studies have developed methods of audience-oriented research.[30] For the most part, their studies involve surveys meant to discover how interpretation is impacted by factors such as the class, gender, racial, ethnic, or sexual identities of different audiences. Such an approach is difficult to adopt in relation to early modern obstetrical treatises;

there is little indication of how the broad audience who encountered the treatises actually responded to them.

Another way to broach the question of reception is to examine early modern modes of responding to visuality. The study of what is now referred to as visual culture investigates historically and culturally specific ways of seeing the world – a visuality distinguished from the biological ability to see.[31] I have already alluded to this approach by indicating that early modern viewers did not necessarily prioritize the identity of artists when evaluating images. There is also evidence of the specific ways of looking at portraiture in early modern France. According to art historian Michel Melot, early modern French portraits were highly deliberate images, with each attribute and gesture rife with political meaning.[32] Concurrent descriptions of portraits indicate that viewers paid careful attention to how the rendering of facial features, hair, costume, and hands represented the character and social status of the individual portrayed.[33] This practice of looking can be taken into consideration when analysing the author portraits in obstetrical treatises. Such concerns coincide with those of semiotics, an approach which understands visual images as signs that communicate meaning when decoded by audiences. Yet it is not easy to recover historical modes of visuality; contemporary viewers bring their own culturally specific ways of looking to images. Instead of denying the impact of the present on viewing the past, scholars can draw attention to how visuality changes over time. In my analysis of early modern images of the unborn, for example, I contend these engravings look different now, in part because of the meanings currently attached to fetal imagery.

This discussion of my interest in visual semiotics and the site of representation implies that I am exclusively interested in the images in French obstetrical treatises. Nonetheless I also examine the written texts in these publications. I arguably pay even more attention to writing, with one chapter devoted entirely to the printed criticism medical practitioners launched at each other. My emphasis on writing is informed by the content of obstetrical treatises. These sources contain more written text than images – text which surrounds the visual representations, providing them with an immediate context. I do not, however, refer to writing in order to explain the images or anchor their meanings. This approach would assume both that images illustrate written texts and that written signs are somehow more reliable and transparent than visual signs.

I am particularly interested in the relationship between the visual and written portions of the treatises, stressing the times they are at odds. In my analysis of images of the unborn, I find that while they seem to depict large children who are both active and detached from the maternal body, written texts paint a different picture; not only do unborn creatures not move at will, their fate is intimately bound up with that of their mothers. In a similar manner, a mixed message is conveyed by the written and visual aspects of the author portrait displayed in the treatise of Bourgeois. While the engraving draws attention to the bodily stature of the midwife, the verse inscribed beneath it alludes to a disjuncture between her body and obstetrical abilities. Rather than attempt to stabilize these and other contradictory messages, I explore them to unsettle beliefs about the subject matter and function of early modern obstetrical treatises.

My commitment to the visual aspects of the treatises extends to their written content. I read the texts with a primary interest in vision, examining written representations of looking and being looked at. The lying-in chamber emerges as a highly visual realm, with authors describing how male and female midwives should present themselves to clients. Surgeon men-midwives also expounded on what fellow practitioners could and could not see. Though the maternal body often remained hidden from view, the unborn child was always invisible, requiring men to rely on touch rather than vision to determine its position in the womb. All the same, when a woman died during labour, these men could perform autopsies, opening her body to view. I consider both the spectacular nature of childbirth and discussions of what remained unseen. In this way, I interpret previously neglected layers of meaning in the treatises, while assessing the importance of visual communication in early modern French culture.

Rethinking Early Modern Childbirth

My analyses are in dialogue with a growing body of scholarship on early modern midwifery. A wide range of scholars study early modern birthing practices, women's as well as men's roles in the lying-in chamber, and social understandings of maternity. Historians of medicine have made especially important contributions to the field. By undertaking careful archival research, they have undermined longstanding assumptions about early modern childbirth. It is no longer possible to presume that female midwives were incompetent, women had no control over conception, and birth itself was extremely dangerous. Hilary Marland, Helen King, Doreen Evenden, and Nina Rattner Gelbart, for example, have studied the record books, treatises, and testimonials produced by women to argue that many female midwives were not only well-educated, respected members of their communities, but they were also able to manage various complications in childbirth.[34] While the stereotype of the bungling female midwife has been solidly refuted, some questions remain about women's knowledge of birth control and abortion. Early modern women are no longer considered victims of their biology, but it is uncertain how many of the numerous contraceptive methods and abortifacients described in recipe books as well as medical texts were actually effective.[35] It is clear, however, that pregnancy and birth were not always linked with death at the time. Although maternal mortality rates are notoriously difficult to calculate, several thorough comparative studies suggest they were much lower than was previously thought. Quantitative research by Roger Schofield and Irvine Loudon places the maternal mortality rate in early modern Europe well below the eight to fifteen per cent estimated by previous scholars.[36] These studies make it more difficult to regard the past from a position of superiority in the present – wondering how hapless early modern women managed to escape the lying-in chamber with their lives.

Research by historians contributes to a broader reconsideration of early modern childbirth, one which extends far beyond mortality rates, the education of birthing assistants, and the techniques employed in the lying-in chamber. Birth is now approached as an important social event both shaped within and significant to early modern culture at large. Several recent collections of essays attest to the expansive nature of current work on early modern reproduction. Editors Valeria Finucci and Kevin Brownlee, for example, bring together essays which consider how discourses of generation and genealogy were articulated in legal, religious, medical, and philosophical literature from antiquity to the early modern period.[37] The volume edited by Naomi J. Miller and Naomi Yavneh converges more specifically on early modern discussions of maternity, but is equally comprehensive, including considerations of literature, art, music, education manuals, and medical treatises.[38] Though these collections are interdisciplinary, most of the scholars who contributed to them are trained in literary studies. They thus bring sophisticated theories of representation, identity, authorship, and metaphor to the study of early modern childbirth.[39]

All of this work would have been unthinkable, however, without the development of women's studies. Since at least the 1970s, feminist theorists have insisted that issues such as childbirth are worthy of analysis.[40] The study of early modern women is now particularly active, with increasing numbers of publications and conferences supported by associations such as the Society for the Study of Early Modern Women.[41] Topics addressed by scholars in this field range from the politics of Queenship to dance rituals, women writers, marriage, and literacy.[42] Now also an established teaching field, textbooks cover all aspects of the lives of early modern women. A notable publication is Merry E. Wiesner's survey of early modern European women in which material is organized under the headings 'The Body,' 'The Mind,' and 'The Spirit.'[43] In this and other studies of early modern women, gender, sexuality, race, ethnicity, social status, and the body are important categories of historical research.

I follow these publications by understanding gender as a crucial category of analysis. I examine articulations of both masculinity and femininity in early modern French obstetrical treatises – in line with practices often labelled gender studies rather than women's studies. Some advocates of women's studies fear that attending to representations of masculinity will return men to the forefront of scholarly work at the expense of women.[44] But as literary scholar Eve Kosofsky Sedgwick argues, men and masculinity should not be conflated, just as women cannot be understood with exclusive reference to femininity.[45] Such rigid associations are actually at odds with the aims of women's studies, solidifying historical conceptions of gender rather than denaturalizing them. Though research on early modern masculinity has increased – with particular reference to English literature and fashion – early modern women have not been displaced as a result.[46] Kathleen P. Long's edited collection of essays on early modern France, for example, shows that masculinity was a concept that fluctuated along with changing notions of femininity; the two terms were typically defined in relation to each other.[47] In my own research, I likewise find that early modern French masculinity was insecure, rather than all powerful. Men-midwives emerge from obstetrical treatises as unsteady figures who, like women, were subject to scrutiny in the lying-in chamber. While reading these sources for representations of how women resisted male power structures, I also contemplate how men strove both to adapt to and change a realm traditionally identified with women, namely the birthing chamber.

My understanding of gender is influenced by theorists Eve Kosofsky Sedgwick and Judith Butler, art historians Griselda Pollock and Abigail Solomon-Godeau, and historian Joan Scott.[48] Readers, however, may be surprised to learn that the work of sociologist Pierre Bourdieu is also important.[49] Bourdieu is certainly better known for his work on class than on gender, about which he wrote relatively little. All the same, theorist Toril Moi makes a convincing case for the feminist appropriation of Bourdieu. She argues that 'one of the advantages of Bourdieu's theory is that it not only insists on the social construction of gender, but that it permits us to grasp the immense *variability* of gender as a social factor.'[50] Moi invokes Bourdieu's concept of field, a spatial metaphor that characterizes the competitive system of social relations between institutions, organizations, and individuals. Although distinct fields (such as the art world or education system) function within broader social structures, they have their own specific logic, including the kinds of symbolic capital (legitimacy within the field) that are recognized.[51] According to Moi, gender is not awarded its own field by Bourdieu, but is instead understood to operate in all fields; it thus permeates every category. It does not follow, however, that gender is the most central power relation at stake in every social situation. Since it operates relationally, gender carries a different weight in different contexts and must be analysed on a case by case basis.[52]

I find Bourdieu's flexible conception of gender particularly appealing for understanding midwifery and childbirth during the early modern period. It helps to undermine simplistic descriptions of the increased practice of male midwives, and concomitant decrease in power of female midwives, as a battle of the sexes in which men prevailed. This understanding of early modern midwifery was proposed by Barbara Ehrenreich and Deirdre English, feminists who argued that women were systematically driven out of medical practice by men, with female midwives persecuted as witches because of their intimate understanding of women's bodies.[53] Ehrenreich and English's claims significantly challenged the idea that men, equipped with specialized medical training and forceps, had marched triumphantly into the lying-in chamber to save the lives of women and children.[54] Yet subsequent research by historians has disproved many of their arguments, particularly the idea that female midwives were identified as witches.[55] More recent examinations of early modern childbirth focus on regional practices, avoiding general narratives that efface differences.

Historian Mary Lindemann notes the 'tyranny of an Anglo-Saxon model,' which saw men dominating obstetrics rather rapidly, influenced the restricted perception of midwifery practice in early modern Europe as a contest between men and women.[56] In much of Europe, men came to displace the traditional female midwife even in regular deliveries by the early twentieth century. This transformation, however, took place most quickly and completely in England, where childbirth became part of medicine between 1720 and 1770, and many men attended normal deliveries, especially those of wealthy urban women, by 1780.[57] In France, male expansion may have begun earlier, but occurred at a slower rate and was always relatively rare in both rural and southern areas. In some ways, eighteenth-century France saw the revival of the female midwife, in the form of Madame du Coudray, hired by Kings Louis XV and Louis XVI to teach her methods throughout the country.[58] In the Netherlands, the female midwife was even more ensconced; the move during the eighteenth century was to regulate and train women, not drive them out of business.[59] Likewise, little effort was made to replace female midwives in eighteenth-century Germany.[60] And, in contrast to the rest of Europe, men never came to dominate the practice of childbirth in Italy. Historian Nadia Maria Filippini attributes this situation to the disapproval of both the Catholic Church and the general populace, but notes that by the eighteenth century the public role of the female midwife had been reduced to attending normal births.[61]

Like these scholars, I concentrate on a limited historical period and region – the seventeenth and early eighteenth centuries in France, especially Paris – to avoid proffering a sweeping pan-European account. I decided to terminate my study at roughly 1730 because scholars of French midwifery Jacques Gélis and Mireille Laget have already undertaken intensive studies of the eighteenth century. Drawing primarily on legal documents and archival records as well as the contents of obstetrical treatises, Gélis contends that traditional midwives were first replaced by better-educated female midwives and then gradually by male practitioners beginning around 1730–1760.[62] He examines the education of midwives, arguing that the increased status of *chirurgiens accoucheurs* was linked with the institutionalization of obstetrical training. At the same time, he proposes that shifting *mentalités* made both state bureaucracies and the average citizen more concerned with preserving populations, turning their attention to saving the lives of labouring women and newborns.[63] Laget likewise places the practice of early modern French childbirth within a broader mental universe, studying it in relation to social structures, politics, and folklore. She contends that after 1760 a new brand of practitioner was more open to using technical innovations and instruments within the lying-in chamber.[64]

Unlike Gélis and Laget, I am not interested in charting the changes in French midwifery over the *longue durée*. I wish to concentrate on the less-studied seventeenth and early eighteenth centuries. The later eighteenth century has received more scholarly attention partly because a substantial number of records survive from the period. The increasing interest in regulating midwifery and measuring populations produced many documents, ultimately encouraging a quantitative and archival approach to the research of eighteenth-century childbirth.[65] Without neglecting the far fewer earlier archival records, my study features seventeenth- and early eighteenth-century obstetrical treatises as a genre of writing and representation rather than one source of information among others; in that sense it is a literary and art-historical project rather than a traditionally historical one.

Investigating this earlier period makes it more difficult to rely on standard explanations of the changes in birthing practices. The forceps, for example, has been considered an important reason for male expansion in childbirth.[66] While no longer described as the key to the lying-in chamber, the forceps continues to be featured in critical studies, especially those emphasizing childbirth in early modern England. Wilson argues that British men-midwives were tolerated only after improving their reputations by performing successful forceps deliveries of live children.[67] He also shows that forceps use was debated among men-midwives in London during the first half of the eighteenth century, and was apparently linked with political affiliations. It is becoming increasingly clear, however, that the instrument did not have the same impact in other countries, where it appeared at a slower rate.[68] Invented in England by the Chamberlen family, and kept as its secret, the forceps was not widely used in France until after 1730; Paris surgeon Grégoire the Younger helped to popularize the forceps in the 1730s, but surgeon André Levret did not publish his design of the curved forceps until 1753.[69] According to French surgeon man-midwife François Mauriceau, Hugh Chamberlen travelled to Paris in 1670, attempting to sell his family's device to the first physician of the King of France. Yet the Englishman's offer was rejected because when Chamberlen applied his instruments to a malformed Parisian woman, he succeeded only in torturing her, and she died undelivered.[70]

Though various scholars search for earlier instances of forceps use in France, I attend to discussions of how surgeons employed other instruments as well as their bare hands in difficult deliveries.[71] Mauriceau argued, for example, that after witnessing Chamberlen's disappointing demonstration, he invented his own tool, the *tire-tête* [head puller], to pull dead children from the womb.[72] In 1694, French surgeon man-midwife Philippe Peu criticized Mauriceau's invention, calling it an instrument of murder, while defending the use of more traditional hooks.[73] The heated exchange that ensued between Mauriceau and Peu indicates that, even as male practice was beginning to expand in France, instrument use remained controversial. In fact, a number of surgeon men-midwives refused to operate with instruments, insisting that their hands were specialized tools capable of managing any delivery.[74] I argue that this emphasis on manual labour was part of attempts by surgeon men-midwives to link themselves with a direct and physical understanding of childbirth – one capable of substituting for women's bodily experience of maternity.

In addition to the invention of the forceps, the quest for social status is associated with the spread of man-midwifery in early modern Europe. Contesting the belief that there was a unified women's culture, Wilson argues that literate, wealthy English women sought to distinguish themselves from the lower orders during the eighteenth century by hiring more costly men-midwives to assist at their deliveries.[75] As Gélis and Laget have argued, the employment of men-midwives spread most rapidly in urban centres in northern France, especially among the wealthy elite.[76] Class distinction was certainly a factor in women's decision to call for male assistance. I do not stress this issue, however, for my book concerns the display of obstetrical authority in early modern French obstetrical treatises, not the motivations of pregnant French women and their families. Nevertheless, unlike previous scholars, I consider how authors of treatises represented distinctions between birthing practitioners. In keeping with the arguments of Wilson, I find that surgeon men-midwives were not a unified group. They articulated their identities both in relation to and distinction from other male practitioners, as well as female midwives.

The increasing criticism of female midwives is perhaps most frequently identified as a factor contributing to the expanding practice of men-midwives. In their weighty survey of early modern French medicine, historians Laurence Brockliss and Colin Jones refer to the 'relentless propaganda campaign' waged against female midwives.[77] Though significant, this criticism has often been considered in isolation, as if female midwives were the only targets. Male midwives, however, additionally attacked each other, male physicians, and so-called charlatans with much fervour in various publications. The rhetoric men employed in these attacks is very similar to that used to malign female midwives. Male authors routinely referred to other male medical practitioners as ignorant, untrained meddlers who posed a danger to women and children alike. The criticism of female midwives was therefore part of a conventional practice in the competitive world of early modern medicine. This book offers a more nuanced vision of medical criticism by analysing the attacks on male practitioners as well as female midwives.

In the end, my goal is not to displace other accounts of early modern midwifery, but to add another layer to them – one that insists on the complexity of early modern French obstetrical treatises without assuming men were destined to take over the practice of midwifery. I understand the treatises as contradictory sites of representation participating in the struggle over both the meaning of childbirth and the identity of medical practitioners. These texts, however, should not be considered mechanisms directly contributing to male expansion, a position that risks overestimating the power of men-midwives. No doubt the treatises had effects. Their escalating rate of publication, as well as the multiple editions and translations of many treatises, indicate they were widely distributed and consumed.[78] Nevertheless, interpretations of the treatises would have varied according to the diverse backgrounds, education, and interests of their audiences. Instead of speculating about how the treatises produced the behaviour and identities they promote, I consider how they construct and exhibit arguments about obstetrical authority.

Chapter 1, 'French Treatises 1550–1730: A Survey,' introduces readers to obstetrical publications, describing their authors, contents, and audiences. The treatises were largely homogeneous throughout this period, providing standardized rather than innovative information. They nevertheless became more specialized during the seventeenth century, concentrating exclusively on childbirth instead of including it among other medical practices. For the most part, differences between treatises can be explained with reference to the author's position within the medical hierarchy of early modern France. Surgeons, for example, stressed their manual interventions in difficult deliveries, while physicians featured the herbal remedies they were authorized to prescribe. Setting the stage for subsequent interpretations of the treatises, this chapter shows that the publications did far more than transmit medical information. They were devoted both to defining and defending the roles of various practitioners within the lying-in chamber.

In Chapter 2, 'Risking Exposure: The Visual Politics of Childbirth,' the focus shifts to how the treatises portray visual exchanges within the lying-in chamber. Linking vision with knowledge and identity, authors described the looking they did when assisting at births. While surgeon men-midwives disapproved of female clients who refused to expose themselves to male practitioners, they praised the occasional woman who did so without hesitation. These men were not, however, always actively inspecting others. They also alluded to the visual scrutiny that male birthing assistants endured within the lying-in chamber. Surgeon men-midwives offered advice to their male colleagues about the dress, facial expressions, and behaviour that would please women within the birthing chamber. Moving beyond an exclusive focus on the male observation of female bodies, this chapter offers a more complete picture of the visual dynamics of the birthing room by considering how women looked back at men. At the same time, it draws attention to how obstetrical treatises made men visible by presenting them to the critical eyes of readers. Striving for a broader understanding of these treatises, the chapter concludes by placing the books within the 'display culture' of early modern France, a period when social hierarchies were both expressed and produced in material ways.

Chapter 3, 'Reading the Midwife's Body: Louise Bourgeois,' examines the representation of the female midwife in obstetrical treatises. During the early modern period descriptions of female midwives were not always derogatory, even in those treatises written by male practitioners. Many manuals outline the characteristics of an admirable midwife, portraying her as courteous, chaste, prudent, well-informed, always cheerful, and of a suitable age. Though inspired by Soranus of Ephesus' second-century publication, early modern French accounts of the ideal midwife distinctively feature her body. Bourgeois certainly drew attention to her own physical qualities, boasting that the Queen only had to look at her to know she was qualified to assume the position of royal midwife. Bourgeois implied that her identity as a skilled midwife was visibly evident in her person. The image of the royal midwife that emerges from Bourgeois' writings is, however, by no means unified. I analyse three selections from her publications which associate the midwife's body with her facility as a midwife, finding they send mixed messages. Bourgeois' author portrait, for example, depicts her as a hybrid figure, fluctuating between efficient female midwife and educated theoretical writer.

Chapter 4, 'Looking the Part: Men-midwives on Display,' turns to the bodily exhibition of the ideal man-midwife, examining descriptions of his proper behaviour, dress, and comportment. The physical qualities and personality traits desired in a female midwife were also those required of a male practitioner. He was urged to dress modestly, have small hands, and treat labouring women with compassion. Though the ideal man-midwife embodied the qualities of the model female midwife, he was supposed to exceed her in training, knowledge, and skill. In keeping with the previous chapter, this study is enriched with interpretations of author portraits – those of *chirurgiens accoucheurs* who wrote obstetrical treatises. The portraits often feature the sitters' hands, linking them visually with learning and surgical skill, as well as a firsthand comprehension of childbirth. This chapter shows that both written descriptions and portraits exhibit the flexible masculinity of surgeon men-midwives in early modern France. Like the portrait of Bourgeois, their images shift between traditionally masculine and feminine characteristics.

In Chapter 5, 'Bodies in Labour: Rhetoric, Rivalry, and Male Maternity,' I consider negative representations of men-midwives. Although better known for their criticism of female midwives, male authors of obstetrical treatises also drew attention to mistakes made by young and inexperienced *chirurgiens accoucheurs*. Authors regularly attacked their own colleagues in print, accusing them of lacking an extensive personal experience with difficult deliveries. In contrast to this contemptuous portrayal of rivals, surgeon men-midwives produced positive images of themselves. Maligning other practitioners was a mode of self-representation in the quest for legitimacy. Notably, male authors referred to their female relatives in these critical accounts, extracting from the experiences of wives, sisters, or mothers to augment their own authority and undermine that of male rivals. The men also described difficult deliveries that exhausted them physically, implying that their own bodily labour substituted for and even surpassed that of the suffering mother. Was this male association with female family members and labouring women informed by a redefinition of masculinity or did it consist of a masculine appropriation of the female body? Striving to answer this question, Chapter 5 considers whether or not arguments made about the identity and authority of surgeon men-midwives were predicated on the concomitant disembodiment of women.

Chapter 6, 'Handling the Unborn: Men-midwives between Vision and Blindness,' examines the images of unborn figures in early modern French obstetrical treatises. Unborn children are shown floating in large wombs next to detailed descriptions of how heroic male practitioners can intervene to save the mother and sometimes child at dangerous deliveries. Although some scholars argue that these engravings begin to present the fetus as a rights-bearing individual, neither the visual nor the written portions of obstetrical treatises portray unborn creatures as autonomous patients. In the images, unborn figures are shown at risk and thus in need of medical assistance. In their treatises, *chirurgiens accoucheurs* described embryos, fetuses, and unborn children as sites for the production of their own identity. The men claimed, for example, that obstetrical emergencies were the most demanding type of surgical procedure precisely because practitioners could see neither the child nor the body of the suffering woman. The surgeon man-midwife was therefore faced with the ultimate test of his dexterity. Why, then, the emphasis on visualizing the unborn child in these texts? I contend the images were not attempts to picture accurately the interior of the female body, but were instead part of the effort to legitimate male intervention in childbirth. Insisting on the complex layers of significance in the images, I relate them to arguments about how the skilled hands and embodied knowledge of medical experts could replace maternal intelligence.

After the initial survey of obstetrical treatises, each chapter considers how a different site of display is articulated in the publications. Beginning with the lying-in chamber, the book goes on to analyse the female midwife's body, the surgeon man-midwife's body, the labouring body (of the mother as well as the surgeon as proxy to her labour), and finally the unborn body. I uniquely examine all characters in the birthing room, including male and female birthing assistants, labouring women, and unborn children. I do so, however, in a very specific way, by investigating representations of the visual and physical exchanges between these characters. My goal is to reveal the imbrication of vision, authority, and knowledge from different angles. I find that bodies, particularly those of midwifery practitioners, were crucial to the exchange of information and establishment of identity in the lying-in chamber. This emphasis on bodily display not only offers a fuller understanding of obstetrical treatises, but also illuminates how the body participated in the negotiation of social status, gender roles, and medical hierarchies in early modern France.

Notes

1.   I follow early modern usage by referring to an unborn child instead of a fetus in the womb. See Chapter 6 for the status of the unborn in early modern France.
2.   François Mauriceau, *Des maladies des femmes grosses et accouchées* (Paris, 1668), 350, wrote that even when the death of a child or labouring woman was not the surgeon's fault, he was treated like a butcher and a hangman. In his preface to the English translation of Mauriceau's treatise, *The Accomplisht Midwife, Treating of the Diseases of Women with Child, and in Child-bed* (London, 1673), Hugh Chamberlen reported that men's use of hooks led to the belief 'that where a man comes, one or both must necessarily dye.' Louise Bourgeois, *Observations diverses sur la stérilité, perte de fruict, foecondité, accouchements et maladies des femmes et enfants nouveaux naiz* (Paris, 1609), 31–2, argued that when called too late by midwives, the surgeon was unfairly likened to a butcher. Unless otherwise indicated, I will henceforth refer only to the more accessible 1652 edition of Bourgeois, prefaced by Françoise Olive and republished in 1992.
3.   See, for example, Hilary Marland, ed., *The Art of Midwifery: Early Modern Midwives in Europe* (London: Routledge, 1993), and Adrian Wilson, *The Making of Man-Midwifery: Childbirth in England 1660–1770* (London: UCL Press, 1995).
4.   My use of the term obstetrical is not meant to invoke a professional branch of medicine, but merely refers to the theme of childbirth featured in the treatises. Though some scholars call similar publications midwifery manuals, the treatises I consider were far more than practical handbooks, as indicated in Chapter 1.
5.   For a recent discussion see Jeanette Herrle-Fanning, 'Figuring the Reproductive Woman: The Construction of Medical Identity in Eighteenth-Century British Midwifery Texts,' Mary M. Lay, et al., eds, *Body Talk: Rhetoric, Technology, Reproduction* (Madison: University of Wisconsin Press, 2000), 29–48.
6.   Brigitte Jordan, 'Authoritative Knowledge and Its Construction,' Robbie E. Davis-Floyd and Carolyn F. Sargent, eds, *Childbirth and Authoritative Knowledge: Cross-Cultural Perspectives* (Berkeley: University of California Press, 1997), 55–79. See also Brigitte Jordan, *Birth in Four Cultures: A Cross-Cultural Investigation of Childbirth in Yucatan, Holland, Sweden and the United States* (Prospect Heights: Waveland Press, 1993).
7.   Eugene Declercq, Raymond DeVries, Kirsi Viisainen, Helga B. Salvesen, and Sirpa Wrede, 'Where to Give Birth? Politics and the Place of Birth,' Raymond DeVries, Cecilia Benoit, Edwin R. van Teijlingen, and Sirpa Wrede, eds, *Birth by Design: Pregnancy, Maternity Care, and Midwifery in North America and Europe* (New York: Routledge, 2001), 7–27, analyses the medicalization of childbirth in the twentieth century, arguing that it proceeded for diverse reasons and at different rates in different Western countries.
8.   Marland, *The Art of Midwifery*, and Wilson, *The Making of Man-Midwifery*.
9.   Ludmilla Jordanova, 'Medical Men 1780–1820,' Joanna Woodall, ed., *Portraiture: Facing the Subject* (Manchester: Manchester University Press, 1997), 101–15.
10.   For recent discussions of Poussin see Katie Scott and Genevieve Warwick, eds, *Commemorating Poussin: Reception and Interpretation of the Artist* (Cambridge:

Cambridge University Press, 1999), and Todd P. Olson, *Poussin and France: Painting, Humanism, and the Politics of Style* (New Haven: Yale University Press, 2002).

11.   Barbara Maria Stafford, *Body Criticism: Imaging the Unseen in Enlightenment Art and Medicine* (Cambridge, MA: MIT Press, 1991), 2–9.

12.   See, for example, Hilary Marland, trans. and ed., *'Mother and Child Were Saved'. The Memoirs (1693–1740) of the Frisian Midwife Catharina Schrader* (Amsterdam: Rodopi, 1987), Wendy Perkins, *Midwifery and Medicine in Early Modern France: Louise Bourgeois* (Exeter: University of Exeter Press, 1996), David Cressy, *Birth, Marriage, and Death: Ritual, Religion, and the Life-Cycle in Tudor and Stuart England* (Oxford: Oxford University Press, 1997), Agnes Risko, *'"Gott Zu Ehren, Dem Neben=Christen Zu Nutz..."': Anna Elisabeth Horenburg's Manual for Midwives'* (Ph.D. Diss., Ohio State University, 1998), and Doreen Evenden, *The Midwives of Seventeenth-Century London* (Cambridge: Cambridge University Press, 2000).

13.   Jordanova, 'Medical Men 1780–1820,' 110.

14.   Ludmilla Jordanova, 'Gender, Generation and Science: William Hunter's Obstetrical Atlas,' W.F. Bynum and Roy Porter, eds, *William Hunter and the Eighteenth-Century Medical World* (Cambridge: Cambridge University Press, 1985), 385–412. See also her *Nature Displayed: Gender, Science and Medicine 1760–1820* (London: Longman, 1999), 183–202.

15.   Pierre Bertrand, 'L'Univers de la naissance en France dans la peinture et la gravure (1550–1700): La poétique de l'image face à la rhétorique médicale' (Mémoire de D.E.A. en histoire de l'art, Paris I, 1990), and Pierre Bertrand, 'Graver la naissance au XVIIe siècle,' *Ethnologie française* 26, 2 (1996), 329–39.

16.   Pierre Bertrand, 'Le portrait de Gabrielle d'Estrées au Musée Condé de Chantilly ou la gloire de la maternité,' *Gazette des beaux-arts* 6, 122 (1993), 73–82.

17.   Jonathan Sawday, *The Body Emblazoned: Dissection and the Human Body in Renaissance Culture* (London: Routledge, 1995). Some historians of medicine have been critical of Sawday's work. See David Harley's review in *Medical History* 40 (1996), 253–4.

18.   Bette Talvacchia, 'Mythology, Sexuality, and Science in Charles Estienne's Manual of Anatomy,' *Taking Positions: On the Erotic in Renaissance Culture* (Princeton: Princeton University Press, 1999), 161–87.

19.   Peter Burke, *Eyewitnessing: The Uses of Images as Historical Evidence* (Ithaca: Cornell University Press, 2001), 12.

20.   Roy Porter, *Bodies Politic: Disease, Death, and Doctors in Britain, 1650–1900* (London: Reaktion Books, 2001), 12.

21.   Lisa Forman Cody suggested this particular criticism to me.

22.   Porter, *Bodies Politic*, 12.

23.   Mieke Bal and Norman Bryson, 'Semiotics and Art History,' *Art Bulletin* 73, 2 (1991), 174.

24.   James Hoopes, ed., *Peirce on Signs: Writings on Semiotic by Charles Sanders Peirce* (Chapel Hill: University of North Carolina Press, 1991). See also Kaja Silverman, *The Subject of Semiotics* (New York: Oxford University Press, 1983), 14–25, and Bal and Bryson, 'Semiotics and Art History,' 188–91.

25.   Gillian Rose, *Visual Methodologies* (London: Sage, 2001), 16–28.

26. *Ibid.*, 17–22.

27. Michel Foucault, 'What is an Author?' Donald Bouchard and Sherry Simon, trans. and Josué V. Harari, ed., *Textual Strategies: Perspectives in Post-Structuralist Criticism* (Ithaca: Cornell University Press, 1979), 141–60. See also Mieke Bal, 'Intention,' *Travelling Concepts in the Humanities: A Rough Guide* (Toronto: University of Toronto Press, 2002), 253–85.

28. For the early modern appreciation of the materiality of art works see Evelyn Welch, *Art and Society in Italy 1350–1500* (Oxford: Oxford University Press, 1997), 37–77. For the lowly status of the artist in early modern France see Donald Posner, 'Concerning the "Mechanical" Parts of Painting and the Artistic Culture of Seventeenth-Century France,' *Art Bulletin* 75 (1993), 583–98.

29. Stuart Hall, 'Encoding, Decoding,' Simon During, ed., *The Cultural Studies Reader* (London: Routledge, 1993), 90–103.

30. Perhaps the most famous example of such audience-oriented research is Ien Ang, *Watching Dallas: Soap Opera and the Melodramatic Imagination* (London: Methuen, 1985).

31. For a recent discussion of visuality see Mieke Bal, 'Visual Essentialism and the Object of Visual Culture,' *Journal of Visual Culture* 2, 1 (2003), 5–32.

32. Michel Melot, Antony Griffiths, Richard S. Field, and André Béguin, *Prints: History of an Art* (New York: Rizzoli, 1981), 79.

33. Emmanuel Coquery, 'Le portrait vu du Grand Siècle,' *Visages du Grand Siècle: Le portrait français sous le règne de Louis XIV, 1660–1715* (Paris: Somogny, 1997), 29.

34. Marland, '*Mother and Child Were Saved*', Hilary Marland, '"Stately and Dignified, Kindly and God-fearing": Midwives, Age and Status in the Netherlands in the Eighteenth Century,' Hilary Marland and Margaret Pelling, eds, *The Task of Healing: Medicine, Religion and Gender in England and the Netherlands 1450–1800* (Rotterdam: Erasmus Publishing, 1996), 271–305, Helen King, '"As if None Understood the Art that Cannot Understand Greek": The Education of Midwives in Seventeenth-Century England,' Vivian Nutton and Roy Porter, eds, *The History of Medical Education in Britain* (Amsterdam: Rodopi, 1995), 184–98, Evenden, *The Midwives of Seventeenth-Century London*, and Nina Rattner Gelbart, *The King's Midwife: A History and Mystery of Madame du Coudray* (Berkeley: University of California Press, 1998). See also the following debate: David Harley, 'Ignorant Midwives – A Persistent Stereotype,' *Society for the Social History of Medicine Bulletin* 28 (1981), 6–9, Adrian Wilson, 'Ignorant Midwives – a Rejoinder,' *Society for the Social History of Medicine Bulletin* 32 (1983), 46–9, and Bernice Boss and Jeffrey Boss, 'Ignorant Midwives – a Further Rejoinder,' *Society for the Social History of Medicine Bulletin* 33 (1983), 71.

35. Angus McLaren, *A History of Contraception: From Antiquity to the Present Day* (Oxford: Blackwell, 1990), John M. Riddle, *Contraception and Abortion from the Ancient World to the Renaissance* (Cambridge, MA: Harvard University Press, 1992), and John M. Riddle, *Eve's Herbs: A History of Contraception and Abortion in the West* (Cambridge, MA: Harvard University Press, 1997). Helen King, *Hippocrates' Woman: Reading the Female Body in Ancient Greece* (London: Routledge, 1998), 144–5, argues that not every ancient recipe designed to 'bring on the menses' was an

abortifacient, as Riddle suspects. Patricia Crawford, 'Sexual Knowledge in England, 1500–1750,' Roy Porter and Mikuláš Teich, eds, *Sexual Knowledge, Sexual Science: The History of Attitudes to Sexuality* (Cambridge: Cambridge University Press,1994), 99, doubts the efficacy of early methods of birth control, given the high incidence of unwanted pregnancies outside of marriage.

36.   Roger Schofield, 'Did the Mothers Really Die? Three Centuries of Maternal Mortality in "The World We Have Lost",' Lloyd Bonfield et al., eds, *The World We Have Gained* (Oxford: Blackwell, 1986), 231–60, Irvine Loudon, 'Deaths in Childbed from the Eighteenth Century to 1935,' *Medical History* 30 (1986), 1–41, Irvine Loudon, *Death in Childbirth: An International Study of Maternal Care and Maternal Mortality 1800–1950* (Oxford: Clarendon, 1992). See also B. M. Willmott Dobbie, 'An Attempt to Estimate the True Rate of Maternal Mortality, Sixteenth to Eighteenth Centuries,' *Medical History* 26 (1982), 79–90, and Adrian Wilson, 'The Perils of Early Modern Procreation: Childbirth With or Without Fear?' *British Journal for Eighteenth-Century Studies* 16 (Spring 1993), 1–19. For similarly low French maternal mortality rates see Alain Bideau, 'Accouchement "naturel" et accouchement à "haut risque",' *Annales de demographie historique* (1981), 4–66.

37.   Valeria Finucci and Kevin Brownlee, eds, *Generation and Degeneration: Tropes of Reproduction in Literature and History from Antiquity to Early Modern Europe* (Durham: Duke University Press, 2001).

38.   Naomi J. Miller and Naomi Yavneh, eds, *Maternal Measures: Figuring Caregiving in the Early Modern Period* (Aldershot: Ashgate, 2000).

39.   For a recent literary study of early modern French childbirth see Holly Tucker, *Pregnant Fictions: Childbirth and the Fairy Tale in Early-Modern France* (Detroit: Wayne State University Press, 2003).

40.   For studies that reclaim childbirth as a feminist issue see Suzanne Arms, *Immaculate Deception: A New Look at Women and Childbirth in America* (Boston: Houghton Mifflin, 1975), Ann Oakley, 'Wisewoman and Medicine Man: Changes in the Management of Childbirth,' Juliet Mitchell and Ann Oakley, eds, *The Rights and Wrongs of Women* (Harmondsworth: Penguin, 1976), 17–58, and Hilda Smith, 'Gynecology and Ideology in Seventeenth-Century England,' Berenice A. Carroll, ed., *Liberating Women's History: Theoretical and Critical Essays* (Urbana: University of Illinois Press, 1976), 97–114.

41.   For more information about the Society for the Study of Early Modern Women, founded in 1994, consult its Web site: www.ssemw.org.

42.   See, for example, Clarissa Campbell Orr, ed., *Queenship in Britain, 1660–1837* (Manchester: Manchester University Press, 2002), Sarah R. Cohen, *Art, Dance, and the Body in French Culture of the Ancien Régime* (Cambridge: Cambridge University Press, 2000), Cristelle L. Baskins, *Cassone Painting, Humanism, and Gender in Early Modern Italy* (Cambridge: Cambridge University Press, 1998), Abby Zanger, *Scenes from the Marriage of Louis XIV: Nuptial Fictions and the Making of Absolutist Power* (Stanford: Stanford University Press, 1997), Susan Broomhall, *Women and the Book Trade in Sixteenth-Century France* (Aldershot: Ashgate, 2002), and Valerie Traub, M. Lindsay Kaplan, and Dympna Callaghan, eds, *Feminist Readings of Early Modern Culture* (Cambridge: Cambridge University Press, 1996).

43. Merry E. Wiesner, *Women and Gender in Early Modern Europe* (Cambridge: Cambridge University Press, 1993).

44. For a discussion of masculinity that does not foreground men see Judith Halberstam, *Female Masculinity* (Durham: Duke University Press, 1998).

45. Eve Kosofsky Sedgwick, 'Gosh, Boy George, You Must be Awfully Secure in your Masculinity!' Maurice Berger, Brian Wallis, and Simon Watson, eds, *Constructing Masculinity* (New York: Routledge, 1995), 11–20. See also Judith Kegan Gardiner, ed., *Masculinity Studies and Feminist Theory* (New York: Columbia University Press, 2002).

46. See, for example, David Kuchta, *The Three-Piece Suit and Modern Masculinity: England, 1550–1850* (Berkeley: University of California Press, 2002), Robin Headlam Wells, *Shakespeare on Masculinity* (Cambridge: Cambridge University Press, 2000), Mark Breitenberg, *Anxious Masculinity in Early Modern England* (Cambridge: Cambridge University Press, 1996), and Michele Cohen, *Fashioning Masculinity: National Identity and Language in the Eighteenth Century* (London: Routledge, 1996).

47. Kathleen P. Long, ed., *High Anxiety: Masculinity in Crisis in Early Modern France* (Kirksville: Truman State University Press, 2002).

48. Eve Kosofsky Sedgwick, *Epistemology of the Closet* (Berkeley: University of California Press, 1990), Judith Butler, *Gender Trouble: Feminism and the Subversion of Identity* (New York: Routledge, 1990), Judith Butler, 'Imitation and Gender Insubordination,' Diana Fuss, ed., *Inside/Out: Lesbian Theories, Gay Theories* (New York: Routledge, 1991), 13–31, Griselda Pollock, *Vision and Difference: Femininity, Feminism and Histories of Art* (London: Routledge, 1988), Abigail Solomon-Godeau, 'Male Trouble,' Maurice Berger, Brian Wallis, and Simon Watson, eds, *Constructing Masculinity*, 68–76, and Joan Wallach Scott, *Gender and the Politics of History* (New York: Columbia University Press, 1999).

49. Pierre Bourdieu, *The Logic of Practice*, Richard Nice, trans. (Stanford: Stanford University Press, 1990).

50. Toril Moi, 'Appropriating Bourdieu: Feminist Theory and Pierre Bourdieu's Sociology of Culture,' *New Literary History* 22 (1991), 1035.

51. Pierre Bourdieu, 'Some Properties of Fields,' *Sociology in Question*, Richard Nice, trans. (London: Sage, 1993), 72–7.

52. At my suggestion, Susan Broomhall also frames her work in this manner. In *Women's Medical Work in Early Modern France* (Manchester: Manchester University Press, 2004), she shows that the healing work performed by religious women in hospitals was not appreciated by male administrators because of their understanding of women's 'natural' duties. In a different context, however, Broomhall finds that women healers were not singled out as outsiders especially worthy of scorn by the Paris Faculté de Médecine. I thank Sue Broomhall for allowing me to consult her text prior to its publication.

53. Barbara Ehrenreich and Deirdre English, *Witches, Midwives, and Nurses: A History of Women Healers* (New York: The Feminist Press, 1973).

54. See, for example, Edwin A. Jameson, *Gynecology and Obstetrics* (New York: Hoeber, 1936), James V. Ricci, *The Genealogy of Gynaecology: History of the Development of Gynaecology throughout the Ages, 2000 B.C.–1800* (Philadelphia: Blakiston, 1943),

Theodore Cianfrani, *A Short History of Obstetrics and Gynecology* (Springfield: Thomas, 1960), Irving Samuel Cutter and Henry R. Viets, *A Short History of Midwifery* (Philadelphia: Saunders, 1964), and Walter Radcliffe, *Milestones in Midwifery* (Bristol: Wright & Sons, 1967).

55.   David Harley, 'Historians as Demonologists: The Myth of the Midwife-witch,' *Journal of the Society for the Social History of Medicine* 3, 1 (1990), 1–26, and Jane P. Davidson, 'The Myth of the Persecuted Female Healer,' *Journal of the Rocky Mountain Medieval and Renaissance Association* 14 (1993), 115–29. Caroline Bicks, *Midwiving Subjects in Shakespeare's England* (Aldershot: Ashgate, 2003), 137–41, and Tucker, *Pregnant Fictions*, 55–75, nevertheless insist that female midwives were represented in literary sources as witches, even if they were not persecuted as such.

56.   Mary Lindemann, 'Professionals? Sisters? Rivals? Midwives in Braunschweig, 1750–1800,' Marland, ed., *The Art of Midwifery*, 176.

57.   Wilson, *The Making of Man-Midwifery*, 2, argues English men-midwives held a 'permanent place' among wealthy, urban clients by the late eighteenth century.

58.   Gelbart, *The King's Midwife*. Despite the increase in male practice throughout the eighteenth century, Jacques Gélis, *La sage-femme ou le médecin: une nouvelle conception de la vie* (Paris: Fayard, 1988), 305, contends that men-midwives exclusively devoted to childbirth remained an exception in France until the nineteenth century, especially in the southern parts of the country, 325. Mireille Laget, *Naissances: L'accouchement avant l'âge de la clinique* (Paris: Seuil, 1982), 211, notes that the practice of female midwives declined primarily in large, urban centres.

59.   Hilary Marland, 'The *"burgerlijke"* Midwife: The *stadsvroedvrouw* of Eighteenth-Century Holland,' Marland, ed., *The Art of Midwifery*, 192–213.

60.   Lindemann, 'Professionals? Sisters? Rivals?' 176–91.

61.   Nadia Maria Filippini, 'The Church, the State and Childbirth: The Midwife in Italy During the Eighteenth Century,' Marland, ed., *The Art of Midwifery*, 152–75.

62.   Gélis, *La sage-femme ou le médecin*, 111–94.

63.   *Ibid.*, 387–487.

64.   Laget, *Naissances*, 240–48, and Mireille Laget, 'Childbirth in Seventeenth- and Eighteenth-Century France: Obstetrical Practices and Collective Attitudes,' Robert Forster and Orest Ranum, eds, *Medicine and Society in France: Selections from the Annales Economies, Sociétés, Civilizations*, vol. 6 (Baltimore: Johns Hopkins University Press, 1980), 137–76. See also Jacques Gélis, Mireille Laget, and Marie-France Morel, *Entrer dans la vie – Naissances et enfances dans la France traditionelle* (Paris: Gallimard, 1978).

65.   Gélis, *La sage-femme ou le médecin*, 67–107, discusses the increasing interest in demography and its impact on midwifery.

66.   Jameson, *Gynecology and Obstetrics*, 67–98, Cianfrani, *A Short History of Obstetrics and Gynecology*, 189–222, Cutter and Viets, *A Short History of Midwifery*, 44–69, and Radcliffe, *Milestones in Midwifery*, 30–45.

67.   Wilson, *The Making of Man-Midwifery*, 97.

68.   Filippini, 'The Church, the State and Childbirth,' 167–8.

69.   Peter M. Dunn, 'The Chamberlen Family (1560–1728) and Obstetric Forceps,' *Archives of Disease in Childhood* 81, 3 (1999), 232–5, Martial Dumont, 'Histoire et

petite histoire du forceps,' *Journal de gynécologie, obstétrique, et biologie* 13, 7 (1984), 743–57. Laurence Brockliss and Colin Jones, *The Medical World of Early Modern France* (Oxford: Clarendon Press, 1997), 615.

70. François Mauriceau, *Observations sur la grossesse et l'accouchement des femmes et sur leurs maladies* (Paris, 1695), 16–18.

71. Eduard Kaspar Jakob von Siebold, *Essai d'une histoire de l'obstétricie*, vol. 2 (Paris: Steinheil, 1891–1892), 84, argues that sixteenth-century surgeon Pierre Franco used his speculum as a kind of forceps. G. Panel, *Jacques Mesnard, chirurgien et accoucheur (1685–1746) et ses oeuvres* (Rouen: Lestringant, 1889), 25, argues that an instrument used by Mesnard, the *tenettes*, was in fact a true forceps.

72. Mauriceau, *Observations sur la grossesse*, 18.

73. Philippe Peu, 'Du tire-tête,' *La pratique des accouchemens* (Paris, 1694), 357–76. I discuss this debate in Chapter 5.

74. Cosme Viardel, *Observations sur la pratique des accouchemens naturels, contre nature & monstrueux* (Paris, 1671), unpaginated preface, argued the surgeon should use his hands alone to assist at deliveries.

75. Wilson, *The Making of Man-Midwifery*, 185–95.

76. See note 58 above.

77. Brockliss and Jones, *The Medical World of Early Modern France*, 613.

78. For the dissemination of European obstetrical treatises see Gélis, *La sage-femme ou le médecin*, 328–32.

Chapter 1

French Treatises 1550–1730:
A Survey

Providing an overview of French obstetrical treatises is challenging because a substantial amount of writing on childbirth was produced during the early modern period. According to my research, French authors composed at least 23 obstetrical treatises and 1 unpublished text between 1550 and 1730, in addition to translations of treatises first published in other languages.[1] By focusing on the broader category of women's health care, historian Alison Klairmont Lingo argues that 22 texts (8 translations and 14 new publications) appeared in French from 1536 to 1636.[2] My figures include, however, only those treatises that originated in France and address multiple aspects of childbirth. I temporarily leave to one side the overtly polemical pamphlets attacking male midwives, tracts describing monstrous births, and sources exclusively concerned with conception or the anatomy of the reproductive organs.[3] Although such topics are frequently present in obstetrical treatises, birth manuals are distinctive in both form and content.

Obstetrical treatises constitute a genre of publication. They are often organized similarly, and include comparable material, advice, and images. Drawing attention to the conventional nature of these treatises counterbalances the tendency to accentuate individual authors. During the early twentieth century, men, usually trained as physicians rather than professional historians, discussed renowned obstetrical treatises in chronological order, noting how specific writers had contributed to the progress of medical knowledge.[4] By insisting that each publication succeeded its predecessor, these writers overlooked the uniformity of the books in favour of their innovative content. At the same time, they assumed that early modern obstetrical treatises were meant both to improve and to transmit knowledge. Considering the homogeneity of the publications not only casts doubt on such assumptions, it encourages us to reexamine the social function of the books.

Various scholars have already begun this process, arguing that obstetrical treatises were involved in producing the reputation of their authors. English professor Isobel Grundy, for example, explores the ways in which Sarah Stone constructed her identity as a skilled midwife in her English treatise of 1737.[5] Historian Nina Rattner Gelbart makes an even stronger case for the role of obstetrical treatises in self-promotion. She argues that the book published by Angélique Marguerite Le Boursier du Coudray in 1759, *Abrégé de l'art des accouchements* [Abridgment of the art of childbirth], validated the midwife's patriotic mission to disseminate her midwifery methods throughout France.[6] Offering sophisticated understandings of obstetrical treatises, these recent studies eschew narratives of medical progress. They nevertheless continue to downplay the generic nature of the books by emphasizing how publications by female midwives diverge from those of their male colleagues.[7] Even as significant differences exist, texts written by women are in many ways akin to those produced by men.

Although approaching obstetrical treatises as a genre of publication diminishes the continuing interest in unique authors, it may also be limiting. Genre analysis risks overemphasizing similarity to create a falsely stable category of evaluation. Genres are, after all, continually in flux as new works are produced. Authors transform genres by reshaping some conventions while adhering to others.[8] It follows that an overly stable definition of a genre can enforce a rigid typology, excluding texts and overlooking differences for apparently indiscriminate reasons. What, then, is the basis for determining the rules for inclusion in a genre? Given the tendency for overlap between genres, such regulations are notoriously difficult to calculate.[9] In the end, it is always possible to find texts that are exceptions to the rules defining a particular genre.[10]

Recognizing these problems, this chapter describes the conventions of early modern French obstetrical treatises, while acknowledging their differences as well as how they changed over time. Addressing issues typically neglected in surveys of medical literature, it considers the material qualities and potential readers of the texts. Without ignoring individual authors, this discussion does not position them as stable points able to anchor interpretations of the treatises. The variations in the publications can often be related to the author's position within the medical hierarchy of early modern France. The books tend to extol the collective identities of physician, surgeon, or midwife, rather than strictly individual beliefs.

It is important to examine early modern French obstetrical treatises because they are less well known than English books. Historian Audrey Eccles, for example, discusses a wide range of English obstetrical texts published before 1740, considering how they portray sexuality, gynaecology, and difficult deliveries.[11] There is no comparable study of the French sources, though scholars recognize that many significant seventeenth- and early eighteenth-century midwifery manuals emanated from France.[12] Historians of medicine are primarily aware of the celebrated French texts written by Ambroise Paré, Louise Bourgeois, Jacques Guillemeau, and François Mauriceau. Eccles pays particular attention to Mauriceau's *Des maladies des femmes grosses et accouchées* [Diseases of women with child and in child-bed], a treatise appearing in four editions during the surgeon man-midwife's lifetime (1668, 1675, 1681, 1694), numerous reprints after his death in 1709, and translations into German, Dutch, Italian, Latin, Flemish, and English.[13] In my own survey, the ambition is not only to increase awareness of such famous sources, but also to extend beyond them, including publications that have previously received little attention from scholars.

It is difficult to determine what, if anything, is specifically 'French' about these obstetrical treatises. The medical hierarchy in early modern France was in some ways distinctive, but considering the publications in terms of national difference is too confining. The international exchange of books and prevalence of translations means that treatises produced in different countries were often in dialogue with each other.[14] The French books must therefore be understood in relation to a range of non-French texts, a process begun here and continued in subsequent chapters.

This chapter is meant to provide a useful starting point for analyses of French obstetrical treatises. Though these texts remain central throughout the book, other kinds of historical materials will also be considered, including pamphlets, medical journals, popular sex manuals, anatomical treatises, and etiquette books. Successive chapters draw on a wide array of sources to highlight the intertextuality of the French treatises, showing how they engage with broader cultural representations of, among other things, maternity, manners, and bodily display.[15] Ultimately, my goal is to achieve a richer understanding of the treatises, without losing sight of them as a genre of publication.

Materiality and the Assessment of Audiences

French obstetrical treatises were typically published in *octavo* dimensions, with pages between 17 and 20 centimetres in length. This relatively small size was in keeping with the trend toward publishing modest, portable books; ponderous folios were meant for learned reading in libraries.[16] French historian Henri-Jean Martin links smaller books with a more popular readership, noting that handbooks in a *duodecimo* format such as physician Philbert Guybert's *Médecin charitable* [The charitable doctor] of 1627 contained recipes and advice for curing everyday ailments.[17] Few obstetrical treatises were this small, though Jean Ruleau's diminutive *Traité de l'opération cesarienne, et des accouchemens difficiles & laborieux* [On the caesarean operation and difficult and laborious deliveries] of 1704 provides an exception. Ruleau, a sworn surgeon in Saintes, claimed that his *duodecimo* book of 276 pages could be conveniently carried and easily read, unlike the 'gros Volumes' written by others.[18] In addition to increasing portability, using less paper as well as smaller type founts made books more affordable, and potentially accessible to a greater number of readers.[19]

The standard use of the vernacular in obstetrical treatises also ensured they addressed a broad audience. According to Klairmont Lingo, authors of early modern publications on women's health care wrote in a comprehensible language to extend their influence beyond elite medical practitioners.[20] In contrast, many anatomical studies continued to be published in Latin, suggesting their authors expected a more specialized audience.[21] This more learned language, however, was not entirely absent from obstetrical treatises. Though Denis Fournier wrote his *L'accoucheur méthodique* [The methodical man-midwife] of 1677 in French, he used Latin to convey remedies designed to expel a dead child or retained afterbirth. The master surgeon, who was born in Lagny but worked in Paris, implied that untrustworthy persons might use the recipes to induce abortion.[22] By inserting Latin into his treatise, Fournier not only preserved certain kinds of medical information for highly educated physicians and surgeons, he also demonstrated his own fluency in the language. In a similar way, the Parisian surgeon man-midwife Mauriceau published the third edition of his treatise, *Des maladies des femmes grosses et accouchées*, in both Latin and French in 1681, revealing his mastery of Latin as well as the intellectual nature of his book.[23]

While the material characteristics of obstetrical treatises suggest something of their intended audiences, authors also specified who would benefit from reading the books. Fournier claimed he meant to teach young surgeons rather than female midwives, echoing the preface written in 1609 by Jacques Guillemeau, royal surgeon to French Kings Charles IX, Henri III, and Henri IV.[24] In contrast to Fournier and Guillemeau, most French authors explicitly included women among potential readers, identifying both female midwives and pregnant women along with male practitioners.[25] These expected audiences did not necessarily correspond, however, to the identities of actual readers. Some modern scholars therefore attempt to calculate the readership of medical books by discovering who owned them, finding that wealthy physicians had the most extensive collections.[26] Yet according to historian Roger Chartier, the possession of books did not circumscribe their access.[27] The practice of lending books and reading them aloud made print available to a range of people, including the illiterate. Nor did the contents of obstetrical treatises necessarily determine their readership. English professor Robert A. Erickson argues that certain audiences for early modern English midwifery books were simply in search of a sex manual.[28] In the end it is difficult to define exactly who encountered obstetrical treatises, but these audiences were likely both diverse and equipped with varying levels of literacy.

Despite attracting a wide range of readers, French obstetrical treatises are almost always lengthy. Averaging 400 pages, the texts are usually divided into three books covering childbirth before, during, and after the delivery. The expanse of these books is not simply required to cover the necessary material. It is also conventional; French novels at the time could appear in volumes of over 1000 pages.[29] Nevertheless, during the early modern period some readers remarked on the verbosity of the French treatises. In the preface to his English translation of Mauriceau's text in 1673, Hugh Chamberlen noted that the author was often 'too prolix; a fault that many of the French affect,' but decided not to cut the French surgeon man-midwife's prose.[30] It seems that in France a substantial tome could be associated with the value of its contents as well as its author. In his surgical publication of 1702, Barthélemy Saviard argued that if he had planned to present himself as a great author he would have produced a more ample book because 'the vulgar are accustomed to regard those who produce thick books as considerable authors, and the creators of small volumes as writers of little merit.'[31]

It follows that Guillaume Mauquest de La Motte's *Traité complet des accouchemens* [Complete treatise of childbirth] of 1721, with its large *quarto* format and more than 900 pages, may have made an impression on early modern audiences before they read it, or even if they neglected to read it altogether. The amount of paper used would certainly have increased the book's material value. The surgeon from Valognes did not enrich his treatise, however, with expensive engraved plates.[32] In contrast, the first edition in 1668 of Mauriceau's *Des maladies des femmes grosses et accouchées* appeared in *quarto* dimensions and was replete with engravings; the gravity and visual presence of this lengthy book likely would have influenced early modern readers. English man-midwife Percival Willughby suggested as much in 1672 when he accused midwives of showing the images in such books to clients in order to establish their own education and ability.[33] While meaning to criticize women, Willughby raised an important possibility for authors and readers alike: the books had symbolic as well as pedagogical import.

Though the materiality of obstetrical treatises contributed to their meaning, it does not usually receive much attention. Early chronological surveys ignore the complex social reception of the texts, implying that audiences read them in an orderly fashion. Yet readers potentially had access to a range of older as well as more recent publications. For example, the three volumes of the obstetrical treatise written by Louise Bourgeois, royal midwife to Queen Marie de Médicis from 1601 to 1609, were published in 1609, 1617, and 1626 respectively, with all the volumes appearing together in 1626, 1634, 1642, and 1652. Latin, German, Dutch, and English translations of Bourgeois' text continued to appear into the early eighteenth century; they were slightly altered and contained different engravings.[34] Clearly, Bourgeois' obstetrical treatise was read alongside or in place of publications by later authors, making it difficult both to establish her book within a publishing sequence, and to secure the meaning of her text in relation to the beliefs and practices of her own lifetime (1563–1636).

The modification of Bourgeois' publication furthermore demonstrates that obstetrical treatises were far from stable. Previous scholars have sometimes assumed that the knowledge contained in these treatises was both rendered permanent and considered trustworthy during the early modern period. However, in his fascinating study of early modern English book publishing, Adrian Johns affirms the reliability of books had to be forged; it was not a quality inherent to print.[35] He casts doubt on Elizabeth Eisenstein's argument that print gave a certain degree of fixity to information.[36] Challenging this belief with references to pirating, Johns demonstrates how difficult it was for early modern authors to control the publication and dissemination of their own books.[37] Mauriceau pointed to this problem in the 'Avertissement' of his second treatise, *Observations sur la grossesse et l'accouchement des femmes* [Observations on women's pregnancy and childbirth], a collection of case studies published in 1695. He warned the public that certain booksellers of Lyon had furtively persisted in publishing the earlier, less perfect volumes of his first treatise.[38] Even one of the most celebrated surgeon men-midwives of the seventeenth century could not regulate the reproduction of his own obstetrical treatises.

The Value of Repetition

Some early historians may have overestimated not only the progressive nature and fixity of obstetrical treatises, but also the status of books in the education of early modern healers. In keeping with models of education in the rest of Europe, French surgeons and female midwives were trained during apprenticeships with experienced practitioners; they learned by means of observation and hands-on practice, not exclusively or even primarily by reading published texts.[39] The French surgeon men-midwives who wrote obstetrical treatises cautioned against depending too heavily on written texts for a comprehensive knowledge of childbirth. They dismissed a strictly theoretical approach to labour and delivery, arguing that hands-on experience was crucial to a full understanding of the lying-in chamber.[40] In a similar way, male authors of English midwifery manuals expressed fears that some readers, especially female midwives, would simply consult a few books and then imagine themselves to be skilled birth attendants, capable of undertaking any obstetrical emergency.[41]

Though the number of medical textbooks increased during the early modern period, it is difficult to say whether or not people used them in a practical way. Several historians of science doubt that written texts provided the principal foundation for knowledge, especially the transmission of manual skills.[42] Even an influential midwifery manual such as Eucharius Rösslin's *Der swangern frawen und he bammen roszgarten* [The rose garden for pregnant women and midwives], first published in 1513, contained little in the way of practical advice. The state physician of Worms and Frankfurt am Main recommended turning malpresenting children for a head-first delivery, but merely alluded to *podalic* version, a method of manipulating the child in the womb for delivery by its feet.[43] In her recent English translation of Rösslin's text, literary scholar Wendy Arons observes the treatise may have marked a decline rather than increase in obstetrical knowledge.[44] Helen King likewise finds that early modern English midwifery manuals combined 'antiquarianism, irrelevance, salaciousness and the blindingly obvious,' offering little useful information to the midwives they ostensibly addressed.[45] King nevertheless insists women could have benefited from reading the English version of Guillemeau's more detailed treatise, first published in 1609 as *De l'heureux accouchement des femmes* [On the happy delivery of women].[46] This Parisian surgeon man-midwife explained how to perform *podalic* version in cases of emergency, advising practitioners to locate the child's feet and, if finding only one, tie a long ribbon around it as a guide before returning it to the womb and searching for the second foot.[47]

Though practical information was contained in early modern French obstetrical treatises, they were typically far from innovative. Scholars overstate the inventive nature of these books when they draw attention to occasional insights such as Bourgeois' recommendation of prompt delivery in cases of premature separation of the placenta, or the manoeuvre used by Mauriceau to flex the unborn child's head by placing one or two fingers in its mouth.[48] Obstetrical treatises were in many ways conservative rather than forward looking. They endorsed theories and methods long after other practitioners had begun to question them. French physicians debated new embryological theories after 1665, and most anatomists recognized the existence of *ova* by 1680 if not earlier.[49] In contrast, French surgeon men-midwives simply reaffirmed the Galenic doctrine until 1714, insisting that conception was caused by the mixture of male and female seed – a subject discussed in Chapter 6.

The lengthy books often reiterated information conveyed in earlier publications. Writers referred to preceding authors, placing themselves within an esteemed publishing tradition that included contemporary writers as well as the Hippocratic corpus and texts by Galen.[50] Early modern authors also apologized, however, for producing books covering familiar material. Guillemeau defensively claimed that though the ancients had already produced great works on childbirth 'there is no less wit and understanding required, to be able to judge of sciences formerly written, than to be the first to shed light on them.'[51] Writing over sixty years later, Cosme Viardel, royal surgeon to French Queen María Teresa, admitted that numerous ancient and modern authors had already written about childbirth, making it necessary for his *Observations sur la pratique des accouchemens naturels, contre nature & monstrueux* [Observations on the practice of natural, unnatural and monstrous childbirth] of 1671 to follow in their footsteps.[52] Mauquest de La Motte was slightly less modest. In the preface to his treatise, the surgeon man-midwife confessed to being intimidated by the learned Mauriceau, but insisted he had discovered a few new things about the art of midwifery.[53] In contrast, Parisian surgeon man-midwife Philippe Peu baldly stated that Mauriceau's obstetrical treatise was repetitive and boring.[54]

Though Peu sought to discredit his rival, his argument was not entirely specious. Authors of obstetrical treatises regularly addressed the same subjects, agreeing about which aspects of pregnancy and birth required attention, the particular illnesses that could arise, and the kinds of treatments necessary. The treatise published in 1561 by ambulatory barber-surgeon Pierre Franco provides the most blatant example of this phenomenon, repeating much of the chapter on childbirth in Paré's *Briefve collection de l'administration anatomique* [Brief collection of anatomical administration] of 1550.[55] Most publications do not include, however, a conspicuous amount of what modern readers would consider plagiarism. All the same, the treatises typically begin by discussing theories of conception, fertility, and sterility, moving on to consider the means of diagnosing pregnancy and determining the sex of an unborn child. Authors described how a woman should behave during her pregnancy, suggesting nourishing foods to eat, and dangerous ones to avoid. They reviewed the nature and treatment of the apparently manifold illnesses that could arise during pregnancy, focusing on the causes of miscarriage. After carefully outlining the signs of 'true' labour, authors provided a brief description of normal delivery, as well as instructions about the diet and baths necessary for the postpartum woman and her child.

The bulk of obstetrical treatises is devoted to those difficult deliveries requiring more intervention on the part of medical practitioners. Authors classified different kinds of birth presentations, explaining how to determine the position of the child's body in the womb. There were certainly differences of opinion expressed in the most difficult cases, particularly with regard to the appropriate use of instruments. Nevertheless, every author endorsed *podalic* version as the primary method for delivering malpresenting children. The process outlined by Guillemeau was described by Soranus of Ephesus in the second century, revived by the French barber-surgeon Paré in his treatise of 1550, and recommended well into the eighteenth century.[56] Authors of obstetrical treatises essentially repeated the instructions offered by Paré, Guillemeau, and Bourgeois throughout the early modern period, though a few disparities can be noted. In his treatise of 1685, *La pratique des accouchemens* [The practice of childbirth], Parisian surgeon man-midwife Paul Portal asserted it was not necessary to discover both feet in order to perform *podalic* version; finding one was often sufficient.[57]

This recapitulation of medical problems and treatments in French obstetrical treatises can be at least partially explained with reference to the ancient theory of the humours that continued to dominate early modern medicine.[58] Authors maintained a similar conception of the body, believing it was constituted by four humours or fluids (yellow bile, blood, phlegm, and black bile) which could become unbalanced and lead to illness. They promoted similar therapies, especially specific foods or lifestyle changes to restore the humoural balance of suffering pregnant women. At the same time, authors advocated the elimination or redirection of offending humours through blood letting, purgatives, sweatings, and diuretics. Before recommending a specific treatment, however, writers noted the humoural composition of the individual woman, as well as her age and social status. The duration of her pregnancy was also regularly taken into consideration. Guillemeau, for example, argued that instead of bleeding women throughout their pregnancies, the procedure should be performed primarily from the fourth to the seventh months.[59]

Early modern educational practices further illuminate the repetition of material in obstetrical treatises. According to historian Mary Lindemann, the examination of medical students was highly ritualized during the medieval and early modern periods.[60] Candidates demonstrated their knowledge by orally expounding on accepted theories of illness as well as methods of treatment. The student's rhetorical style was of primary importance. Displaying individual or original ideas about medical treatment was not a priority and could even lead to the reduction rather than enhancement of authority. In keeping with these traditional methods of exhibiting knowledge, authors of obstetrical treatises concentrated on reiterating accepted information, making intermittent references to novel ideas and techniques.

This preference for repetition was apparently extended to the images included in obstetrical treatises. While more than half of the French publications contain illustrations, at least 10 of them feature unborn figures in awkward positions, hovering in wombs detached from the maternal body. Like much of the written content of the treatises, these images harken back to ancient precedent.[61] The earliest surviving examples of unborn figures inside transparent wombs are found in the ninth-century version of the manuscript by Muscio, a Latin translation of the influential *Gynaecology* written by Soranus of Ephesus in the second century[62] (Figure 1.1). Muscio's images were later adopted in the sixteenth-century text by Rösslin (Figure 1.2), and were recopied in subsequent versions, including the 1586 French translation by physician Paul Bienassis (Figure 1.3). Comparable representations of unborn figures remained standard fare in European obstetrical treatises into the eighteenth century.

There is no evidence, however, that the plates used to produce the images in French publications were recycled from one book to the next. The few sixteenth-century woodcuts and numerous later engravings often have similar compositions and subject matter, but are not identical. Despite differences in detail and style, authors of obstetrical treatises sometimes claimed that rivals had duplicated their images. Mauriceau, for example, accused Peu of copying the images of both pessaries – forms used to support a prolapsed uterus – and unborn children from his treatise. Peu responded that pessaries belonged to all authors, denying any ownership of their visual image. The surgeon man-midwife used a different tactic, however, to defend his commonplace engravings of the unborn. Peu claimed to have directed an artist to draw from a collection of small puppets he had arranged to show some of the possible postures of the child in the womb.[63]

Peu's assertions provide a rare reference to the production of obstetrical images, indicating it was a collective rather than individual effort. During the early modern period, engravings were produced collaboratively; usually the book's publisher would

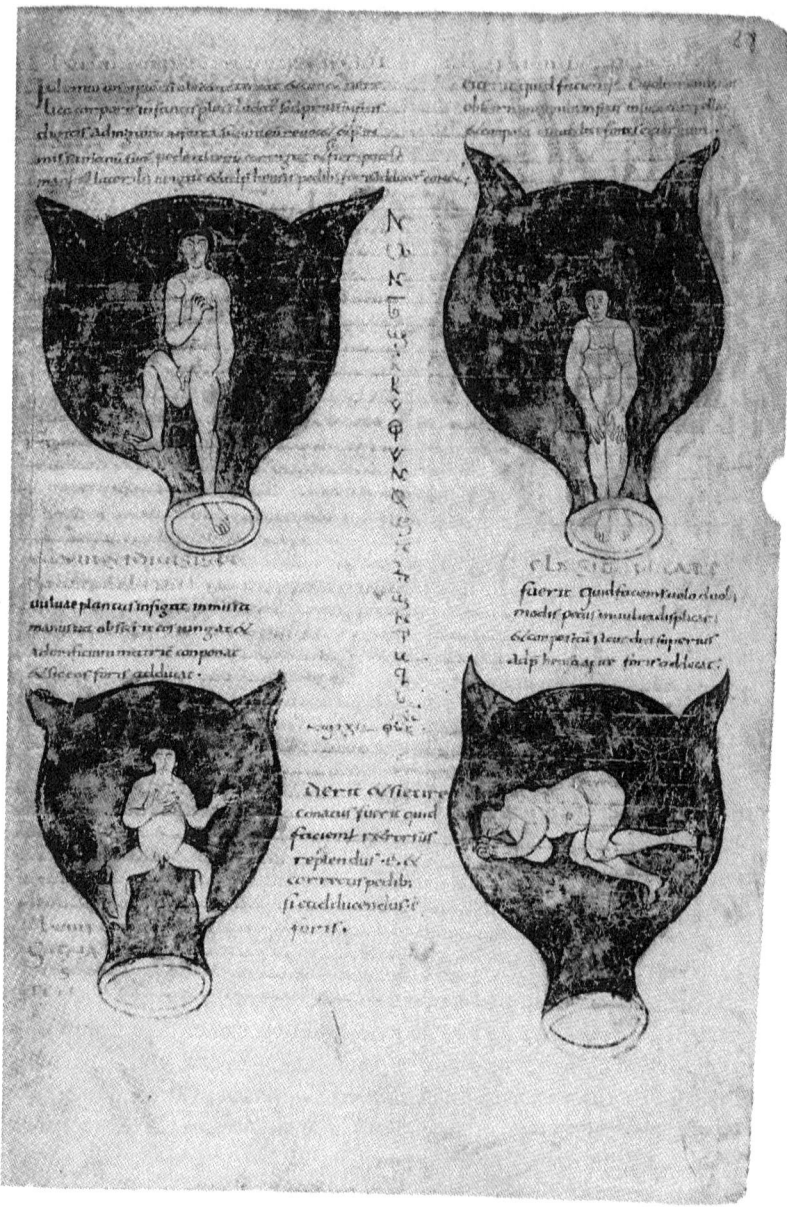

Figure 1.1   Unborn figures, from Muscio's Ms. 3701–15, 9th century, Folio 28.
Copyright Bibliothèque royale de Belgique

Der frawen

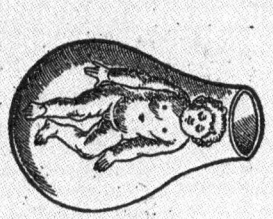

Roßgarten

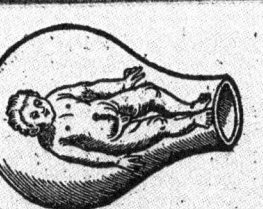

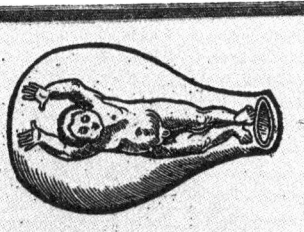

Figure 1.2 Unborn figures, from Eucharius Rösslin's *Der swangern frawen und he bammen roszgarten*, 1513, Argentine. Copyright Bibliothèque nationale de France, Paris

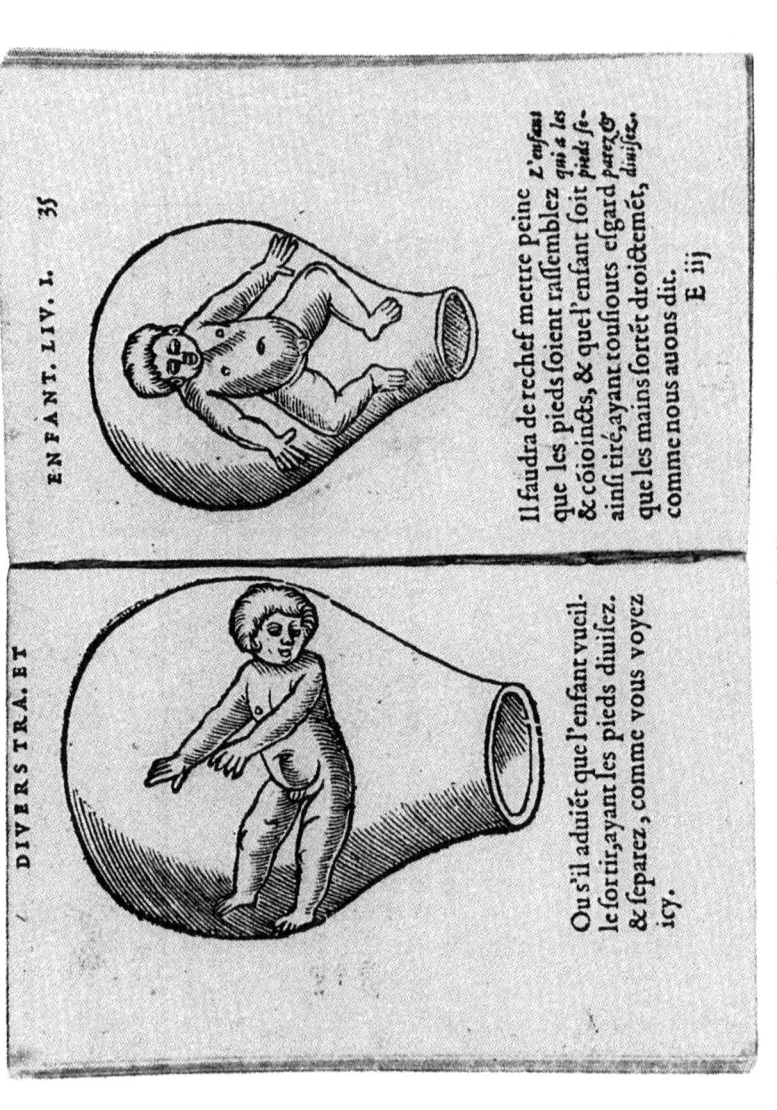

Figure 1.3 Unborn figures, from Eucharius Rösslin's *Des divers travaux et enfantements des femmes*, Paul Bienassis, trans., 1586, Paris. Copyright Bibliothèque nationale de France, Paris

Le Propagatif

L.

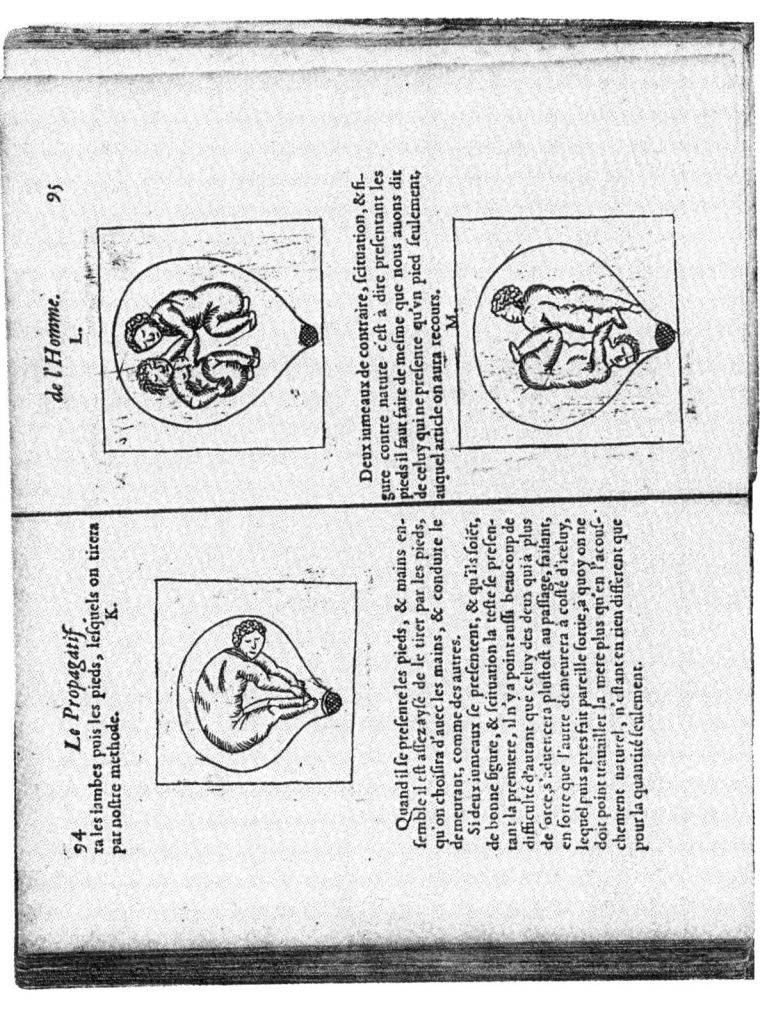

94

ra les jambes puis les pieds, lesquels on tirera par nostre methode. K.

Deux iumeaux de contraire, situation, & figure contre nature c'est à dire presentant les pieds il faut faire de mesme que nous auons dit de celuy qui ne presente qu'vn pied seulement, auquel article on aura recours.

M.

Quand il se presente les pieds, & mains ensemble il est assez aysé de le tirer par les pieds, qu'on choisira d'auec les mains, & conduire le demeurant, comme des autres.

Si deux iumeaux se presentent, & qu'ils soiet, de bonne figure, & situation la teste se presentant la premiere, il n'y a point aussi beaucoup de difficulté d'autant que celuy des deux qui à plus de force, s'aduencera plustost au passage, faisant, en sorte que l'autre demeurera à costé d'iceluy, lequel puis apres fait pareille sortie, a quoy on ne doit point trauailler la mere plus qu'en l'accouchement naturel, n'estant rien different que pour la quantité seulement.

Figure 1.4 Unborn figures, from Jacques Bury's *Le propagatif de l'homme*, 1623, Paris. Copyright Bibliothèque nationale de France, Paris

commission an engraver to inscribe the drawing of another artist, but authors could also participate.[64] It is therefore difficult to link obstetrical images exclusively with the intentions of authors, although in one unusual case a surgeon man-midwife decided to bypass artists to produce images 'by his own hand.' Jacques Bury claimed the engravings in his *Le propagatif de l'homme* [The propagation of man] of 1623 'refer[red] to the diverse postures held by children entering the world'[65] (Figure 1.4). Though badly drawn, the figures resemble the representations found in many other treatises, pointing to a longstanding genre of publication more than to the author himself.

Changing Traditions

There were, of course, differences between the treatises. Authors sometimes expressed distinct opinions about controversial medical practices. Not every writer agreed, for example, that it was reckless to undertake the caesarean operation on a living woman. Guillemeau's warnings against the procedure were echoed in the treatise written by surgeon Jacques Duval in 1612, *Traité des hermaphrodits, parties génitales, accouchemens des femmes* [On hermaphrodites, genitalia, childbirth]. Duval, a native of Évreux who worked in Rouen, argued that a surgeon should not even consider the operation until after the woman had taken her last breath, in the hopes of baptizing a living child.[66] Mauriceau, Viardel, Peu, and Pierre Dionis concurred, but Ruleau insisted women could survive the operation.[67] He drew on arguments made in 1581 by François Rousset, a French physician claiming to have witnessed the successful performance of the caesarean operation.[68] Ruleau went even further, however, by affirming he had practised it on living women with his own hands, and that the women had not only survived, but had flourished long afterward.

Other disparities in the treatises were due more to change over time. The presentation of the texts varied after the sixteenth century. Most early publications on childbirth, such as Paré's *Deux livres de chirurgie, de la génération de l'homme* [Two books of surgery, on the generation of man] of 1573, were included among a wide array of medical topics. The barber-surgeon's account of pregnancy and birth was coupled with a book on monsters in the 1573 edition, and constituted just one of the 27 chapters in his monumental surgical tome, *Les oeuvres de M. Paré* of 1575. Following the same pattern, Franco's *Traité des hernies contenant une ample déclaration de toutes leurs espèces, et autres excellentes parties de la chirurgie* [On hernias, including an ample enumeration of all their types, and other excellent parts of surgery] featured a chapter on childbirth sandwiched between writings on amputation and diseases of the eyes. In his *Erreurs populaires* [Popular errors] of 1578, physician Laurent Joubert launched a lengthy defence of the practice of medicine by physicians before debunking misconceptions about menstruation, conception, birthmarks, and the cravings women had during pregnancy.[69]

Instead of displaying the breadth of their medical knowledge, seventeenth- and eighteenth-century authors devoted treatises exclusively to pregnancy and childbirth. In some ways, this change marked a return to ancient precedents such as Soranus' *Gynaecology* or the medieval Trotula, texts featuring female physiology and parturition.[70] Yet the transformation was also in keeping with broader trends in medical publication. According to Martin, by the late seventeenth century medical compendiums were replaced by books addressing single aspects of disease, such as fever or anatomy.[71] Obstetrical treatises similarly indicated that assisting at deliveries was not simply one kind of medical activity among others; it required distinctive knowledge and unique forms of practice.

Most of these increasingly specialized texts divided childbirth into a series of stages with attendant problems, featuring chapters on sterility, miscarriage, difficult labour, and intractable afterbirths. Three books covered the material, however, in a string of questions and answers. According to Lindemann, this format dated from the Middle Ages, when many medical texts were composed as catechisms, encouraging students to supply the correct answers to rote questions.[72] One of the earliest French obstetrical treatises to follow this pattern was *L'eschole méthodique et parfaite des sages-femmes* [Midwives' methodical and perfect school], published in 1650 by Parisian physician Charles de Saint-Germain. The author focused on problems that could precede, accompany, and follow birth, posing pointed questions such as 'what is sterility?' 'what are the illnesses during pregnancy?' and 'what are the signs of a difficult labour?' In each case, Saint-Germain had a fictional female midwife answer a physician. Though he portrayed the midwife as well-informed, she was clearly subservient to the man interrogating her.[73] Given this hierarchy, it seems likely that Saint-Germain's treatise was meant to prepare midwives for the kinds of questions physicians would ask during their official examination. When the earliest known statute regulating French midwives appeared in 1560, it specified that before being licensed, midwives had to be examined by two surgeons, one physician, and two *matrones jurées* – older women who had already undergone the examination and taken the official oath at the legal courts of Châtelet in Paris.[74]

According to Jacques Gélis such catechisms were designed for midwives barely able to read.[75] Yet even if Saint-Germain claimed female midwives as his primary audience, the question and answer format was not always reproduced with women in mind. Pierre Amand, a surgeon man-midwife who enjoyed a substantial reputation in his day, used a similar arrangement in his *Nouvelles observations sur la pratique des accouchemens* [New observations on the practice of childbirth] in 1714, addressing both surgeons and midwives.[76] Nor were such texts necessarily more simplistic than other obstetrical treatises, for they covered much of the same material.

While Saint-Germain provided detailed descriptions of the anatomy of the male and female reproductive organs, Amand described difficult deliveries as well as how to remove a stubborn afterbirth by hand.[77]

Amand's text also included case studies, in keeping with a further change in obstetrical treatises. As the texts became more specialized, they increasingly featured descriptions of authors' personal experiences in the lying-in chamber. Paré's early publications made only a few references to his hands-on practice of childbirth, but by 1695 Mauriceau's treatise consisted of 700 tales about his encounters with suffering female clients.[78] Authors such as Mauriceau claimed to record actual experiences, offering them up for both the public good and for younger colleagues to contemplate as well as emulate.[79] The stories nevertheless conform to a narrative pattern.[80] They typically begin by stating the date of the incident and providing information about the client, such as her husband's occupation. The tales then give an overview of the woman's physical condition, stressing its dire nature while referring to the one or more previous practitioners who had only made it worse through mismanagement. The surgeon man-midwife's heroic entrance into the lying-in chamber is thereby positioned as a turning point; his intelligent interventions bring the woman, and sometimes even her child, back from the brink of death.

The increasing importance of case studies had much to do with the fact that surgeons produced 16 of the obstetrical treatises published in France between 1550 and 1730. According to historian Nancy Siraisi, personal anecdotes were a longtime feature of surgeons' books, serving to portray authors as successful practitioners who treated patients of some social distinction.[81] The stories in obstetrical treatises certainly cast surgeon men-midwives in a positive light, typically associating them with the preservation rather than destruction of life. At the same time, the tales established the authors as men whose knowledge was founded on hands-on experience and not simply book learning.

This emphasis on manual skill differentiated the treatises written by surgeon men-midwives from those produced by physicians. Four of the five obstetrical treatises written by French physicians before 1730 refer more to theoretical knowledge and the ancient texts attributed to Hippocrates and Galen than to the manual activities performed by surgeons. The early publication by Joubert, for example, neglects to include the kinds of hands-on advice found in the treatises of Paré and Franco. Books by physicians Jean Liébault in 1582 and Charles Saint-Germain in 1655 – his *Traité des fausses couches* [Of miscarriages] – continue to offer theoretical information, describing conditions such as menstrual suppression or miscarriage in general, and then making dietary recommendations or relating remedies to be taken internally.[82] Not surprisingly, publications by physicians exclude the engravings of unborn figures in the womb often found in books by surgeon men-midwives. Such images usually accompany descriptions of how to intervene in difficult labours by performing *podalic* version or using surgical tools.[83] Though physicians recognized the need for manual interventions in certain cases, they usually advised calling on surgeons to undertake them. In contrast, Jacques Fontaine, a physician who worked in Avignon for 20 years and was a professor of medicine at the university in Aix, claimed to have pulled children from the womb with his own hands, without recourse to surgeons.[84] His treatise of 1611 is, however, at odds with the emphasis on prescribed treatments found in most publications by physicians.

The differences between texts written by surgeons and physicians can be related to the hierarchical nature of the early modern medical world, which consisted of practitioners of both sexes with varying degrees of education and status. Healers were gradually separated (as physicians, surgeons, barber-surgeons, or apothecaries) into royally ordained fraternities or guilds that protected the rights and privileges of members, regulated apprenticeships, and controlled licensing. While the foundation of such organizations took place during the fourteenth and fifteenth centuries (and in Italy first), much medical practice was corporatized rather slowly, between 1500–1650 in France, and even later in England.[85] The specific structure of guilds, as well as their degree of independence from each other, varied in the different regions of Europe. All of the institutions contributed, however, both to the construction and policing of boundaries between licit and illicit medical practice. Disagreements over these boundaries could lead to conflict between different guilds. During the seventeenth century, for example, the physicians of the Faculté de Médecine in Paris regularly charged the surgeons belonging to the Confrérie Saints Côme et Damien des Chirurgiens de Paris [Saint-Côme] with attempting to usurp the rights accorded to physicians by teaching publicly, diagnosing illness, and wearing long robes.[86]

Authors of obstetrical treatises expressed some disagreement about who should have the most authority within the birthing chamber, while attempting to delineate the activities appropriate to each kind of medical practitioner. French surgeons, equipped with less university training, were associated with 'lowly' manual labour as opposed to theoretical knowledge. They were therefore expected to defer to physicians both within and outside of the birthing room because physicians were fluent in Latin as well as ancient medical theories. In cases of difficult childbirth, physicians were officially empowered to offer advice and prescribe remedies. According to Fournier, these men confirmed the necessity of any surgical intervention about to be undertaken.[87] Other surgeon men-midwives, however, were less willing to acknowledge the status of physicians within the lying-in chamber. Amand described physicians who simply agreed with his own recommendations, while both Mauriceau and Dionis claimed that a theoretical knowledge of childbirth could not compare with surgeons' practical understanding of it.[88]

Surgeons eagerly claimed assisting at difficult deliveries as their exclusive domain. Mauriceau asserted:

> There are many who believe it is not very difficult to deliver women, because women usually take care of it. In effect, there is no great mystery, when all things come naturally: But when the birth is contrary to nature, it is most certain that it is the most difficult and labourious and the most dangerous of all surgical operations, as is well known to those who have practiced it.[89]

The surgeon man-midwife was rather defensive, insisting that extraordinary surgical skills were required in difficult cases. His claims not only elevated the status of manual labour, but also implied that not just any medical man could perform in the lying-in chamber. This position is at odds with Fontaine's assertions as well as the obstetrical treatises published in other parts of Europe. Some English and Italian publications, for example, were written by physicians who nevertheless included accounts of the physical manipulations required to deliver malpresenting children.[90]

Mauriceau clearly wanted to claim intervening in difficult births as both an exclusively surgical and properly masculine activity. He carefully distinguished what surgeons did from mere women's work, arguing that the activities usually undertaken by female midwives were unskilled. This disparagement of women's traditional occupation in the lying-in chamber is a standard feature in obstetrical treatises written by men. It is important to note, however, that during the early modern period, surgeon men-midwives were not attempting to drive female midwives out of the lying-in chamber. Instead, male authors separated what they deemed natural from unnatural births, relegating the former to women and claiming the latter for themselves. Surgeon men-midwives consistently described natural birth as an event occurring when, after the appropriate length of time, and through the mutual efforts of mother and unborn child, the child emerged head first, its body following.[91] They exhorted female midwives to avoid interfering with this natural process, to await the birth with patience, ensure the afterbirth was completely discharged, and then cut the navel string of the newborn. Surgeon men-midwives claimed that unnatural births – cases of obstruction, malpresentation, or monstrous birth – required inserting the hand into the labouring woman's womb, an action only the boldest midwife would undertake.[92] The treatises written by these men are littered with stories about reckless female midwives who, when faced with a malpresenting child, inevitably mistake one body part for another, or thoughtlessly pull on an extended limb, severing it in the process.[93]

Despite their differences, both French surgeons and physicians agreed that the role of female midwives should be limited to straightforward births. Describing difficult labours as medical events in their treatises, the men designated the work of female midwives as less important than their own, constructing a rigid medical hierarchy that excluded women. According to historian Susan Broomhall, the Paris Faculté de Médecine considered midwifery 'non-medical when it was performed by women.'[94] For the most part, female midwives were urged to recognize when something was awry, and promptly call for the assistance of a man.[95] Even men who argued that female midwives should be better educated were primarily concerned with narrowing women's role in the lying-in chamber. In the first treatise by Saint-Germain, for example, the physician insisted female midwives should have a good understanding of both anatomy and unnatural births. He hoped, however, that women would thereby be able to make accurate reports to physicians, and would defer to male expertise in difficult cases.[96]

In contrast to these arguments, publications by female midwives insist that women could handle difficult labours. French midwives produced three obstetrical texts before 1730, though one remained unpublished during the early modern period. The most famous treatise penned by a French woman is undoubtedly Bourgeois' *Observations diverses sur la stérilité, perte de fruit, foecondité, accouchements et maladies des femmes et enfants nouveaux naiz* [Various observations on sterility, miscarriage, fertility, childbirth and diseases of women and newborns], already mentioned above. In her study of this fascinating treatise, literary scholar Wendy Perkins places Bourgeois' medical practices firmly within the humoural theories dominant at the time, while noting the midwife sometimes revised the beliefs of Hippocrates and Galen.[97] The royal midwife's treatise covered a range of familiar topics such as sterility, miscarriage, and unnatural births. It is in many ways similar to the treatises produced by men, though Bourgeois affirmed that female midwives were able to manage various kinds of difficult labours, especially when equipped with a working knowledge of anatomy.[98] She even implied that women could use instruments – legally the preserve of surgeons – by describing a case in which she borrowed her husband's *pincette* [tweezers] to remove an obstruction from a client's urinary tract.[99] Though Bourgeois had access to such instruments because her husband, Martin Boursier, was a surgeon, it was not unheard of for women to apply surgical tools to their clients. The seventeenth-century Dutch midwife Catharina Schrader, for example, recorded using a *crochet* in six cases of obstructed delivery.[100]

Bourgeois discussed her use of the *pincette* in a case study portraying her as an inventive midwife capable of handling any problem. The royal midwife included numerous personal narratives in her treatise, emphasizing her hands-on experiences of childbirth as well as the social status of her clients. She drew particular attention to the way in which French Queen Marie de Médicis recognized her capacity to become the royal midwife, a topic explored in Chapter 3. Like surgeon men-midwives, Bourgeois emerges from her case studies as a heroic saviour of women and children, more skilled than most female midwives as well as male practitioners.

The second obstetrical text produced by a French woman is far less well-known than that of Bourgeois. In a lengthy unpublished letter written in 1671, Mademoiselle Baudoin transmitted her knowledge to Dr. Vallant, at his request. Calling it a small treatise, Baudoin hoped her discussion of 'good' and 'bad' [natural and unnatural] deliveries would be ordered, embellished and eventually published by the esteemed physician.[101] Baudoin was a reputed midwife in her own day, working in Paris before moving to Clermont in Auvergne. She was apparently well educated after undergoing three months of training in the *salle des accouchées* [lying-in room] at the Hôtel-Dieu in Paris under the watchful eye of the *maîtresse sage femme* [head midwife], Madame Le Vacher.[102] Although almost exclusively focusing on difficult deliveries rather than the regime of pregnant women or illnesses they might suffer, Baudoin's letter generally adheres to the conventions of obstetrical treatises – treatises she clearly read, citing 'our authors' as well as at least one technique advocated by Mauriceau.[103] The midwife explained what to do in various malpresentations, advising *podalic* version without referring to specific case studies. When the unborn child was dead, Baudoin recommended the use of *crochets* to remove it from the womb. She was cautious, however, arguing that the death of an unborn child was very difficult to ascertain; sometimes its mother did not expel excrements or have bad breath, two signs of death noted by Paré.[104] Echoing Bourgeois, Baudoin considered female midwives capable of remedying such difficult situations by inserting their hands into the womb.[105]

In keeping with texts by her female predecessors, Marguerite de La Marche's treatise of 1677 both deferred to and disagreed with male authorities. La Marche was the head midwife at the Hôtel-Dieu from 1670 to 1686, long after the retirement of Baudoin's teacher.[106] Her brief book, *Instruction familière et très utile aux sages-femmes pour bien pratiquer les accouchemens* [Well-known and very useful lessons for midwives to manage deliveries well], covered the usual material, including theories of generation, descriptions of the parts of the womb, and advice for managing both natural and unnatural births. Like the 1650 treatise by Saint-Germain, the midwife presented this information in the form of a catechism, asking questions and providing brief responses. La Marche claimed to write at the behest of the male physicians who administered the Hôtel-Dieu.[107] She nevertheless distanced herself from physicians, arguing that her book included the 'useless theoretical questions' these men tended to ask midwives at the required examination.[108] The head midwife favoured a more practical understanding of childbirth, insisting the hands-on material in her treatise stemmed from her own experiences.[109]

La Marche's book begins with engraved illustrations showing unborn children floating in opened wombs (Figure 1.5). These standardized representations place her work within an established publishing tradition, aligning it with books produced by surgeons. Her text also boasts, however, two engravings of a bizarre 'double womb'

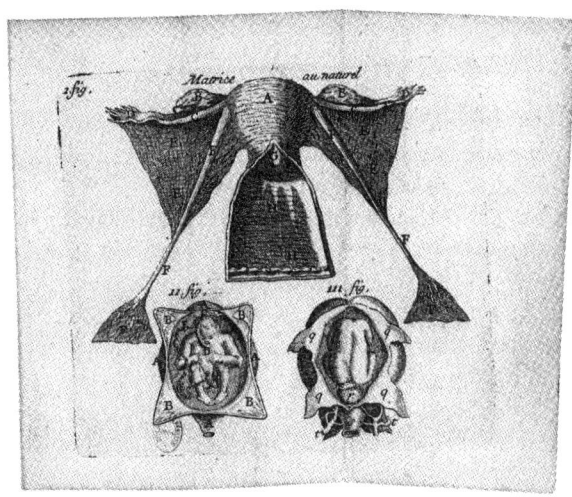

Figure 1.5   Uterus and unborn figures, from Marguerite de La Marche [du Tertre]'s *Instruction familière et très utile aux sages-femmes pour bien pratiquer les accouchemens*, 1710, orig. 1677, Paris. Copyright Bibliothèque nationale de France, Paris

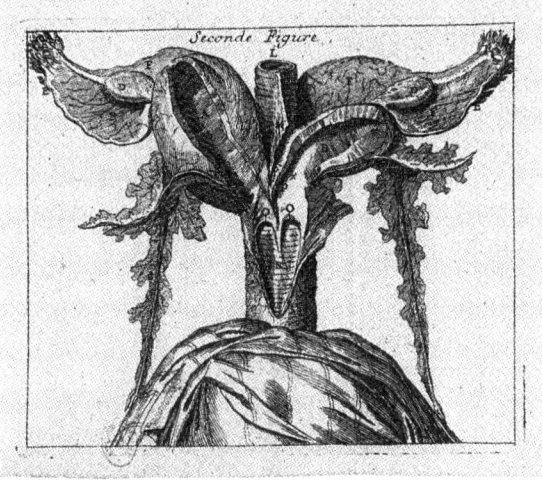

Figure 1.6   Double uterus, from Marguerite de La Marche [du Tertre]'s *Instruction familière et très utile aux sages-femmes pour bien pratiquer les accouchemens*, 1710, orig. 1677, Paris. Copyright Bibliothèque nationale de France, Paris

she claimed to have dissected in the presence of female midwifery students at the Hôtel-Dieu[110] (Figure 1.6). Though other obstetrical treatises discuss reproductive anatomy, only four of them include images of dissected organs, focusing on normal cases.[111] La Marche's treatise includes one image of a normal womb, but the other engravings are unusual, invoking the conventions of both popular and anatomical tracts rather than only those of obstetrical treatises. In 1673, a certain Germain L'Honoré, for example, published a description of a monster born in Rouen, complete with vivid illustrations.[112] Yet such pamphlets were also produced by established medical men. In 1681, the anatomist and surgeon man-midwife Dionis published *Histoire anatomique d'une matrice extraordinaire* [Anatomical tale of an extraordinary womb], delineating his dissection of a woman whose death was mysterious (though likely caused by a tubal pregnancy), and including images of her tattered womb.[113] By displaying her own discovery of an extraordinary womb, La Marche insisted she was able both to perform the dissections usually associated with male practitioners and to comprehend the realm of unnatural births.

Conclusions

This survey showed that French obstetrical treatises cover a succession of issues related to childbirth in more or less chronological order, emphasizing the difficulties associated with pregnancy, labour, and postpartum care, while suggesting appropriate treatments. Though the consistency of the organization and substance of these books is remarkable, discrepancies also emerged. The books changed over time, becoming more specialized, and including an increasing number of case studies. The treatises furthermore advanced different arguments depending on whether the author was trained as a surgeon, physician, or midwife. While physicians emphasized their theoretical understanding of illness, both surgeons and female midwives stressed the practical knowledge learned by interacting with clients. Women uniquely insisted on the extensive capabilities of the well-trained midwife, a position at odds with male authors who strove to delimit her role. Yet the distinctive nature of writing by female midwives should not be overstated; these women reshaped but did not eschew the established genre of obstetrical publication.

Despite striving to discover the conventions of obstetrical treatises, the survey was not a traditional one, with attendant claims to mastery and completion. Differences were strategically highlighted, portraying the instability of the genre as well as how it could potentially be expanded. A few books hovered at the edges of the genre. Rousset's treatise of 1581, for example, provides an early case of specialization because it is exclusively concerned with the caesarean operation. Though Ruleau's treatise also favours the operation, it is more conventional, including descriptions of the womb, normal births, and a host of difficult birth presentations. Other books could not be classified as obstetrical treatises. The publication by Saviard, a surgeon who worked at the Hôtel-Dieu in Paris for 17 years, contains only a few case studies pertaining to childbirth among numerous discussions of head wounds, gangrene, and tumours. In addition, the pamphlets describing a monstrous birth and a damaged womb are extremely brief, cover a single case, and do not offer advice about how to treat suffering women. These tracts were nevertheless related to obstetrical treatises to indicate that despite adhering to conventions, birth manuals are complex publications with multiple layers of meaning.

This chapter provides the basis for thinking differently about early modern French obstetrical treatises, opening them up to analysis. Clearly, the books neither simply delivered information about childbirth, nor revealed actual medical practices. Obstetrical treatises were venues for authors to represent both themselves and others. Writers drew on the conventional format and content of the publications to make arguments about obstetrical identity and authority. They attempted to establish their own expertise in the lying-in chamber, while differentiating themselves from other kinds of medical practitioners. This activity involved more than asserting gendered distinctions between men and women, for male physicians and surgeons also demarcated the appropriate activities of each other. The treatises presented complex arguments about how knowledge of childbirth could be displayed, evaluated, and accumulated in the lying-in chamber.

Notes

1. For a list of these treatises see my bibliography.
2. Alison Klairmont Lingo, 'Print's Role in the Politics of Women's Health Care in Early Modern France,' Barbara B. Diefendorf and Carla Hesse, eds, *Culture and Identity in Early Modern Europe (1500–1800): Essays in Honor of Natalie Zemon Davis* (Ann Arbor: The University of Michigan Press, 1993), 203.
3. For these kinds of sources see, for example, Philippe Hecquet, *De l'indécence aux hommes d'accoucher les femmes* (Paris, 1708), François Bayle, *Histoire anatomique d'une grossesse de 25 ans* (Toulouse, 1678), Louys de Serres, *Discours de la nature, causes, signes et curation des empeschemens de la conception, et de la stérilité des femmes* (Lyon, 1625), and Claude Brunet, *Traité raisonné sur la structure des organes des deux sexes destinez à la génération* (Paris, 1696).
4. See, for example, Edwin A. Jameson, *Gynecology and Obstetrics* (New York: Hoeber, 1936), James V. Ricci, *The Genealogy of Gynaecology: History of the Development of Gynaecology throughout the Ages, 2000 B.C.–1800 A.D.* (Philadelphia: Blakiston, 1943), Theodore Cianfrani, *A Short History of Obstetrics and Gynecology* (Springfield:

Thomas, 1960), Irving Samuel Cutter and Henry R. Viets, *A Short History of Midwifery* (Philadelphia: Saunders, 1964), Walter Radcliffe, *Milestones in Midwifery* (Bristol: Wright, 1967), and Harold Speert, *Obstetric and Gynecologic Milestones Illustrated* (New York: Parthenon, 1996).

5.   Isobel Grundy, 'Sarah Stone: Enlightenment Midwife,' *Clio Medica* 29 (1995), 131.

6.   Nina Rattner Gelbart, *The King's Midwife: A History and Mystery of Madame du Coudray* (Berkeley: University of California Press, 1998).

7.   Grundy, 'Sarah Stone: Enlightenment Midwife,' 139, argues that Stone related one case study after another because as a female midwife her identity was unstable, yet this chapter shows that many men did exactly the same thing. Gelbart, *The King's Midwife*, 77–8, overstates the innovative nature of du Coudray's book by claiming the midwife's abridgement presented a new genre, generating a fad for question-and-answer catechisms on childbirth. My survey indicates that French birth manuals had been published in this format since at least 1650; Madame de La Marche's text of 1677 is even shorter than that of du Coudray. Gelbart, 130–31, further exaggerates the originality of the images in du Coudray's book. See Chapter 6 for my analysis of these plates.

8.   David Duff, 'Introduction,' David Duff, ed., *Modern Genre Theory* (Harlow: Pearson Education Limited, 2000), 7–8. See also John M. Swales, *Genre Analysis* (Cambridge: Cambridge University Press, 1990), 36.

9.   Christine Gledhill, 'History of Genre Criticism,' Pam Cook, ed., *The Cinema Book* (London: British Film Institute, 1985), 59–60.

10.   Stephen Neale, 'Genre and Cinema,' Tony Bennett et al., eds, *Popular Television and Film* (London: British Film Institute/Open University Press, 1981), 9. For other discussions of the complexities of genres see Robert Stam, *Film Theory: An Introduction* (Oxford: Blackwell, 2000), 123–30, and Richard Coe, Lorelei Lingard, and Tatiana Teslenko, eds, *The Rhetoric and Ideology of Genre* (Cresskill: Hampton, 2002).

11.   Audrey Eccles, *Obstetrics and Gynaecology in Tudor and Stuart England* (London: Croom Helm, 1982).

12.   *Ibid.*, 12, 16.

13.   For Mauriceau's biography see D. Ficheux, 'François Mauriceau, accoucheur sous le Roi Soleil' (Thèse pour le doctorat en médecine, Université d'Amiens, 1985).

14.   Jacques Gélis, *La sage-femme ou le médecin: une nouvelle conception de la vie* (Paris: Fayard, 1988), 330, argues that between 1668 and 1815, more than 400 editions of some 245 obstetrical treatises were published in 13 different European countries.

15.   For a discussion of intertextuality see Graham Allen, *Intertextuality* (London: Routledge, 2000), as well as my Chapter 6.

16.   Henri-Jean Martin, *Print, Power, and People in 17th-Century France*, David Gerard, trans. (Metuchen: Scarecrow, 1993), 566.

17.   *Ibid.*, 567. For other discussions of printing in early modern France see Robert Darnton, 'Reading, Writing, and Publishing in Eighteenth-Century France: A Case Study in the Sociology of Literature,' *Daedalus* (Winter 1971), 214–56, Henri-Jean Martin, Roger Chartier and Jean-Pierre Vivet, *Histoire de l'édition française* (Paris:

Promodis, 1982), and Roger Chartier, *The Cultural Uses of Print in Early Modern France*, Lydia G. Cochrane, trans. (Princeton: Princeton University Press, 1987).

18. Jean Ruleau, *Traité de l'opération cesarienne, et des accouchemens difficiles & laborieux* (Paris, 1704), 113.

19. Henri-Jean Martin, *The History and Power of Writing*, Lydia G. Cochrane, trans. (Chicago: University of Chicago Press, 1994), 237–9.

20. Lingo, 'Print's Role in the Politics of Women's Health Care,' 203. See also Matthew Ramsey, 'The Popularization of Medicine in France, 1650–1900,' Roy Porter, ed., *The Popularization of Medicine, 1650–1850* (New York: Routledge, 1992), 97–133.

21. See, for example, Jacques Dubois [Jacobus Silvius], *De mensibus mulierum, et hominis generatione* (Paris, 1555), and Caspar Thomesen Bartholin, *De ovariis mulierum et generationis historia epistola anatomica* (Rome, 1677).

22. Denis Fournier, *L'accoucheur méthodique* (Paris, 1677), 213. For his biography see Nicolas-François-Joseph Éloy, *Dictionnaire historique de la médecine ancienne et moderne*, vol. 1 (Mons: H. Hoyois, 1778), 259, and Amédée Dechambre, ed., *Dictionnaire encylopédique des sciences médicales* (Paris: Masson, 1879), ser. 4, vol. 3, 767.

23. François Mauriceau, *Des maladies des femmes grosses et accouchées* (Paris, 1681), François Mauriceau, *De mulierum praegnantium, parturientium et puerperarum morbis tractatus* (Paris, 1681).

24. For male authors who name male surgeons as their intended audience, see the prefaces in Fournier, *L'accoucheur méthodique*, and Jacques Guillemeau, *De l'heureux accouchement des femmes* (Paris, 1609), as well as François Rousset, *Traitté nouveau de l'hysterotomotokie, ou enfantement caesarien* (Paris, 1581), Jacques Fontaine, *Deux paradoxes, appartenant à la chirurgie, le premier contient la façon de tirer les enfans du ventre de leur mère par la violence extraordinaire* (Paris, 1611), and Jacques Bury, *Le propagatif de l'homme* (Paris, 1623). For the biographies of Guillemeau and his son, Charles, see François Poulain, *La vie et l'oeuvre de deux chirurgiens: Jacques Guillemeau (1550–1613) et Charles Guillemeau (1588–1656)* (Université de Montpellier I, Faculté de Médecine, 1993).

25. Jacques Duval, *Traité des hermaphrodits, parties génitales, accouchemens des femmes* (Rouen, 1612), François Mauriceau, *Des maladies des femmes grosses et accouchées*, Paul Portal, *La pratique des accouchemens* (Paris, 1685), Pierre Amand, *Nouvelles observations sur la pratique des accouchements* (Paris, 1714), name female midwives as potential readers, as do the treatises written by female midwives, noted below.

26. Martin, *Print, Power, and People in 17th-Century France*, 361. Françoise Lehoux, *Le cadre de vie des médecins parisiens aux XVIe et XVIIe siècles* (Paris: Picard, 1976), studies the inventories and wills of 66 doctors in Paris from the early sixteenth century to around 1665. For other discussions of book ownership see Natalie Zemon Davis, 'Printing and the People,' *Society and Culture in Early Modern France* (Stanford: Stanford University Press, 1975), 211–13, and Mary E. Fissell, 'Readers, Texts, and Contexts: Vernacular Medical Works in Early Modern England,' Roy Porter, ed., *The Popularization of Medicine 1650–1850* (London: Routledge, 1992), 72–96.

27.   Roger Chartier, *The Order of Books: Readers, Authors, and Libraries in Europe between the Fourteenth and Eighteenth Centuries*, Lydia G. Cochrane, trans. (Stanford: Stanford University Press, 1994), 19. For another discussion of the French reading public see Henri-Jean Martin, *Le livre français sous l'Ancien Régime* (Paris: Promodis, 1987), 149–223. For early modern French literacy and reading practices see Roger Chartier, 'The Practical Impact of Writing,' Roger Chartier, ed., *A History of Private Life, vol. 3, Passions of the Renaissance*, Arthur Goldhammer, trans. (Cambridge, MA: Harvard University Press, 1989), 111–59.

28.   Robert A. Erickson, '"The Books of Generation": Some Observations on the Style of the British Midwife Books, 1671–1764,' Paul-Gabriel Boucé, ed., *Sexuality in Eighteenth-Century Britain* (Manchester: Manchester University Press, 1982), 74–94.

29.   Thomas DiPiero, *Dangerous Truths and Criminal Passions: The Evolution of the French Novel, 1569–1791* (Stanford: Stanford University Press, 1992), 41.

30.   Hugh Chamberlen, trans. *The Accomplisht Midwife, Treating of the Diseases of Women with Child, and in Child-bed* (London, 1673), unpaginated preface.

31.   Barthélemy Saviard, *Nouveau recueil d'observations chirurgicales* (Paris, 1702), unpaginated preface: 'le vulgaire aïant coûtume de regarder ceux qui font de gros Livres, comme des Auteurs d'une grande consideration; & les faiseurs de petits volumes, comme des Ecrivains d'un léger merite.'

32.   For Mauquest de La Motte see Jacques Gélis, *Accoucheur de campagne sous le Roi-Soleil: Le traité des accouchements de G. Mauquest de La Motte* (Paris: Imago, 1989).

33.   Percival Willughby, *Observations on Midwifery*, Henry Blenkinsop, ed. (Wakefield: S. R. Publishers, 1972; orig. manuscript 1863), 341. Willughby's book includes case studies from 1640–70. See also David Cressy, 'Books as Totems in Seventeenth-Century England and New England,' *Journal of Library History* 21 (1986), 92–106.

34.   For a list of Bourgeois' publications in French see François Rouget and Colette H. Winn's edition, *Récit véritable de la naissance de messeigneurs et dames les enfans de France* (Geneva: Droz, 2000), 45.

35.   Adrian Johns, *The Nature of the Book: Print and Knowledge in the Making* (Chicago: University of Chicago Press, 1998).

36.   Elizabeth Eisenstein, *The Printing Press as an Agent of Change*, vol. 1 (Cambridge: Cambridge University Press, 1979), 113–26.

37.   Johns, *The Nature of the Book*, 6–28, 181–2, 634–5.

38.   François Mauriceau, 'Avertissement,' *Observations sur la grossesse et l'accouchement des femmes* (Paris, 1695), unpaginated preface.

39.   For the training of female midwives in France see Henriette Carrier, *Origines de la Maternité de Paris. Les maîtresses sages-femmes et l'office des accouchées de l'ancien Hôtel Dieu (1378–1796)* (Paris: Steinheil, 1888), Marcel Fosseyeux, 'Sages-femmes et nourrices à Paris au XVIIIe siècle,' *Revue de Paris* 19 (October 1921), 535–54, and Evelyne Berriot-Salvadore, *Les femmes dans la société française de la renaissance* (Geneva: Droz, 1990), 251–3. For the training of surgeons see Jeanne Rigal, *La communauté des maîtres-chirurgiens jurés de Paris au XVIIe et au XVIIIe siècle* (Paris: Vigot Frères, 1936), Pierre Franco, *Chirurgie*, E. Nicaise, intro. (Geneva: Slatkine Reprints, 1972; orig. 1561), xxxvi–xlviii, Laurence Brockliss and Colin Jones,

The Medical World of Early Modern France (Oxford: Clarendon Press, 1997), 188–92, and Toby Gelfand, *Professionalizing Modern Medicine: Paris Surgeons and Medical Science and Institutions in the 18th Century* (Westport: Greenwood, 1980), 85–90.

40. Pierre Dionis, *Traité général des accouchemens* (Paris, 1718), x, argued that the art of delivery did not require great arguments, but depended on the hand of the surgeon. Portal, *La pratique des accouchemens*, 2, claimed to offer in his treatise only that which he had seen, and had learned through experience. Philippe Peu, *La pratique des accouchemens* (Paris, 1694), 1, argued that his treatise was limited to treating things based on his own experience, avoiding theoretical materials.

41. Helen King, '"As if None Understood the Art that Cannot Understand Greek": The Education of Midwives in Seventeenth-Century England,' Vivian Nutton and Roy Porter, eds, *The History of Medical Education in Britain* (Amsterdam: Rodopi, 1995), 190.

42. For knowledge as inescapably social and learned through personal interaction, not by following instructions, see Harry M. Collins, *Changing Order: Replication and Induction in Scientific Practice* (London: Sage, 1985), 55–7. Christopher Lawrence, 'Incommunicable Knowledge: Science, Technology and the Clinical Art in Britain 1850–1914,' *Journal of Contemporary History* 20 (1985), 503–20, argues that nineteenth-century physicians defended their natural qualities as gentlemen against the incursion of a more practical and scientific education.

43. Wendy Arons, trans. and intro., *Eucharius Rösslin: When Midwifery Became the Male Physician's Province* (Jefferson: McFarland, 1994), 19, 56.

44. *Ibid.*, 10.

45. King, '"As if None Understood the Art that Cannot Understand Greek",' 189.

46. *Ibid.*, 189. Guillemeau's treatise was published as *Child-Birth or, the Happy Deliverie of Women* in 1612.

47. Guillemeau, *De l'heureux accouchement des femmes*, 277–8.

48. Cutter and Viets, *A Short History of Midwifery*, 74–5, Pierre Huard and Mirko Drazen Grmek, *La chirurgie moderne. Ses débuts en occident XVIe–XVIIe–XVIIIe siècles* (Paris: Dacosta, 1968), 91–2, and Radcliffe, *Milestones in Midwifery*, 25.

49. Laurence Brockliss, 'The Embryological Revolution in the France of Louis XIV: The Dominance of Ideology,' G. R. Dunstan, ed., *The Human Embryo: Aristotle and the Arabic and European Traditions* (Exeter: University of Exeter Press, 1990), 162–9, and Jacques Roger, *The Life Sciences in Eighteenth-Century French Thought*, Robert Ellrich, trans. (Stanford: Stanford University Press, 1997), 215.

50. See, for example, Guillemeau, *De l'heureux accouchement des femmes*, unpaginated preface, Cosme Viardel, *Observations sur la pratique des accouchemens naturels, contre nature & monstrueux* (Paris, 1671), unpaginated preface, and Dionis, *Traité général des accouchemens*, preface.

51. Guillemeau, *De l'heureux accouchement des femmes*, unpaginated preface: 'qu'il n'ya pas moins d'esprit, ny d'entendement, de pouvoir bien juger les sciences cy devant escrites, que de les avoir des premiers mises en lumière.'

52. Viardel, *Observations sur la pratique des accouchemens naturels, contre nature & monstrueux*, unpaginated preface. For Viardel's biography see Émile Placet,

L'obstétrique aux XVIIe et XVIIIe siècles. Viardel, Portal, et Mauquest de La Motte (Paris: Baillière, 1892).

53.   Guillaume Mauquest de La Motte, *Traité complet des accouchemens* (Paris, 1729; orig. 1721), vi.

54.   Philippe Peu, *Réponse de M. Peu aux observations particulières de M. Mauriceau sur la grossesse et l'accouchement des femmes* (n.l., n.d.), 25. For Peu's biography see Éloy, *Dictionnaire historique de la médecine ancienne et moderne*, vol. 2, 271–2, and Dechambre, ed., *Dictionnaire encylopédique des sciences médicales*, ser. 2, vol. 23, 772.

55.   Book 5, 'Accouchements.– Maladies des femmes' of Pierre Franco's *Traité des hernies contenant une ample déclaration de toutes leurs espèces, et autres excellentes parties de la chirurgie* (Lyon, 1561) borrows portions from Ambroise Paré, 'La manière de extraire les enfans tant mors que vivans hors le ventre de la mère,' the discussion of childbirth appended to his *Briefve collection de l'administration anatomique* (Paris, 1550), 88–96. For Franco's biography see Franco, *Chirurgie*, lxxxiii–lxxxix. For Paré's biography see, among other sources, Paule Dumaitre, *Ambroise Paré: chirurgien de quatre rois de France* (Paris: Librairie Académique Perrin Fondation Singer-Polignac, 1986).

56.   Beryl Rowland, *Medieval Woman's Guide to Health: The First English Gynecological Handbook* (Kent: Kent State University Press, 1981), 21, argues that Soranus is credited with originating the *podalic* method. Henri Stofft, 'Ambroise Paré, accoucheur,' *Histoire des sciences médicales* 32, 4 (1998), 399–407, affirms that Paré invented it. See Paré, 'La manière de extraire les enfans tant mors que vivans hors le ventre de la mère,' 92.

57.   Portal, *La pratique des accouchemens*, 59. For Portal's biography see François Duchatel, 'Paul Portal (1630?–1er juillet 1703): Un accoucheur méconnue du XVIIe siècle,' *Histoire des sciences médicales* 14, 4 (1980), 407–18.

58.   See Mary Lindemann, 'Sickness and Health,' *Medicine and Society in Early Modern Europe* (Cambridge: Cambridge University Press, 1999), 8–36, Roy Porter, *Medicine: A History of Healing* (New York: Marlowe, 1997), 20–21, and Nancy G. Siraisi, *Medieval and Early Renaissance Medicine: An Introduction to Knowledge and Practice* (Chicago: University of Chicago Press, 1990), 104–6. The uniformity of French obstetrical treatises cannot be explained with reference to publishers because many different publishers participated in producing the books.

59.   Guillemeau, *De l'heureux accouchement des femmes*, 45.

60.   Lindemann, *Medicine and Society in Early Modern Europe*, 95.

61.   This visual similarity does not mean, however, that the images had the same meanings over time. See Chapter 6 for my analysis of images of the unborn.

62.   E. Ingerslev, 'Rösslin's "Rosegarten": Its Relation to the Past (the Muscio Manuscripts and Soranos), particularly with regard to Podalic Version,' *The Journal of Obstetrics and Gynaecology of the British Empire* 15, 1 (1909), 1–25.

63.   Peu, *Réponse de M. Peu aux observations particulières de M. Mauriceau sur la grossesse et l'accouchement des femmes*, 94.

64. For a discussion of engravings in medical books see André Hahn, Paule Dumaitre, and Janine Samion-Content, *Histoire de la médecine et du livre médical* (Paris: Olivier Perrin, 1962), 207–9. For the differences between woodcuts and engravings see Robert Brun, *Le livre français* (Paris: Larousse, 1948), 65–6, and Lucien Febvre and Henri-Jean Martin, *The Coming of the Book*, David Gerard, trans. (London: Verso, 1976), 85–6, and Michel Melot, Antony Griffiths, Richard S. Field, and André Béguin, *Prints: History of an Art* (New York: Rizzoli, 1981).

65. Bury, *Le propagatif de l'homme*, unpaginated preface.

66. Guillemeau, *De l'heureux accouchement des femmes*, 328–34. Duval, *Traité des hermaphrodits, parties génitales, accouchemens des femmes*, 202–12. For Duval's biography see Éloy, *Dictionnaire historique de la médecine ancienne et moderne*, vol. 2, 121, and Dechambre, ed., *Dictionnaire encyclopédique des sciences médicales*, ser. 1, vol. 30, 726. See also Kathleen Long, 'Jacques Duval on Hermaphrodites,' Kathleen Long, ed., *High Anxiety: Masculinity in Crisis in Early Modern France* (Kirksville: Truman State University, 2002), 107–38.

67. Mauriceau, *Des maladies des femmes grosses et accouchées*, 356–67, Viardel, *Observations sur la pratique des accouchemens naturels, contre nature & monstrueux*, 172–80, Peu, *La pratique des accouchemens*, 322–36, and Dionis, *Traité général des accouchemens*, 310–18. Ruleau, *Traité de l'opération cesarienne, et des accouchemens difficiles & laborieux*, 75.

68. Rousset, *Traitté nouveau de l'hysterotomotokie, ou enfantement caesarien*, 16–30.

69. Laurent Joubert, *Erreurs populaires* (Bordeaux, 1578). See also Natalie Zemon Davis, 'Proverbial Wisdom and Popular Errors,' *Society and Culture in Early Modern France*, 227–67.

70. Soranus of Ephesus, *Gynecology*, Owsei Temkin, trans. and intro. (Baltimore: The Johns Hopkins University Press, 1956), and Monica H. Green, ed. and trans., *The Trotula: A Medieval Compendium of Women's Medicine* (Philadelphia: University of Pennsylvania Press, 2001).

71. Martin, *Print, Power, and People in 17th-Century France*, 566.

72. Lindemann, *Medicine and Society in Early Modern Europe*, 95.

73. Charles de Saint-Germain, *L'eschole méthodique et parfaite des sages-femmes* (Paris, 1650). Saint-Germain also wrote *Traité des fausses couches* (Paris, 1655).

74. Richard L. Petrelli, 'The Regulation of French Midwifery during the *Ancien Régime*,' *Journal of the History of Medicine* 27 (1971), 276–92, Gélis, *La sage-femme ou le médecin*, 21–64, and *Statuts et reiglemens ordonnez pour toutes les matronnes, ou saiges femmes de la ville, faulxbourgs, prevosté, et vicomté de Paris* (Paris, n.d.). See also my discussion of female midwives in Chapter 3.

75. Gélis, *La sage-femme ou le médecin*, 99, 329.

76. For his biography see Éloy, *Dictionnaire historique de la médecine ancienne et moderne*, vol. 1, 105, and Dechambre, ed., *Dictionnaire encyclopédique des sciences médicales*, ser. 1, vol. 3, 483.

77. Amand, *Nouvelles observations sur la pratique des accouchements*, 13–14, and 215.

78. Mauriceau, *Observations sur la grossesse et l'accouchement des femmes*.

79. See the unpaginated prefaces in Mauriceau, *Observations sur la grossesse et*

l'accouchement des femmes, and Portal, *La pratique des accouchemens*, as well as Mauquest de La Motte, *Traité complet des accouchemens*, xii–xiii.

80. Gélis, *La sage-femme ou le médecin*, 312.
81. Siraisi, *Medieval and Early Renaissance Medicine*, 170–72.
82. Jean Liébault, *Thrésor des remèdes secrets pour les maladies des femmes* (Paris, 1582), is a French translation of Liébault's Latin version of Giovanni Marinelli, *Le medicine partenenti alle infermità delle donne* (Venice, 1574), leading me to exclude it from my list of French obstetrical treatises. I also excluded Théodore Turquet de Mayerne's *La pratique de médecine...avec le régime des femmes grosses* (Lyon, 1693), published long after his death in 1655 by his godson, Théodore des Vaux, who gleaned material from the unpublished casebooks his godfather produced in England. The Huguenot physician was born near Geneva and trained in Montpellier, serving King Henri IV of France before becoming the first physician to a number of English Kings. Selections of Mayerne's notes on childbirth appeared in *The Compleat Midwife's Practice Enlarged*, 3rd edn (London, 1663), and the treatise published in France differs primarily in its attention to difficult cases requiring surgical intervention. Unlike texts written by French physicians, Mayerne's book advocates controversial chemical remedies as a last resort, after the unsuccessful application of conventional treatments. See Brian Nance, *Turquet de Mayerne as Baroque Physician: The Art of Medical Portraiture* (Amsterdam: Rodopi, 2001).
83. These images, however, should not be considered illustrations of the womb and its contents, a point made in Chapter 6.
84. Jacques Fontaine, *Deux paradoxes, appartenant à la chirurgie*. For his biography see Éloy, *Dictionnaire historique de la médecine ancienne et moderne*, vol. 2, 250.
85. Brockliss and Jones, *The Medical World of Early Modern France*, 170–229, 480–552.
86. Joseph Lévy-Valensi, *La médecine et les médecins français au XVIIe siècle* (Paris: Baillière, 1933), François Millepierres, *La vie quotidienne des médecins au temps du Molière* (Paris: Hachette, 1964), 169–87, Rigal, 'Démêlés avec la Faculté de Médecine, 1600–1655,' *La communauté des maîtres-chirurgiens jurés de Paris*, 25–42, and Gelfand, *Professionalizing Modern Medicine*, 21–57.
87. Fournier, *L'accoucheur méthodique*, 3.
88. Amand, *Nouvelles observations sur la pratique des accouchements*, 184, Mauriceau, *Des maladies des femmes grosses et accouchées*, unpaginated preface, and Dionis, *Traité général des accouchemens*, 291.
89. Mauriceau, *Des maladies des femmes grosses et accouchées*, 269:

> Il y a bien des gens qui croyent qu'il n'y a pas grande difficulté à pratiquer les accouchemens, puisque ce sont des femmes qui s'en meslent ordinairement; En effet, il n'y a pas grand mystere, quand toutes choses viennent naturellement: Mais quand l'accouchement est contre nature, il est tres-certain, que c'est la plus difficile & laborieuse, & la plus dangereuse de toutes les operations de Chirurgie, ce qu'ils connoîtroient bien facilement s'ils l'avoient pratiquée.

90. See, for example, William Sermon, *The Ladies Companion, or the English Midwife* (London, 1671), and Girolamo Mercurio, *La commare o riccoglitrice* (Venice, 1601).

91. See, for example, Mauriceau, *Des maladies des femmes grosses et accouchées*, 194–5, and Portal, *La pratique des accouchemens*, 7.

92. Mauriceau, *Des maladies des femmes grosses et accouchées*, 207–8, Viardel, *Observations sur la pratique des accouchemens naturels, contre nature & monstrueux*, 29, Fournier, *L'accoucheur méthodique*, 166, 262, Peu, *La pratique des accouchemens*, 257–62, and Dionis, *Traité général des accouchemens*, 247.

93. Portal, *La pratique des accouchemens*, 212, described a woman pulling limbs from a child, and Viardel, *Observations sur la pratique des accouchemens naturels, contre nature & monstreux*, 114–15, described a case in which a young midwife mistook a child's cheeks for its buttocks.

94. Susan Broomhall, *Women's Medical Work in Early Modern France* (Manchester: Manchester University Press, 2004), 55.

95. Mauriceau, *Des maladies des femmes grosses et accouchées*, 243, decried presumptuous midwives who avoided calling surgeons. Portal, *La pratique des accouchemens*, 9, claimed that women would be saved if midwives called men in time. Peu, *La pratique des accouchemens*, 261, argued that timid midwives did not call for help because of their pretended abilities.

96. Saint-Germain, *L'eschole méthodique et parfaite des sages-femmes*, 4, 211.

97. Wendy Perkins, *Midwifery and Medicine in Early Modern France: Louise Bourgeois* (Exeter: University of Exeter Press, 1996), 11.

98. Louise Bourgeois, *Observations diverses sur la stérilité, perte de fruict, foecondité, accouchements et maladies des femmes et enfants nouveaux naiz*, Françoise Olive, ed. (Paris: Côté-Femmes, 1992; orig. 1652), 104–7.

99. *Ibid.*, 110.

100. G. J. Kloosterman, 'Some Obstetric Remarks on Vrouw Schrader's Notebook and Memoirs,' *'Mother and Child Were Saved'. The Memoirs (1693–1740) of the Frisian Midwife Catharina Schrader*, Hilary Marland, trans. (Amsterdam: Rodopi, 1987), 37.

101. Baudoin's 'Lettre sur les accouchements' is reproduced in Paul-Émile Le Maguet, *Le monde médical parisien sous le Grand Roi, suivi du portefeuille de Vallant* (Paris: Maloine, 1899), 314–40. Baudoin addressed her letter to Monsieur Vallant, the doctor of Mademoiselle de Guise and Madame de Sablé, indicating she did so at his request, in the hope that he would publish what she wrote to him.

102. *Ibid.*, 313. Biographical information about the older midwife is lacking, but according to historian Henriette Carrier the surgeon man-midwife Philippe Peu worked with Le Vacher in 1646. See Carrier, *Origines de la Maternité de Paris*, 8.

103. Baudoin, 'Lettre sur les accouchements,' 323.

104. *Ibid.*, 336. Paré discusses the signs of death in Chapter 31, 'De la génération de l'homme,' itself part of *Les oeuvres de M. Paré* (Paris, 1575).

105. Baudoin, 'Lettre sur les accouchements,' 320.

106. Marguerite de La Marche [du Tertre], *Instruction familière et très utile aux sages-femmes pour bien pratiquer les accouchemens* (Paris, 1710; orig. 1677). For her biography see A. Delacoux, *Biographie des sages-femmes célèbres, anciennes,*

modernes, contemporaines (Paris: Trinquart, 1833), 107.

107.   La Marche [du Tertre], *Instruction familière*, unpaginated preface. Most authors of obstetrical treatises claimed to write at the behest of others, usually friends and colleagues.

108.   *Ibid.*, unpaginated preface.

109.   *Ibid.*, unpaginated preface.

110.   *Ibid.*, caption of 'Premiere Figure.'

111.   For other images of dissected wombs that do not feature malpresenting unborn children in them see Duval, *Traité des hermaphrodits, parties génitales, accouchemens des femmes*, Mauriceau, *Des maladies des femmes grosses et accouchées*, Fournier, *L'accoucheur méthodique*, and Dionis, *Traité général des accouchemens*. Dionis' treatise also features an engraved image of a tubal pregnancy.

112.   Germain L'Honoré, *Description d'un monstre dont une femme de la ville de Rouen accoucha le mois d'octobre 1672* (Rouen, 1673).

113.   Pierre Dionis, *Histoire anatomique d'une matrice extraordinaire* (Paris, 1683), 19, dissected the womb without cutting it too much so that artists could draw it. This example indicates that anatomical practices could be dictated by the desire for images, at odds with the commonplace notion that such images were secondary, and simply reflected the appearance of dissections.

Chapter 2

Risking Exposure:
The Visual Politics of Childbirth

In 1617 royal midwife Louise Bourgeois offered advice to her daughter. Publishing an open letter in Volume 2 of her well-known treatise, *Observations diverses sur la stérilité, perte de fruict, foecondité, accouchements et maladies des femmes et enfants nouveaux naiz*, Bourgeois cautioned the younger midwife against experimenting with remedies, withholding the caul that sometimes covered the head of an infant, and receiving women into her own home.[1] Entitled *Instruction à ma fille* [Lessons for my daughter], the letter also bitterly denounced the 'effrontery' of those women who summoned men to assist them in normal labours. Bourgeois nevertheless suggested how to cope with the increasing demand for male intervention by describing an episode from her past:

> One day I found myself at the lying-in of a young noblewoman, a good friend of mine whose husband was away; she was being helped by three or four of her friends, who asked me what was the state of her delivery. I told them that the child was coming poorly, but that I would have it, helping God, without danger to either mother or child. They asked me to be so kind as to have a surgeon see her. To relieve them, I conceded, provided that she did not see him, for I knew that that might cause her to die of dread and shame. I persuaded her to slip down to the foot of her bed. I put the cushion in the middle of the bed and lowered the bed curtains on the side which he had to pass by and at the foot. He touched her as I spoke, she did not see him, and gave birth with neither artificial intervention nor help other than that of God and nature.[2]

In the name of protecting her client against both a frightening vision and an infringement on female modesty, the clever midwife ensured that when the surgeon man-midwife appeared in the lying-in chamber, he simultaneously disappeared.

Bourgeois' anecdote offers the modern scholar a glimpse at how one midwife negotiated, or at least claimed to have negotiated, the entry of a male medical practitioner into what was traditionally a feminine realm. We see signs of some disagreement between the women in the birthing room although, according to this account, it was ultimately the midwife's decision to call for male assistance. The story lends support to recent arguments, by Adrian Wilson and Hilary Marland among others, that early modern European women were not simply passive victims of male midwives, but rather actively participated in their employment.[3] At the same time, the tale exhibits the female midwife's resistance to this intrusion. Even as Bourgeois admitted a male practitioner was sometimes wanted in dangerous deliveries, she demanded 'that the woman neither see him nor have knowledge of his presence, and that the surgeon not see her either.'[4] The midwife was apparently less concerned with the man's manual interventions than with who would be seen by whom.

In this chapter, I explore what I think is the most important aspect of Bourgeois' didactic narrative: the visual politics of early modern French childbirth. I analyse how authors of obstetrical treatises described the visual exchanges occurring in the lying-in chamber, examining the meanings associated with acts of looking and being looked at. How did writers articulate the relationship between vision and the acquisition of obstetrical expertise? According to Bourgeois, acts of looking were far from neutral. She claimed that both seeing and being seen by a male surgeon could have negative consequences for her labouring client. Bourgeois' narrative nevertheless suggests she was concerned with more than the woman's well-being. By reserving visual access to the client for herself, the royal midwife asserted control of the lying-in chamber and reaffirmed the early modern belief that it was inappropriate for men to cast their eyes on the female genitalia.[5]

Bourgeois portrayed the dangers of male looking at a time when male practitioners were urging women to shed their 'false modesty' and allow men to assist at difficult deliveries. Male authors of early modern French obstetrical treatises argued that men entered the lying-in chamber solely to help women and children. They praised female clients who agreed to be examined by men; by recognizing male medical expertise, these women increased their chances of survival. In contrast, women who refused to be seen or touched were portrayed by male authors as rashly more concerned with maintaining social conventions that safeguarding their own lives.

Modern scholars have analysed both how men claimed the right to look at female bodies, and the effects of that looking. Some historians argue that once women surmounted old-fashioned taboos against men-midwives, childbirth became safer.[6] Others are more sceptical about the benefits of men's scrutiny of women, linking it with male efforts to control the lying-in chamber. Feminist scholar Lynne Tatlock, for example, contends that male looking was crucial to men's eventual appropriation of childbirth from female midwives.[7] According to her analysis of early modern German obstetrical treatises, the vaginal speculum opened the female body to a male gaze, changing the field of obstetrics and gynaecology forever. She contends that once women's bodies were exposed to invasive observation, they became objects of masculine medical knowledge.

Tatlock's argument is informed by the theory of the medical gaze developed by philosopher and historian Michel Foucault. He claimed that during the eighteenth and nineteenth centuries, physicians were associated with the ability to see the hidden truth of the body.[8] Their powerful gaze examined the body, inside and out, producing it as a passive entity subject to discipline and alteration. Yet for Foucault power was never exclusively repressive in its effects. The medical gaze also transformed the body into a discrete object, equipped with new possibilities and perceptions.

Though Foucault was not primarily interested in gender, his theory has been important to feminist scholars who insist the male scrutiny of women's bodies was increasingly institutionalized after the early modern period, reaching its apogee in twentieth-century obstetrics and gynaecology. In a recent study, health educator Terri Kapsalis argues that modern gynaecology was founded on efforts to master the female body by making it both visible and knowable. She notes, however, that visibility itself is neither inherently good nor evil; instead 'making spectacles is about power, about who has the power to render visible and who has the power to look.'[9] According to Kapsalis, the gaze is typically identified with the medical practitioner (or technological substitute) and directed toward the patient. The doctor is not usually portrayed as subject to the patient's gaze, a kind of looking that is less powerful in modern contexts given the prestige regularly accorded to physicians. Kapsalis nevertheless wonders what would happen if practitioners were exposed to visual examination during medical procedures.[10] Striving to change the power dynamics of the pelvic exam, she suggests that if female patients looked back at clinicians – returning their gaze – women might become participants rather than passive objects.

Kapsalis' scenario in which women gaze upon medical personnel resonates with the early modern period. For despite Tatlock's claims, male midwives did more than use instruments to peer at female clients; the men were themselves on display in the birthing room. Male authors of obstetrical treatises described their own inspection by those gathered in the lying-in chamber – witnesses who might be quick to condemn the man-midwife if something went wrong. Though authors did not always identify the members of this audience, during the early modern period the birthing chamber was populated primarily by women; in cases of emergency, male family members and additional medical practitioners may also have been present.[11]

Wilson maintains that the process of visual evaluation was crucial to the man-midwife's reputation. According to him, once early modern English men-midwives revealed they could deliver live children with their forceps, they shattered the 'self-perpetuating cycle of fear, craniotomy and death.'[12] No longer principally associated with the use of hooks to remove dead children from the womb, men were called to emergency situations sooner. Wilson claims that male midwives thus had more opportunities to exhibit their skills. Those satisfied customers who viewed successful deliveries would likely spread the news to other potential clients, promoting the expansion of man-midwifery.

Wilson's arguments provide another plausible explanation for Bourgeois' careful concealment of the surgeon called to aid her client; she did not want this man to be identified with the positive outcome of the birth. The visual exchanges occurring inside the early modern lying-in chamber involved more, however, than the straightforward observation and description implied in Wilson's account. Looking is an historical and cultural activity deserving of careful analysis. Scholars including Norbert Elias and Louis Marin have already shown that presenting oneself to be looked at was central to identity formation in early modern France.[13] Their scholarship sheds new light on the accounts of looking contained in obstetrical treatises, suggesting that childbirth practitioners participated in the early modern French 'culture of display.'

Exploring the significance of this display ultimately leads to a new understanding of the treatises themselves. The books emerge as sites of display that made authors visible. This display, however, did not necessarily contribute to an increase in prestige. The books written by male authors, for example, constructed images of men-midwives meant to be evaluated by others. Though these authors urged audiences to provide favourable appraisals, they also guarded against negative reactions. Their texts indicate that putting oneself on display could be both an empowering and intimidating experience.

Mediating the Male Gaze

Men had to defend their presence in the birthing room well into the eighteenth century. They were not readily endowed with a powerful gaze that could 'unlock' the female body. On the contrary, obstetrical treatises written by both male and female midwives portray women who resist being seen and touched by male practitioners. The surgeon man-midwife Guillaume Mauquest de La Motte reported, for example, that when he was called to attend the labouring wife of a pewter worker in 1691, the young woman begged him not to touch her.[14] Though the author regularly linked female opposition with immaturity, he also noted that older women could express an aversion to male assistance.[15] Mauquest de La Motte's description of these women's 'ill-founded modesty' resembles claims made by surgeon man-midwife Philippe Peu in 1694. Peu accused women of possessing an excess of false modesty, causing them to wait until the last minute before allowing men to enter the lying-in room.[16] In contrast, François Mauriceau placed the blame on female midwives. According to him, these women deliberately ruined men's reputations by encouraging clients to fear male practitioners.[17]

Even when men were permitted to touch clients, they were normally denied direct visual access to women's bodies. Throughout the early modern period, labouring women were heavily draped in order both to deter cold from entering their wombs and to uphold social convention. In 1561 Pierre Franco advised fellow surgeons to 'take a warm double sheet, and put it on the patient,' a custom still endorsed by Mauquest de La Motte in 1729.[18] The surgeon from Valognes advocated covering women's legs and thighs to prevent cold as well as for decency's sake.[19] Women were sometimes draped specifically to avert male looking, as in the case outlined by Bourgeois above. Yet the indiscriminate exposure of the female body reflected badly on everyone in the lying-in chamber. In 1612 surgeon Jacques Duval argued that neglecting to cover a labouring woman's buttocks and knees would bring as much shame to the female birthing assistants as to the woman herself.[20] Women were not necessarily eager to reveal their bodies to other women, and occasionally even refused to be seen by a female midwife. Bourgeois described one difficult client who would not allow the midwife to evaluate her condition, claiming to prefer the assistance of a male surgeon. According to Bourgeois, this stubborn woman died undelivered, something the royal midwife could have prevented.[21]

Such cases were nevertheless unusual. For the most part, looking at women's genitals remained the prerogative of female midwives throughout the early modern period in France. In his treatise of 1609, royal surgeon Jacques Guillemeau argued that midwives' traditional duties included inspecting women to make legal determinations about whether or not they were with child.[22] According to surgeon Jacques Bury in 1623, female midwives performed a similar role in the lying-in chamber by examining the genitals of suffering women, and describing them to male practitioners.[23] In 1677 Marguerite de La Marche reaffirmed that female midwives could serve as the 'eye' of physicians by providing them with accurate accounts of women's genital parts.[24] She claimed every female midwife should be familiar with the location and function of the external orifice of the womb, including the mount of Venus, lips, and clitoris, in case a client's modesty prevented her exposure to a man.[25] These authors agreed that male looking could be mediated through the eyes of female midwives, rendering it more socially acceptable.

Men's lack of direct visual access to women's bodies was offset in various ways. Male authors delineated, for example, their visual examination of the upper bodies of women, an activity not proscribed by social mores. In his treatise on miscarriage, Saint-Germain advised fellow physicians to consider the client's complexion, as well as her temperament, age, and particular constitution.[26] Guillemeau's insistence that surgeons perform a comparable evaluation of the labouring woman's face was echoed in Pierre Dionis' treatise of 1718.[27] Dionis explained that if a woman was pale, or looked dejected, the surgeon should think carefully before performing any operation she would be unable to survive.[28] This advice followed the Hippocratic corpus, which stressed the value of observing the countenance of the patient, as well as Galen's emphasis on determining the patient's humoural balance in order to arrive at a correct diagnosis. According to Helen King, the absence of human dissection led ancient practitioners to base arguments about the interior of the body on its exterior.[29] A similar insistence on reading the external signs of the body – correlating the seen with the unseen – was retained throughout the early modern period. It may have had particular relevance in the lying-in chamber, where men were not only frequently prohibited from seeing women's lower bodies but were also unable to see the unborn child within her.

Surgeon men-midwives attempted to portray their restricted vision in a positive light, arguing that visual access to the lower bodies of female clients was unnecessary. According to them, assisting at unnatural labours was a challenging surgical practice precisely because men could see neither the body of the draped woman, nor the unborn child in her womb. Guillemeau boasted:

> As for dexterity, there is no comparison with other operations; for there are no other works in surgery, where it is not necessary to see clearly, whether by daylight or candle light, and that the part that one treats and touches is not visible and revealed to the eye. In contrast, in this operation...it is necessary to search for the child in whatever position it [may be], without being able to see it.[30]

Later authors agreed that surgeon men-midwives had to be equipped with especially skilled hands in order to discern the position of the child in the womb by touch instead of sight.[31] Drawing attention to the manual labour of obstetrical surgeons, they implied that it surpassed visual perception. At the same time, surgeon men-midwives insisted that their physical manipulation of the womb enabled them to envision the unborn child. The men frequently argued that when called to assist at a gruelling delivery, they performed a manual examination to 'see' what was wrong, 'discover' the state of labour, 'look for' the distressed child, and 'observe' its posture. Peu argued, for example, that in one case he slid his hand along the body of an unborn child, finally recognizing its feet.[32] In these accounts vision was simultaneously replaced and enabled by the hands of male practitioners.[33]

This emphasis on perceptive touching continued even in descriptions of the speculum, a tool now associated with the ability to see inside the female body. During the early modern period the speculum assumed different forms, but often had three extensions that could be inserted into the vagina and then opened using a screw mechanism.[34] Though illustrated in the early publications of Ambroise Paré, Franco, and a few later sources, the instrument is rarely mentioned in French obstetrical treatises.[35] When discussed, however, the speculum is associated with physical rather than exclusively with visual access to the female body. In 1561 Franco even claimed to apply traction to the head of an unborn child with the three long blades of his *speculum matricis*, portraying the instrument as an extension of the surgeon's hand, not his eyes.[36] Later authors reported using the speculum to enable the surgical hand to enter women's wombs. When in 1671 surgeon man-midwife Cosme Viardel, for example, discovered a 'callosity' in the vagina of his childless female client, he employed a speculum to dilate the neck of her womb in order to insert his remedy inside it.[37]

This association of the speculum with physical manipulation is at odds with Tatlock's account of men's use of the tool. She argues that during the early modern period in Germany, touching remained the preserve of female midwives, but men could look at women's genitals with the aid of specula.[38] According to her, men's powerful looking ultimately led to touching; after men were permitted to inspect women's bodies with medical instruments, they began to handle those bodies and eventually appropriated the traditional role of the female midwife. Yet French obstetrical treatises tell a different story. Many male authors reported touching women's bodies without looking at them, and several described the speculum enabling their manual access to parturient women. These books suggest a more complex relationship between touching and looking, one that did not prioritize vision over physical manipulation. Of course, elevating the status of hands-on operations was in the interests of those *chirurgiens accoucheurs* traditionally identified with manual activities. Their books nevertheless imply that although male touching was not always welcomed in the lying-in chamber, it was more tolerable than the male scrutiny of female genitals.

Desiring Direct Vision

Despite proclaiming the merits of perceptive touch, surgeon men-midwives valued vision. Their books regularly conflate seeing with knowing, an association scholars have identified with the epistemological foundations of modern science.[39] Even the manner in which surgeon men-midwives drew attention to their manual labour emphasized the status of visual perception. They characterized the activities of surgical hands inside the womb as a kind of seeing, while insisting that women's bodies remained hidden from view. The efforts of surgeon men-midwives to discover the concealed womb correspond with arguments made by Ludmilla Jordanova about depictions of women's bodies in scientific and medical discourse. She argues that during the eighteenth and nineteenth centuries the modestly hidden female body was considered both dangerous and unknowable, exciting the desire to expose it.[40] French obstetrical treatises produced by men communicate a similar longing to unveil the usually hidden female body, revealing it to the eyes of male practitioners.

Authors occasionally described cooperative female patients eager to expose themselves to men. Mauquest de La Motte claimed that in 1692 he had eased a suffering woman by inserting a catheter to drain almost nine pints of fluid from her bladder. Afterwards, the grateful client raised her shift to request a clyster, saying: 'Monsieur, you that see all, and from whom nothing is hid, as you have made me void on this side, do the same to that.'[41] With this anecdote Mauquest de La Motte invoked the popular Greek story of Agnodike, a virgin who broke ancient law by dressing as a man to obtain medical training. When called to assist labouring women, Agnodike performed the gesture of *anasyrmos* – lifting her tunic to expose her body – in order to reassure her female clients that she was a woman who could protect their modesty.[42] In the surgeon man-midwife's early modern version, however, it is the female client who enacts this gesture to reassure the male attendant; she reveals her lower body to demonstrate that his practice is both appropriate and acceptable to women. Her act is portrayed as a flattering display of trust in the male practitioner, at odds with both Duval's association of exposed buttocks with shame, and contemporary legal cases in which bare bottoms were considered provocative.[43] Mauquest de La Motte's compliant woman is an ideal female client contrasting with the recalcitrant women who populate other case studies.

Most descriptions of the male gaze did not include the active participation of women. Female cooperation was in fact unnecessary because surgeons and physicians looked directly at the passive bodies of women who had died while pregnant or suffering from gynaecological conditions.[44] Autopsies were regularly performed to determine the cause of death, especially at the Hôtel-Dieu in Paris, a public hospital that delivered poor women free of charge.[45] In a case occurring in 1573, Paré claimed that after a woman suddenly died of pleurisy, he used surgical tools to open her body 'observing and marking everything very diligently,' but finding only a hard, callous body instead of a womb.[46] Paul Portal described seeing another autopsy performed at the Hôtel-Dieu in 1653, on the body of a woman who had died after giving birth. The procedure revealed a dangerous condition – parts of the afterbirth remained in the womb – but the physician present surprised everyone by proclaiming the female midwife was not to blame because the patient's melancholy temperament had caused the placenta to adhere to her womb.[47] In a similar case, surgeon man-midwife Philippe Peu claimed to have opened a woman who had died in childbirth in order to discover what had happened.[48] Making a long incision in the middle of her belly, Peu revealed a livid, dead child in an awkward position, legs askew.

Authors linked viewing such autopsies with the acquisition of true and direct knowledge of the female body.[49] Mediated vision was endowed with less authority. One striking example of this point is provided by a medical dispute involving Barthélemy Saviard, a surgeon who worked at the Hôtel-Dieu in Paris, attending difficult deliveries as well as other demanding cases. In 1696, Saviard published a report entitled *Récit exact d'une grossesse extraordinaire à l'Hôtel-Dieu de Paris* [Accurate report of an extraordinary pregnancy at the Hôtel-Dieu in Paris] in the scholarly *Journal des Sçavans*, describing the plight of a woman who had died in

October of the same year with her unborn child growing in her belly but outside her womb. The account was quickly attacked in print by an anonymous physician. According to the critic, Saviard did not see the woman before her death, and at the autopsy his observations were hindered by the shoulders of other spectators.[50] In his lengthy response, the outraged surgeon insisted that he had indeed had a clear view of the woman's opened corpse, enabling him to publish reliable statements about it.[51]

Male physicians and surgeons saw relatively fewer anatomical dissections of the female body. Whereas autopsies opened the body to search for abnormalities, anatomies demonstrated beliefs about the location and function of various organs, veins, and cavities. Anatomy was increasingly crucial to medical education during the early modern period, but corpses were difficult to obtain. The dissection of the female body, especially the pregnant female body, was rare.[52] Authors of obstetrical treatises nevertheless argued that those who practised midwifery required extensive anatomical knowledge. Mauriceau began his influential treatise of 1668 with a discussion of female anatomy, claiming it was impossible to understand his subsequent teaching without a perfect comprehension of the reproductive parts.[53] The engravings accompanying his anatomical chapter resemble those found in contemporary anatomical treatises, portraying female trunks with their viscera peeled back to reveal clearly defined internal organs.[54] Mauriceau's chapter also contains a rare external view of the female genitalia, labeled *la partie honteuse* [the shameful part] (Figure 2.1). This image focuses exclusively on the genitals, magnifying them to achieve legibility rather than accuracy.[55] Widely spread legs reveal an open vagina, with drapery pushed back over the woman's pregnant belly to frame her lower body rather than shield it from view. Admitting the engraving might be considered indecent, Mauriceau affirmed it provided necessary information by displaying what normally remained hidden.[56]

Mauriceau's image of unimpeded visual access to the female body is echoed in the 1673 edition of Viardel's treatise, *Observations sur la pratique des accouchemens naturels, contre nature & monstrueux* (Figure 2.2). In one engraving, the entire body of an anatomized woman is shown lying on a bed with her feet drawn close to her buttocks and knees wide apart, the posture recommended by many authors as most convenient for performing an internal examination.[57] The scene presents an uncovered and utterly available female figure, with her open vagina finding its corollary in the gaping hole of her abdomen. Layers of viscera have been removed to reveal an unborn child in a natural position, ready to emerge head first, though impeded by the umbilical cord wrapped around its neck. The woman's open arms heighten her passivity, while her downcast eyes fail to confront the viewer, and may connote death.

Both engravings present women even more submissive than the ideal client celebrated by Mauquest de La Motte. With their secret parts revealed, the figures confirm the link between seeing the female body and having knowledge of it.[58]

Though found in obstetrical treatises, these images recall the wax anatomical 'Venuses' proliferating during the early modern period. The three-dimensional reclining female figures are highly sexualized, with their identity as women associated with their reproductive capacity.[59] The engravings in the treatises of Mauriceau and Viardel similarly objectify and sexualize the female body, opening it to a penetrating gaze. Apparently lending support to feminist arguments about the development of modern gynaecology, they imply that early modern obstetrics depended on the spectacle of women's exposed and vulnerable bodies.[60]

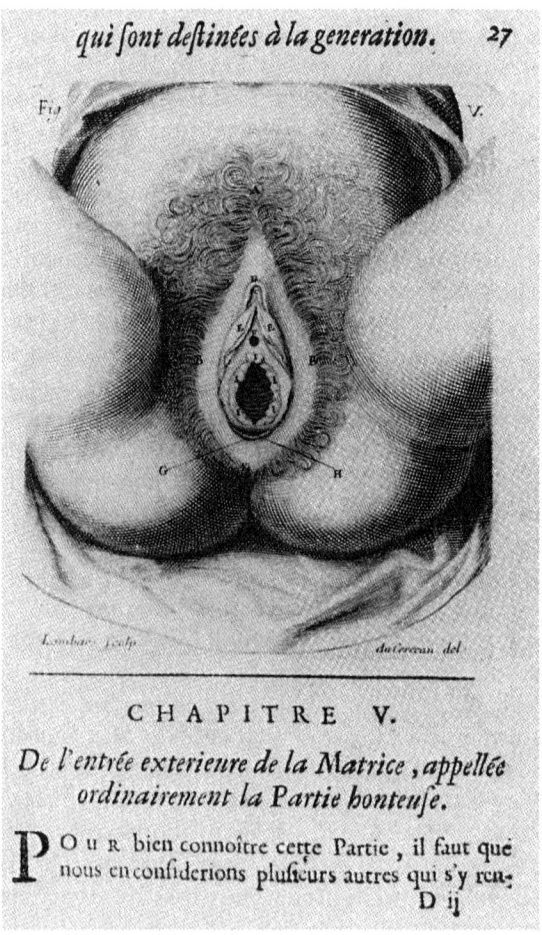

Figure 2.1   Female genitalia, from François Mauriceau's *Des maladies des femmes grosses et accouchées*, 1668, Paris. Courtesy of the Edward G. Miner Library, University of Rochester Medical Center, Rochester, NY

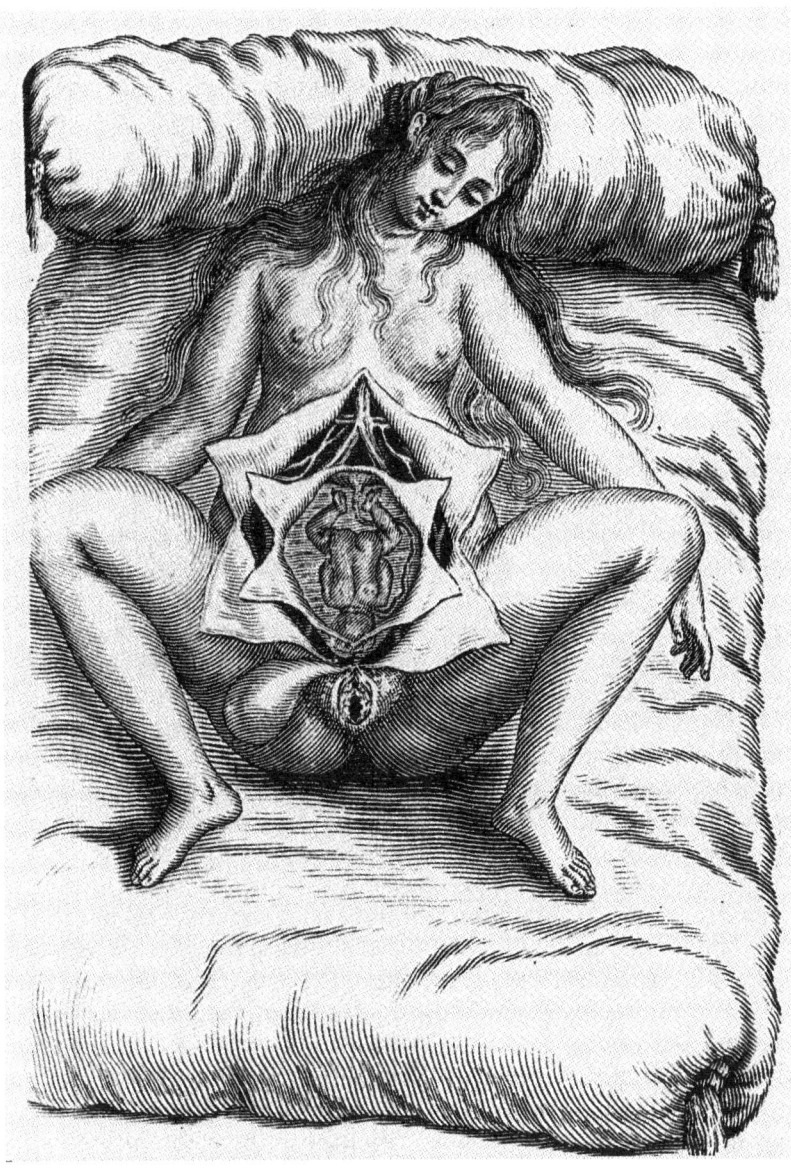

Figure 2.2   Anatomized woman, from Cosme Viardel's *Observations sur la pratique des accouchemens naturels, contre nature & monstrueux*, 1673, Paris. Courtesy of the National Library of Medicine, Bethesda, MD

This interpretation of the images is nevertheless partial. It overlooks the fact that comparable representations of female genitals are rarely found in French obstetrical treatises. Only a handful of the books feature anatomical discussions with accompanying illustrations.[61] Hugh Chamberlen excluded Mauriceau's anatomical chapter from his English translation of the surgeon man-midwife's book, arguing that 'here and there a passage...might offend a chaste English Eye.'[62] Clearly, such images were at odds with the continuing taboo against uninhibited looking. Instead of reflecting what men normally saw, the images portray the kind of visual access men were denied, except when women cooperated or were subject to autopsy after death. The engravings can therefore be considered both another method of compensating for the limited nature of men's scrutiny of the female body, and representations of male desire for unimpeded visual access.

Returning the Gaze

Male practitioners were faced with more than women's resistance to their looking in the lying-in chamber. They were also subjected to an inquisitive and potentially judgmental gaze. Men were not alone with clients, but rather operated before an audience that included the relatives, friends, and neighbours of labouring women. Of course, male physicians and surgeons were not asked to expose their naked bodies to viewers. Nevertheless their descriptions of being on display in the birthing room revolve around a similar dynamic of veiling and unveiling. Aware they were being looked at, authors of obstetrical treatises urged fellow practitioners to expose what should be seen and hide what could cause shame and embarrassment. Even as they outlined strategies for demonstrating dexterity, they explained how to avert negative displays able to ruin the male midwife's reputation.

Mauriceau encouraged the surgeon man-midwife to avoid using instruments if at all possible when called to assist at difficult labours, particularly if the death of the unborn child was uncertain. He asked 'What a horrible spectacle would it be if he brought [out]...a poor child that was still alive after having cut off its arms?'[63] Dionis similarly argued that removing a child piece by piece created a deplorable spectacle, noting that instruments themselves could be terrifying for clients and other bystanders to look at.[64] According to some authors, men did not habitually carry hooks or 'head pullers' with them to the homes of labouring women. Portal, Peu, and Mauquest de La Motte reported sending assistants to collect their *crochets* only after realizing tools were needed in challenging cases.[65] At the same time, they advised male practitioners to hide such instruments in order to preclude an unpleasant display for those gathered in the lying-in chamber. In these cases, the draperies covering women's bodies may have benefited male practitioners, concealing both their potentially frightening instruments and destructive operations.

Male authors insisted that the man-midwife should furthermore disguise his emotions in the lying-in chamber. Expressions of fear were particularly forbidden. Displaying a carefully controlled demeanour, the ideal male practitioner was encouraged to remain calm at all times in order to comfort rather than frighten his clients and their assistants.[66] Part of his responsibility included reassuring labouring women by adopting the behaviour, comportment, manners, and clothing most appropriate to the feminine realm of the birthing room.[67] Peu was especially concerned about these issues, boasting of his own ability to maintain a courageous outlook even when confronted with suffering women on the brink of death.[68]

While concealing both his dangerous operations and expressions, the surgeon man-midwife was nevertheless required to display his manual skills in the lying-in chamber. His reputation depended on demonstrating a concerted effort to help women, as well as the successful completion of any operation. One opportunity to exhibit dexterity revolved around the afterbirth of parturient women. Bourgeois voiced a commonplace belief when she insisted that a woman was not fully delivered until her afterbirth had been removed.[69] Encouraging male surgeons to have patience when dislodging a retained afterbirth, Bourgeois explained that a torn placenta was terrible to behold because a single piece left in the womb could prove fatal to the new mother. Mauriceau advocated displaying the afterbirth to the witnesses gathered in the lying-in chamber, while Peu and Dionis specified it should be placed on a plate to facilitate its visual examination.[70] If this act determined the afterbirth was healthy and whole, the practitioner would be protected from blame should the newly-delivered woman subsequently fall ill or expire. In contrast, a damaged afterbirth could ruin the reputation of male and female midwife alike.[71]

Authors of obstetrical treatises frequently worried about being held responsible for injuries and deaths occurring both during and after childbirth. Sometimes these practitioners deserved the hostility of clients, including the hapless surgeon described in Peu's treatise, who stole away with a child's severed foot hidden in his pocket.[72] For the most part, however, authors feared false accusations. They encouraged fellow practitioners to invite additional practitioners to witness the interventions they performed. Both male and female midwives reported seeking the assistance of two or even three other practitioners in especially difficult cases. These assistants did more than provide additional medical information; they also protected each other. Peu, for example, undertook dangerous operations with a physician standing by in case misinformed bystanders attributed the child's death to the surgeon.[73] Mauquest de La Motte similarly called for a physician's help when he feared receiving blame.[74] Even respected midwife Madame de La Marche encouraged female midwives to defer to physicians in order to avoid condemnation for deaths occurring in the lying-in chamber.[75]

Witnesses might not always be supportive. Male authors frequently labelled female midwives bunglers responsible for the sorry state of the labouring women they encountered; these men also regularly condemned the operations of any male practitioner called to assist before their arrival.[76] At the same time, surgeon men-midwives accused female midwives of calling for their help only to shift the blame to innocent men. In the first volume of her treatise, Bourgeois agreed that male practitioners were sometimes used by female midwives in this manner.[77] In contrast to her description of the dangers of male looking, this reference indicates that the male gaze was not always prohibited in the lying-in chamber, and that it could occasionally benefit female midwives.

According to obstetrical treatises, male practitioners could be vulnerable in the birthing room, an arena pervaded by complex visual exchanges. Despite their university training, men were not automatically respected.[78] They needed to be recognized as capable birth attendants. Because visual display and identity were inextricably linked, seeing the practitioner meant knowing both his capabilities and character. Male attempts to create positive spectacles were risky, and could potentially invoke condemnation from the audience rather than increased authority. All the same, being looked at was crucial to men-midwives' construction of a good reputation, and arguably carried more weight than their sporadic scrutiny of female bodies.

The significance of being on display was not exclusive to the birthing room, but infused early modern French culture. Scholars studying this period usually emphasize the spectacular court of Louis XIV at Versailles, where the political function of display reached a kind of climax. Sociologist Norbert Elias, for example, argues that in this courtly culture the compulsive display of one's rank in effect constituted that rank. The higher a person's status, the greater the obligation to present that identity in outward appearances, especially the prudent regulation of bodily gestures.[79] Art historian Norman Bryson labels this carefully fashioned image the courtly body. He contends that French courtiers attempted to obliterate revealing signs from their bodies, transforming potential sites of betrayal into legible surfaces consisting 'only of eyes, hands, and impassive facial muscles.'[80]

Though the powerful Sun King kept a watchful eye on potentially rebellious nobles at Versailles, he too was on display. Various scholars analyse his exposure to the gaze during courtly pageants as well as in the official constructions of his image that were distributed throughout the realm. Semiotician Louis Marin considers how ubiquitous images of Louis XIV in official histories, medals, and portraits both produced and rendered palpable his absolutist power.[81] In a related study, historian Peter Burke examines the constantly renewed image of the King in paintings, sculptures, plays, and ballets.[82] Concentrating on images of Louis XIV before his declaration of personal rule, literary scholar Abby Zanger argues that engravings of the royal family in almanacs from 1658 to 1659 do not portray the King as the autonomous and confidently regal figure pictured in his later portraits.[83] During a period when Louis XIV's career was in flux, the images contain contradictory references to his virility as well as feminine passions and the threat of sterility.

This scholarship sheds light on the demands male practitioners faced within the lying-in chamber. Their efforts to present an appealing spectacle conformed to broader cultural practices in France, where display was associated with increased social status and power. At the same time, the careers of male midwives were far less stable than that of the young Louis XIV, and exposing themselves to scrutiny was rife with anxiety. Male midwives needed especially to appeal to female clients and their attendants, offering them spectacles of appropriate behaviour and comportment. According to Elias, this emphasis on appealing to others was common throughout Europe.[84] Using etiquette manuals as his primary sources, the sociologist notes that regulations related to eating, drinking, coughing, and natural bodily functions increased from the Middle Ages through the early modern period. He contends that as centralized states came to monopolize the use of physical force, the populace was obligated to master bodily impulses. Emotional outbursts also became less acceptable as an extensive web of 'inter-group interdependencies' necessitated paying more attention to the opinions of one's peers.[85]

Evidence of male efforts to produce an appropriate spectacle in the lying-in chamber is primarily found in those obstetrical treatises written by men-midwives. Attending to the early modern culture of display sheds new light on the function of these books. Like theatrical spectacles at Versailles and representations of Louis XIV, the images of male midwives in these treatises were designed to impress audiences. The visual modes of persuasion in the publications include not only descriptions of the ideal male midwife but also the images within them, especially the author portraits that regularly acted as frontispieces. Art historians argue that portraits should not be approached solely as the unique creation of artists, nor as mere reflections of their subjects' lives and physical appearance. According to Marcia Pointon, portraiture is best understood 'as a shaping and defining mechanism in terms of class, rank and gender.'[86] The frontispiece author portraits in obstetrical treatises herald the nature of their written contents, which exhibit representations rather than records of practitioners. In many ways, obstetrical treatises were themselves sites of display that made male midwives visible.

French men-midwives were not the only medical practitioners to participate in the early modern culture of display. Historian Lisa Forman Cody argues that by the 1720s male midwives in England were spectacular figures.[87] By lecturing publicly, giving testimony on reproductive issues in court, discoursing in coffeehouses, and advertising their services, these men put themselves on display. Obstetrical treatises played a role in the increasing legitimation of male obstetrics. Only six English women published treatises between 1671 and 1798, while dozens of male authors produced more than 200 texts during the same period.[88] Cody concludes that the increasing visibility of the man-midwife both in print and in public contributed to their rising authority, resulting in the concomitant loss by female midwives of their special public status in relation to birth.

The eighteenth-century English man-midwife was, however, arguably more ensconced than his French counterpart. Reaffirming the uncertain nature of their display, French surgeon men-midwives worried about how their texts would be perceived. In the prefaces to their treatises, authors regularly feared they would receive criticism for daring to publish. Male as well as female midwives deflected charges of immodesty by claiming to become authors solely for the public good, and in order to instruct young practitioners.[89] They also sought powerful protectors, dedicating their books to a royal physician or other person of elevated rank. Although such prefaces were conventional, authors' fears were not unfounded. As already indicated by the case involving Saviard, medical publications often provoked intense criticism. Publishing was not necessarily a predictable way in which to produce and promote a desired self-representation.

Conclusions

Obstetrical treatises portray the vagaries of vision, linking it with danger, exposure, reliable knowledge, and protection from blame. These sources present the early modern French lying-in chamber as a complex realm in which labouring women both revealed and concealed themselves. Yet even as looking at women's bodies was associated with powerful knowledge, the publications written by male physicians and surgeons rarely portray a masterful male gaze that dominated women. Instead, these men regularly referred to their own display within the lying-in chamber. Being looked at was crucial to the production of rank and identity in early modern French culture, and may have held particular importance in the birthing room, a realm that traditionally excluded men. Male practitioners needed to be seen in a positive light in order to augment their authority, but could be excluded or rendered invisible to clients in the manner described by Bourgeois.

When scholars insist that women were increasingly exposed to an aggressive male gaze during the early modern period, they ignore the exhibition of male medical practitioners. Achieving a partial understanding of the visual politics of childbirth, they award male physicians and surgeons more power than they actually possessed during the early modern period. This scholarship threatens to erase women from the picture by implying they were voiceless, passive objects lacking the power to resist. Obstetrical treatises written by both male and female authors depict, however, pregnant women who refuse to be seen. The also portray female midwives who intervene to mediate and even prevent male looking. Obstetrical publications neither identify women exclusively with corporeality, nor associate men with a detached, bodiless gaze. These sources suggest that women's ability to look back, scrutinizing the bodies of male practitioners, should not be underestimated.

Exploring references to the representation of the man-midwife's body provides a fuller picture of the visual exchanges occurring in the lying-in chamber. At the same time, it contributes to a richer understanding of the early modern French culture of display, moving beyond studies of the Sun King and his court. Historians Sara E. Melzer and Kathryn Norberg have already remarked that 'if the king's body had great political significance, so too did the bodies of his subjects.'[90] Scholars have therefore begun to consider a wider range of French bodies, including those of slave women and eighteenth-century feminists.[91] The presentation of the bodies of male midwives in obstetrical treatises are equally worthy of study, and it is precisely this kind of display that interests me in subsequent chapters.

This chapter has nevertheless raised a host of additional issues requiring further examination. Were female midwives also subjected to the critical gaze of clients in the birthing room? How were their bodies understood and evaluated in early modern France? And what was the status of male touching in the lying-in chamber? Have scholars overlooked the importance of men's tactile manipulations by focusing on their visual acquisition of knowledge? Ensuing chapters respond to these questions by considering the visual presentation of both female and male midwives, as well as various representations of the surgeon man-midwife's perceptive hands.

Notes

1. Louise Bourgeois, *Observations diverses sur la stérilité, perte de fruict, foecondité, accouchements et maladies des femmes et enfants nouveaux naiz*, Françoise Olive, ed. (Paris: Côté-Femmes, 1992; orig. 1652), 176–7.
2. Bourgeois, *Observations diverses*, 187:

> Je me trouvais un jour à l'accouchement d'une honnête demoiselle de mes bonnes amies, de laquelle le mari était absent; elle était assistée de trois ou quatre de ses amies, lesquelles me demandèrent l'état de son accouchement, je leur dis que l'enfant venait mal, mais que je l'aurais, aidant Dieu, sans danger de la mère ni de l'enfant; elles me prièrent d'avoir agréable de la faire voir au chirurgien; pour leur décharge, je leur accordai, pourvu qu'elle ne le vît point, d'autant que je savais que cela était capable de la faire mourir d'appréhension, et de honte. Je la persuadai de se glisser aux pieds de son lit. Je mis le chevet au milieu du lit et abattis le tour du lit du côté qu'il devait passer, et aux pieds: il la toucha comme je parlais, elle ne le vît point, et accoucha sans artifice ni aide, que de Dieu et de la nature.

Jean Donnison, *Midwives and Medical Men* (New York: Schocken Books, 1977), 11, refers to a similar incident in 1658 when man-midwife Percival Willughby entered a lying-in chamber on all fours to avoid detection. See Percival Willughby, *Observations on Midwifery*, Henry Blenkinsop, ed. (Wakefield: S. R. Publishers, 1972; orig. manuscript 1863), 135.

3.   Adrian Wilson, *The Making of Man-Midwifery: Childbirth in England, 1660–1770* (London: UCL Press, 1995), 191–2, and Hilary Marland, 'Introduction,' Hilary Marland, ed., *The Art of Midwifery: Early Modern Midwives in Europe* (London: Routledge, 1993), 8. David Harley, 'Provincial Midwives in England: Lancashire and Cheshire, 1660–1760,' Hilary Marland, ed., *The Art of Midwifery*, 43, argues that by the mid-eighteenth century husbands may have increasingly selected the man-midwife.

4.   Bourgeois, *Observations diverses*, 187: 'que la femme ne le voie ni ne le sache, et que le chirurgien ne la voie non plus.'

5.   For discussions of the impropriety of male midwives see: Philippe Hecquet, *De l'indécence aux hommes d'accoucher les femmes* (Paris, 1708), and Roy Porter, 'A Touch of Danger: The Man-Midwife as Sexual Predator,' G. S. Rousseau and Roy Porter, eds, *Sexual Underworlds of the Enlightenment* (Chapel Hill: University of North Carolina Press, 1988), 206–32.

6.   For positive accounts of male entry into the lying-in chamber see Theodore Cianfrani, *A Short History of Obstetrics and Gynecology* (Springfield: Thomas, 1960), Irving Samuel Cutter and Henry R. Viets, *A Short History of Midwifery* (Philadelphia: Saunders, 1964), Walter Radcliffe, *Milestones in Midwifery* (Bristol: Wright & Sons, 1967), and Audrey Eccles, *Obstetrics and Gynaecology in Tudor and Stuart England* (London: Croom Helm, 1982).

7.   Lynne Tatlock, 'Speculum Feminarum: Gendered Perspectives on Obstetrics and Gynecology in Early Modern Germany,' *Signs* 17, 4 (1992), 725–60.

8.   Michel Foucault, *The Birth of the Clinic: An Archaeology of Medical Perception*, A. M. Sheridan Smith, trans. (New York: Vintage, 1975).

9.   Terri Kapsalis, *Public Privates: Performing Gynecology from Both Ends of the Speculum* (Durham: Duke University Press, 1997), 7.

10.   *Ibid.*, 179.

11.   For descriptions of the early modern lying-in chamber see Mireille Laget, *Naissances: L'accouchement avant l'âge de la clinique* (Paris: Seuil, 1982), 128–37, Adrian Wilson, 'The Ceremony of Childbirth and its Interpretation,' Valerie Fildes, ed., *Women as Mothers in Pre-Industrial England* (London: Routledge, 1990), 68–107, and David Cressy, *Birth, Marriage, and Death: Ritual, Religion, and the Life-Cycle in Tudor and Stuart England* (Oxford: Oxford University Press, 1997), 50–59, 82–7. For fictional accounts of the celebration following births see Édouard Fournier, *Les caquets de l'accouchée* (Paris: Jannet, 1855), and Domna C. Stanton, 'Recuperating Women and the Man Behind the Screen,' James Grantham Turner, ed., *Sexuality and Gender in Early Modern Europe: Institutions, Texts, Images* (Cambridge: Cambridge University Press, 1993), 247–65.

12.   Wilson, *The Making of Man-Midwifery*, 97.

13.   Norbert Elias, *The Court Society*, Edmund Jephcott, trans. (Oxford: Blackwell, 1983), and Louis Marin, *Portrait of the King*, Martha M. Houle, trans. (Minneapolis: University of Minnesota Press, 1988).

14. Guillaume Mauquest de La Motte, *Traité complet des accouchemens* (Paris, 1729; orig. 1721), 145, and 152, 163.
15. *Ibid.*, 184.
16. Philippe Peu, *La pratique des accouchemens* (Paris, 1694), 168.
17. François Mauriceau, *Des maladies des femmes grosses et accouchées* (Paris, 1668), 243.
18. Pierre Franco, *Chirurgie*, E. Nicaise, ed. (Geneva: Slatkine, 1972; orig. 1561), 234: 'prendre un drap chauld double, et le mettre sur la patiente.'
19. Mauquest de La Motte, *Traité complet des accouchemens*, 107.
20. Jacques Duval, *Traité des hermaphrodits, parties génitales, accouchemens des femmes* (Rouen, 1612), 195.
21. Bourgeois, *Observations diverses*, 149–50.
22. Jacques Guillemeau, *De l'heureux accouchement des femmes* (Paris, 1609), 150. Female midwives traditionally had many legal duties. For an overview see Erwin H. Ackerknecht, 'Midwives as Experts in Court,' *Bulletin of the New York Academy of Medicine* 52 (1976), 1224–8.
23. Jacques Bury, *Le propagatif de l'homme* (Paris, 1623), 70–71.
24. Marguerite de La Marche [du Tertre], *Instruction familière et très utile aux sages-femmes pour bien pratiquer les accouchemens* (Paris, 1710; orig. 1677), 15.
25. For the same argument see Charles de Saint-Germain, *L'eschole méthodique et parfaite des sages-femmes* (Paris, 1650), 4.
26. Charles de Saint-Germain, *Traité des fausses couches* (Paris, 1655), 42.
27. Guillemeau, *De l'heureux accouchement des femmes*, 221–2.
28. Pierre Dionis, *Traité général des accouchemens* (Paris, 1718), 249–50. See also Peu, *La pratique des accouchemens*, 44.
29. Helen King, *Hippocrates' Woman: Reading the Female Body in Ancient Greece* (London: Routledge, 1998), 26.
30. Guillemeau, *De l'heureux accouchement des femmes*, unpaginated preface:

    > Or pour la dexterité, il n'y a rien de comparaison avec les autres orations [sic]: car il ne se faict aucunes oeuvres en Chirurgie, où il ne soit necessaire de voir clair, soit par la lumiere, qui nous est donnee du jour, ou de la chandelle, & que la partie que l'on traicte & manie, ne soit apparente & manifeste à l'oeil. Au contraire, en ceste operation...il faut chercher l'enfant en quelque situation qu'il soit, sans le pouvoir voir.

31. For the same argument see Dionis, *Traité général des accouchemens*, 247–8. English men-midwives associated touch with both intellectual and manual authority according to Eve Keller, 'The Subject of Touch: Medical Authority in Early Modern Midwifery,' Elizabeth D. Harvey, ed., *Sensible Flesh: On Touch in Early Modern Culture* (Philadelphia: University of Pennsylvania Press, 2003), 62–80.
32. Peu, *La pratique des accouchemens*, 408: 'Je la glissai le long du corps pour découvrir l'épine & le ventre, & reconnoître ensuite lequel des deux pieds.'
33. Portal, *La pratique des accouchemens*, 2, 5, 53, 79, linked touching with recognizing, examining and observing. Mauquest de La Motte, *Traité complet des accouchemens*,

192, conflated touching with seeing, or verifying the truth. Pierre Amand, *Nouvelles observations sur la pratique des accouchemens* (Paris, 1714), 163–4, described his hand touching and recognizing the contents of a woman's womb. I analyse this association of hands with vision in Chapter 6.

34.   For the limited use of the speculum before 1821 see King, *Hippocrates' Woman*, 2–3.

35.   Ambroise Paré, *Les oeuvres de M. Paré* (Paris, 1575), 798–9, Franco, *Chirurgie*, 260, Mauriceau, *Des maladies des femmes grosses et accouchées*, 368, and Dionis, *Traité général des accouchemens*, 309.

36.   Franco, *Chirurgie*, 259–60. Eduard Kaspar Jakob von Siebold, *Essai d'une histoire de l'obstétricie*, vol. 2 (Paris: Steinheil, 1891–1892), 84, argues that Franco therefore used his speculum as a kind of forceps.

37.   Cosme Viardel, *Observations sur la pratique des accouchemens naturels, contre nature & monstrueux* (Paris, 1671), 83.

38.   Tatlock, 'Speculum Feminarum,' 759.

39.   See, for example, Jonathan Crary, 'Modernity and the Problem of the Observer,' *Techniques of the Observer: On Vision and Modernity in the Nineteenth Century* (Cambridge, MA: MIT Press, 1998), 1–24, and Ludmilla Jordanova, *Sexual Visions: Images of Gender in Science and Medicine between the Eighteenth and Twentieth Centuries* (New York: Harvester Wheatsheaf, 1989), 90–92.

40.   Jordanova, 'Nature Unveiling Before Science,' *Sexual Visions*, 87–110.

41.   Mauquest de La Motte, *Traité complet des accouchemens*, 90–91. The surgeon man-midwife referred to this story in order to respond to Hecquet's claim in *De l'indécence aux hommes d'accoucher les femmes* that women should prefer death to male assistance in childbirth.

42.   For the Agnodike myth in medical texts see Helen King, 'Agnodike and the Profession of Medicine,' *Proceedings of the Cambridge Philological Society* 32 (1986), 53–77, and her *Hippocrates' Woman*, 181–7.

43.   For a discussion of the cultural meaning of the display of the buttocks in early modern France see Jeffrey Ravel, 'Le Derrière du cocher: une soirée interrompue au XVIIIe siècle,' unpublished communication presented in January 2003 at the École normale supérieure, Paris.

44.   For a sophisticated analysis of this kind of looking, albeit in the nineteenth century, see Elisabeth Bronfen, *Over Her Dead Body: Death, Femininity, and the Aesthetic* (New York: Routledge, 1992), 3–14.

45.   Portal, a *compagnon chirurgien ordinaire* at the Hôtel-Dieu from 1650–1663, claimed to have performed many autopsies on the dead bodies of newly-delivered women. See his *La pratique des accouchemens*, 339. He also reported, 285, using the caesarean operation to open a dead woman's body at least once, but this operation was likely rare. Though Renate Blumenfeld-Kosinski, *Not of Woman Born: Representations of Caesarean Birth in Medieval and Renaissance Culture* (Ithaca: Cornell University Press, 1990) argues the caesarean operation enabled men to enter the lying-in chamber, specialists claim men were usually called too late to perform it. See Mireille Laget, 'La césarienne ou la tentation de l'impossible: XVIIe et XVIIIe siècle,' *Annales de bretagne et des pays de l'ouest* 86 (1979), 177–89.

46.   Paré, *Les oeuvres de M. Paré*, 773.

47. Portal, *La pratique des accouchemens*, 87–8. For other autopsies he had either undertaken himself or attended see 103, 128, 148, 178, 190, and 324–5.

48. Peu, *La pratique des accouchemens*, 340.

49. For example, Mauriceau, *Des maladies des femmes grosses et accouchées*, 309, argued that he would not have believed the amount of water emanating from the belly of a woman's dropsical unborn child if he 'had not seen it for [himself].'

50. Anon., *Récit exact d'une grossesse extraordinaire á l'Hôtel-Dieu de Paris* (n.l., n.d.), reproduces the report originally written by Saviard and then refutes it point by point.

51. Barthélemy Saviard, *Réponse de M. Saviard,…á la critique de l'extrait de sa lettre* (Paris, 1698). The anonymous author of the earlier critique cited eye-witness accounts from both the head midwife at the Hôtel-Dieu, Madame de Goüey, and a surgeon who also worked there, Monsieur Joüy. In his response, Saviard nevertheless claimed the true author of the entire critique was the person who wrote what he called *Progrez de la medecine*. Presumably, he was referring to physician Claude Brunet, who published *Le progrès de la médecine* (Paris, 1697).

52. For the role of anatomy in medical education see Mary Lindemann, *Medicine and Society in Early Modern Europe* (Cambridge: Cambridge University Press, 1999), 71–5, and 86–7, and Toby Gelfand, *Professionalizing Modern Medicine: Paris Surgeons and Medical Science and Institutions in the 18th Century* (Westport: Greenwood, 1980), 52–4. For more general discussions of anatomy see Andrea Carlino, *Books of the Body: Anatomical Ritual and Renaissance Learning* (Chicago: University of Chicago Press, 1999), Andrew Cunningham, *The Anatomical Renaissance: The Resurrection of the Anatomical Projects of the Ancients* (Aldershot: Ashgate, 1997), and K. B. Roberts and J. D. W. Tomlinson, *The Fabric of the Body: European Traditions of Anatomical Illustrations* (Oxford: Clarendon, 1992).

53. Mauriceau, *Des maladies des femmes grosses et accouchées*, 1.

54. Anatomical treatises with similar plates include Charles Estienne, *La dissection des parties du corps humain* (Paris, 1546), and Adriaan van den Spieghel, *De humani corporis fabrica* (Venice, 1627).

55. Lindemann, *Medicine and Society in Early Modern Europe*, 95, argues that medieval anatomical illustrations acted as mnemonic devices rather than accurate depictions. Ludmilla Jordanova, 'Gender, Generation and Science: William Hunter's Obstetrical Atlas,' W.F. Bynum and Roy Porter, eds, *William Hunter and the Eighteenth-Century Medical World* (Cambridge: Cambridge University Press, 1985), 385–412, undermines the traditional narrative of increasing accuracy in anatomical illustration.

56. Mauriceau, *Des maladies des femmes grosses et accouchées*, 26.

57. This posture is described in nearly every treatise but see, for example, Guillemeau, *De l'heureux accouchement des femmes*, 225–6.

58. For the association of women's bodies with secrets see Susan Broomhall, '"Women's Little Secrets": Defining the Boundaries of Reproductive Knowledge in Sixteenth-Century France,' *Social History of Medicine* 15, 1 (2002), 1–15, and Cathy McClive, 'The Hidden Truths of the Belly: The Uncertainties of Pregnancy in Early Modern Europe,' *Social History of Medicine* 15, 2 (2002), 209–27.

59. Jordanova, *Sexual Visions*, 44–50, and Mary D. Sheriff, *The Exceptional Woman:*

Elisabeth Vigée-Lebrun and the Cultural Politics of Art (Chicago: University of Chicago Press, 1996), 13–19.

60. For a standard feminist argument about the link between vision and gynaecology see Roberta McGrath, *Seeing Her Sex: Medical Archives and the Female Body* (Manchester: Manchester University Press, 2002).

61. As indicated in Chapter 1, only five early modern French obstetrical treatises include conventional anatomical plates: Duval, *Traité des hermaphrodits, parties génitales, accouchemens des femmes*, Mauriceau, *Des maladies des femmes grosses et accouchées*, Denis Fournier, *L'accoucheur méthodique* (Paris, 1677), La Marche [du Tertre], *Instruction familière et très utile aux sages-femmes pour bien pratiquer les accouchemens*, and Dionis, *Traité général des accouchemens*.

62. Hugh Chamberlen, trans. *Accomplisht Midwife, Treating of the Diseases of Women with Child, and in Child-bed* (London, 1673), unpaginated preface by the translator.

63. Mauriceau, *Des maladies des femmes grosses et accouchées*, 315: 'Quel horrible spectacle seroit-ce s'il amenoit...un pauvre enfant encore vivant, aprés [sic] luy avoir ainsi tronçonné les bras.'

64. Dionis, *Traité général des accouchemens*, 294, and 305.

65. Portal, *La pratique des accouchemens*, 21, described instrument use as a last resort and, 114, sent a woman's husband to fetch his instruments. Peu, *La pratique des accouchemens*, 99, said in one difficult case there was not enough time to fetch his instruments. Mauquest de La Motte, *Traité complet des accouchemens*, 460, sent for a *crochet* when it was needed.

66. Peu, *La pratique des accouchemens*, 64–5, and Mauquest de La Motte, *Traité complet des accouchemens*, preface, 169, 310, and 367.

67. See my discussion of the ideal French man-midwife in Chapter 4.

68. Peu, *La pratique des accouchemens*, 428.

69. Bourgeois, *Observations diverses*, 80.

70. Mauriceau, *Des maladies des femmes grosses et accouchées*, 279, Peu, *La pratique des accouchemens*, 496, and 555, and Dionis, *Traité général des accouchemens*, 222, and 228. Mauquest de La Motte, *Traité complet des accouchemens*, 590–91, uniquely argued that displaying the afterbirth served no purpose.

71. When royal physicians performed an autopsy on the body of Madame de Bourbon-Montpensier in 1627, they claimed that portions of the placenta remained in the womb, and Bourgeois considered herself blamed for the death of her client. I discuss this case at the end of Chapter 5.

72. Peu, *La pratique des accouchemens*, 426.

73. *Ibid.*, 62–3, and 125. For other accounts of surgeons fearing blame see Mauriceau, *Des maladies des femmes grosses et accouchées*, 350–51, and Portal, *La pratique des accouchemens*, 23, 163, 191–2, 275, and 349.

74. Guillaume Mauquest de La Motte, *A General Treatise of Midwifry*, Thomas Tomkyns, trans. (London, 1746), 534.

75. La Marche [du Tertre], *Instruction familière et très utile aux sages-femmes pour bien pratiquer les accouchemens*, 75.

76. For a discussion of such medical criticism see Chapter 5.

77. Bourgeois, *Observations diverses*, 55, described how midwives unfairly likened surgeons to butchers. For her changing relationship with male practitioners see Wendy Perkins, *Midwifery and Medicine in Early Modern France: Louise Bourgeois* (Exeter: University of Exeter Press, 1996), 99–120. Men also tried to shift blame to other men. Peu, *La pratique des accouchemens*, 110, for example, claimed that the male practitioner called before him falsely accused Peu of causing a woman's death.

78. Isobel Grundy, 'Sarah Stone: Enlightenment Midwife,' *Clio Medica* 29 (1995), 139, overestimates male status in the lying-in chamber when she claims that men's authority was institutional or conferred by degree, whereas that of female midwives was based on experience.

79. Elias, *The Court Society*, 63–4.

80. Norman Bryson, 'The Legible Body: LeBrun,' *Word and Image: French Painting of the Ancien Régime* (Cambridge: Cambridge University Press, 1981), 41.

81. Marin, *Portrait of the King*, 125.

82. Peter Burke, *The Fabrication of King Louis XIV* (New Haven: Yale University Press, 1992). See also Jean-Marie Apostolidès, *Le Roi-machine: spectacle et politique au temps de Louis XIV* (Paris: Minuit, 1981).

83. Abby Zanger, *Scenes from the Marriage of Louis XIV: Nuptial Fictions and the Making of Absolutist Power* (Stanford: Stanford University Press, 1997), 13–36.

84. Norbert Elias, *The Civilizing Process, vol. 1, The History of Manners*, Edmund Jephcott, trans. (New York: Urizen Books, 1978). See also Michael Wolfe, ed., *Changing Identities in Early Modern France* (Durham: Duke University Press, 1996).

85. Elias, *The Civilizing Process, vol. 1*, xv–xvi, 81–2, 137–43.

86. Marcia Pointon, *Hanging the Head: Portraiture and Social Formation in Eighteenth-Century England* (New Haven: Yale University Press, 1993), 4.

87. Lisa Forman Cody, 'The Birth of the Nation: Man-Midwifery and the Conception of Eighteenth-Century Britain' (unpublished manuscript, forthcoming from Oxford University Press), 24–9. I thank Lisa Cody for allowing me to consult her manuscript in progress. See also her 'The Politics of Reproduction: From Midwives' Alternative Public Sphere to the Public Spectacle of Man-Midwifery,' *Eighteenth-Century Studies* 32, 4 (1999), 477–95.

88. Cody, 'The Politics of Reproduction,' 486.

89. Prefaces were conventional in obstetrical treatises written by both men and women. Authors regularly claimed to write only at the behest of friends and colleagues. See, for example, the unpaginated prefaces in Bury, *Le propagatif de l'homme*, Viardel, *Observations sur la pratique des accouchemens naturels, contre nature & monstrueux*, Mauquest de La Motte, *Traité complet des accouchemens*, as well as Peu, *La pratique des accouchemens*, 3–9, 299.

90. Sara E. Melzer and Kathryn Norberg, eds, *From the Royal to the Republican Body: Incorporating the Political in Seventeenth- and Eighteenth-Century France* (Berkeley: University of California Press, 1998), 3.

91. Joseph Roach, 'Body of Law: The Sun King and the Code Noir,' *From the Royal to the Republican Body*, Melzer and Norberg, eds, 113–30, and Elizabeth Colwill, 'Sex, Savagery, and Slavery in the Shaping of the French Body Politic,' *From the Royal to the Republican Body*, Melzer and Norberg, eds, 198–223.

Chapter 3

Reading the Midwife's Body:
Louise Bourgeois

In 1601 the Queen of France, Marie de Médicis, was pregnant with her first child and looking for a new royal midwife. She refused to be delivered by the established Madame Dupuis – her husband's choice for the position – because that elderly midwife had attended several labours of Gabrielle d'Estrées, King Henri IV's mistress. Learning of the Queen's discontent, a number of royal physicians recommended Louise Bourgeois. Though not yet 40 years of age, this midwife was rapidly becoming a favourite birth assistant among the wealthy elite in Paris. One of Bourgeois' clients, Madame la Duchesse d'Elbeuf, spoke with Marie de Médicis about her own delivery, answering the Queen's questions about the midwife's age and *façon* [external appearance or manner]. Noting how well the Queen received this information, the Duchess advised Bourgeois to find a way to be presented to Marie de Médicis. After complicated negotiations, Bourgeois arranged to be at the *maison* of the influential Gondi family when the King and Queen were dining there. The Queen was already inside her carriage, preparing to depart, however, by the time Bourgeois was brought forward. Marie de Médicis looked at the midwife very briefly and did not address her. Nevertheless, the following day Bourgeois received notice that no one but she would touch the Queen during the delivery.

Bourgeois' account of her promotion to the rank of royal midwife appeared in her *Récit véritable de la naissance de messeigneurs et dames les enfans de France* [True account of the births of the Lords and Ladies of France], published in 1617 and included in Volume 2 of her treatise, *Observations diverses sur la stérilité, perte de fruict, foecondité, accouchements et maladies des femmes et enfants nouveaux naiz.*[1] In this striking narrative, Bourgeois maintained that the definitive evidence of her suitability for the role of royal midwife was provided by her physical presence. Reports of the midwife's skill from her satisfied noble customers were apparently not sufficient evidence for Marie de Médicis.[2] The Queen needed to *see* the potential royal servant. Bourgeois had already alluded to the visual determination of her competence in her written address to the Queen at the beginning of Volume 1 of her treatise, first published in 1609. She noted that though some people had considered her too young and inexperienced to deliver Marie de Médicis:

Your Majesty having seen me, from the first time, had the circumspection to recognize the faithful disposition that I had to provide you with a true, attentive service, and that I did not have a manner so imprudent as to dare to introduce myself, and to offer my ability to harvest such a precious fruit without damaging it or the branch which would provide it.[3]

What exactly did the Queen look for as she regarded Bourgeois? The midwife provided few details about the preliminary encounter, noting only that she curtsied to the Queen.[4] Marie de Médicis clearly found Bourgeois agreeable; the commonplace belief that a labouring woman would be adversely affected if she disliked her midwife was what enabled the Queen to overrule King Henri IV's selection of the royal servant.[5] According to Bourgeois, the Queen's preference was confirmed during an encounter which did not require the exchange of words. The midwife's body was the medium of communication verifying her skill. Yet by not elaborating on the visual signs of her obstetrical ability, Bourgeois implied there was something natural or explicit about them.

This chapter investigates what Bourgeois' narrative takes for granted, namely the bodily display and visual assessment of the early modern French midwife. It poses the questions: what was the status of the midwife's body? How was the relationship between her body and her obstetrical abilities articulated? What kinds of arguments were made about her physical presence in the lying-in chamber? In order to formulate some answers, I continue to focus on the writings of Bourgeois, a midwife famous in her own day and now increasingly studied by historians of childbirth.[6] In addition to holding the post of royal midwife to Queen Marie de Médicis from 1601 to 1609, Bourgeois was the first French woman to write an obstetrical treatise. I analyse three selections from her publication which associate the midwife's body with her facility as a midwife. First, I consider Bourgeois' description of the appropriate behaviour, education, and physical qualities of the ideal midwife, then I examine the author portrait of the royal midwife which served as the frontispiece to her treatise (Figure 3.1), and finally I explore Bourgeois' account of her performance at the birth of the future Louis XIII.

Throughout her treatise, Bourgeois described her own experiences assisting at deliveries both straightforward and complicated. Emphasizing her hands-on practices and comportment on these occasions, she offered herself as a model midwife worthy of emulation. In Volume 2 Bourgeois additionally provided a detailed enumeration of the qualities desirable in a female midwife, emphasizing her preferred religious beliefs and moral standing. Bourgeois' account of the ideal midwife was rather conventional, in keeping with the official statutes for Parisian midwives as well as descriptions penned by male authors of obstetrical treatises. Male writers differed, however, by representing the midwife's female body as a limitation to her acquisition of theoretical knowledge, whereas Bourgeois featured the embodied knowledge women gained from their personal experiences of childbirth, claiming that this intelligence formed the basis of midwives' extensive abilities. The royal midwife reaffirmed the traditional belief that women were naturally suited to the practice of midwifery, while challenging the idea that female midwives were incapable of acquiring a masculine understanding of theoretical subjects such as anatomy.

In line with this emphasis on the embodied experience of women, the engraved author portrait of Bourgeois draws attention to the bodily stature of the midwife. More than a decorative addition to the treatise, it is part of the ideal depiction of the royal midwife. The verse inscribed beneath the portrait suggests, however, a mismatch between Bourgeois' body and her ability. It notes the midwife's appearance cannot do justice to her mind or spirit – the substance that produced an esteemed obstetrical treatise. The author portrait thus invokes the gendered distinction associating women with body and men with intellect during the early modern period. Ostensibly designed to flatter Bourgeois, the differentiation between body and mind positions her as an exceptional woman able to surpass the limitations of her feminine physique to succeed in such masculine endeavours as writing. In contrast to her written delineation of the ideal midwife, the portrait implies that the royal midwife's mind is at odds with her body, not an extension of it.

The third representation of Bourgeois is different again, portraying the courtly body of the midwife. The royal midwife described her role at the first labour of Queen Marie de Médicis, drawing attention to her careful execution of gestures and statements rather than her embodied knowledge of maternity. Emphasizing her maintenance of self-control – considered a manly quality during the early modern period – Bourgeois claimed to have avoided displaying the emotional, feminine responses expected of her during the royal birth. The visible demonstration of her status and ability as a midwife therefore entailed the display of her masculine character. Like her author portrait, this account of Bourgeois' controlled body presents her as an exceptional woman who managed to surmount her womanly nature. Yet even as she portrayed midwifery as a practice requiring traits considered unusual in women, Bourgeois continued to describe the lying-in chamber as a feminine realm in which her body conveyed accurate information exclusively to the female attendants of the Queen, not the King and his male courtiers.

The royal midwife emerges from my analyses of the representation of her body as a contradictory figure who shifts between gendered categories, not a stable character standing 'behind' the texts. By emphasizing the politics of display, I reshape scholarly understandings of Bourgeois, enriching studies that feature her medical theories and interaction with male practitioners. My arguments also extend beyond the royal midwife. Striving for the bigger picture, I compare and contrast the contents of her publications with treatises written by both male and female midwives, as well as an array of early modern discussions of women in physiognomy manuals, conduct literature, and the *querelle des femmes*, an ongoing debate about the status of women. My analysis considers how various accounts of the ideal female midwife both adhere to and depart from the gendered norms expounded in other discourses. In the end, I contend that the midwife's body was an unstable terrain during the early modern period, providing a simultaneously substantial and dangerous foundation for arguments about her authority.

Delineating the Ideal Midwife

Bourgeois' obstetrical treatise features a letter to her daughter, offering the younger midwife advice about the proper behaviour of women in their line of work. Drawing on her own experiences and knowledge, Bourgeois created an image of the ideal midwife that reflected rather well on herself. She insisted that a midwife's character be based on standard Christian morals such as charity, honesty, and humility.[7] According to Bourgeois, a midwife who trusted in God would be equipped with a tranquil spirit able to face with composure even the most unexpected situations in the lying-in chamber. This Christian midwife should refuse to provide abortive remedies, but be sure to offer poor women as much care as wealthy clients. Bourgeois affirmed that any monetary losses resulting from such charitable actions would ultimately be rewarded by God.[8] She nevertheless counseled fellow midwives against the practice of delivering desperate single women in their own homes – a mistake she had made in the past – warning that this seemingly generous act could sustain prostitution. If a midwife decided to deliver such women, Bourgeois advised her to do so in an honest place, while admonishing her clients to avoid falling into error again.[9] Though Bourgeois' ideal midwife upheld moral order, she also knew when it was appropriate to reveal information. A good midwife guarded the secrets of her deserving clients, but never acted like a charlatan by withholding useful remedies from doctors or other wise people.[10] With this claim, Bourgeois portrayed her own publications as the work of a sage and generous midwife intent on helping others, reaffirming arguments already made in her preface.[11]

The royal midwife's emphasis on the religious qualities of the ideal female midwife was not unusual. Similar values were inscribed in the legal statutes pertaining to midwifery throughout Europe. Early modern Dutch midwives had to be respectable as well as conformists in religion, while English midwives were subject to ecclesiastical licensing by the Church of England.[12] The 25 clauses of the Parisian regulations for midwives, first devised in 1560, similarly emphasized the moral and religious duties of female midwives, exhorting women to conduct themselves prudently, without recourse to dissolute words or gestures.[13] The royal document issued by the King's parliament paid little attention to the education of midwives, apart from insisting they train under another midwife, and attend an annual anatomy of a female body performed by sworn surgeons. The statutes primarily urged Parisian midwives to 'live as good and honourable women,' reporting the degenerate behaviour of fellow midwives. This allusion to the scrutiny of sinful women accords with Bourgeois' instructions for reestablishing the moral standing of fallen clients. Both instances support arguments made by historian Jacques Gélis, who claims French midwives increasingly performed a role of social surveillance, serving the state by, for example, urging labouring women to name the fathers of their illegitimate children.[14]

Though the regulation of midwives varied in different parts of France, the content of subsequent statutes remained consistent until 1730, when questions of conduct were replaced by a concern with licensing fees.[15] In order to be certified, Parisian midwives had to be examined by a physician and two senior midwives as well as two surgeons, but the women both paid their fees to and were registered by Saint-Côme, the surgeon's guild.[16] Female midwives were not really considered members of the corporation, and not allowed to attend its functions. It seems the primary goal was to make Parisian midwives subservient to surgeons, in accordance with the intensifying regulation of female midwives in other parts of France.[17] Yet attempts to control these women were not always successful. Archival records show that even in 1730 criminal charges were laid against women who continued to practice without being examined and then sworn in at the legal courts of Châtelet in Paris.[18]

The only women who could officially escape the examination process were those who studied at the Hôtel-Dieu in Paris, an institution accepting female students for midwifery instruction since at least 1630.[19] These women observed deliveries for six weeks before assisting for an additional six weeks at the labours of those poor women who gave birth at the hospital. Though such training was prestigious throughout Europe, the number of skilled midwives produced was not substantial because the hospital accepted no more than four female students at a time. Despite stressing the necessity of hands-on training in midwifery, administrators of the Hôtel-Dieu continued to enforce moral standards. The regulations of 1693 demanded that women wishing to occupy the position of head midwife demonstrate scrupulous moral qualities, while dressing modestly 'without buckles and without coloured ribbons.' In addition, each potential apprentice midwife had to present her marriage certificate and a document attesting to her exemplary morals before gaining admittance.[20]

As well as institutional and legal sources, written texts produce a conventional image of the ideal female midwife. Like Bourgeois, most early modern authors of obstetrical treatises recommended that the female midwife have an agreeable disposition, strong belief in God, and desire to help women apart from considerations of monetary reward. According to Helen King, this picture of the excellent midwife ultimately derived from Soranus of Ephesus' second-century *Gynaecology*, an important text surviving in various translations, abbreviations, and compilations.[21] While Soranus portrayed a midwife who was sober, circumspect, and free from superstition, he also drew attention to her physical characteristics. She had to have full use of her senses, sound limbs, a robust constitution, and long, slim fingers with short nails in order to 'touch a deep lying inflammation without causing too much pain.'[22] At the same time, Soranus stressed the intellectual capacity of the female midwife, beginning his catalogue of ideal traits by insisting she be literate, able to comprehend theory, and have a good memory. Soranus' ideal midwife was extremely well-rounded, combining strength of body and mind with an extensive learning in all three branches of therapy: diet, surgery, and drugs.[23]

In France, female writers were most faithful to Soranus' vision, describing midwives who were spiritually, physically, and intellectually suited to their role in the birthing chamber. Though Bourgeois emphasized the character of the exemplary midwife, she also insisted that female midwives required extensive learning, including a knowledge of anatomy. She nevertheless noted that women often lacked the necessary theoretical training. Sometimes dangerously incompetent midwives mistook the womb for the afterbirth, attempting to pull out women's organs.[24] The royal midwife broached the topic of ignorant midwives, however, to argue in favour of their education, not to restrict their activities. She urged doctors to provide women with anatomical instruction, implying that sworn surgeons were not allowing midwives to attend anatomies as required in the regulations of 1560.[25] There is evidence that the surgeons of Saint-Côme were continually reluctant to instruct women in anatomy, failing to notify senior midwives on those occasions when a female body was dissected. After losing a legal suit launched by juried female midwives in 1732, Saint-Côme was ordered to admit female midwifery students to anatomical demonstrations.[26] The surgeons apparently refused to comply, for in 1737 they again defended themselves against the demands of female midwives, claiming these women did not require anatomical knowledge, and would only provide an indecent distraction for male students already crowding the amphitheatre.[27]

Although it is unclear whether or not female midwives ever attended anatomies performed by the surgeons of Saint-Côme, women could receive such training at the Hôtel-Dieu in Paris. According to the reminiscences of established midwife Mademoiselle Baudoin in 1671, her midwifery teacher at the hospital, Madame Le Vacher:

> Had all the excellent qualities that a midwife should have, judgement, wit, memory, the resolve and firmness to undertake important operations when they presented themselves. She spoke very well of her profession, understanding anatomy well, particularly [that] of the lower abdomen; several times I saw her open women with much skill and give us excellent lessons on everything that we demanded of her.[28]

Such instruction was mandated by the Bureau of the Hôtel-Dieu; a deliberation issued in 1657 ordered the head midwife to perform a dissection for her apprentices every six weeks, though it also specified the physician responsible for the *salle des accouchées* had to be present to correct or augment her statements.[29] The head midwife at the hospital between 1670 and 1686 drew attention to her own performance of such dissections. In her obstetrical treatise of 1677, Marguerite de La Marche reaffirmed that midwives should fear God, have pure hearts, keep secrets, and refuse to provide abortives.[30] She also claimed to have dissected a misshapen double uterus for the instruction of her apprentice midwives, as described in Chapter 1.[31]

Though female authors insisted on the theoretical learning of women, their accounts of the ideal female midwife diverged from that of Soranus in one significant aspect. He affirmed the experience of childbirth was not requisite to a good midwife, and that even a woman who had not borne children could sympathize with a mother in pain.[32] In contrast, many female midwives contended that a personal, first-hand knowledge of maternity was crucial to midwifery practice. Bourgeois implied midwives required an intimate bodily experience of childbirth in her discussion of the *culbate* or somersault the unborn child made in preparation for its birth. Referring to her own perceptions of pregnancy, the royal midwife argued this movement sometimes occurred long before the delivery, and could not be considered a sign of impending labour. Avowing 'I say truthfully [that I] have carried one turned for six weeks, undertaking my vocation every day,' Bourgeois maintained the work of both her body and her occupation were mutually informing, even inseparable.[33] She continued to invoke a personal, fleshly knowledge of the subject when she identified with other women to comment on 'our pains.'[34] Most significant, however, was Bourgeois' mockery of young women who had given birth only once or twice and yet discoursed on the subject in the presence of older, wiser women.[35] According to the royal midwife, authority in the female realm of lying-in chamber was based on an abundant personal experience of childbirth.

Beliefs in the natural abilities of women to assist in childbirth were the epistemological grounds used by other female authors to defend women's exclusive right to the practice of midwifery. In her obstetrical treatise of 1671, *The Midwives Book*, English midwife Jane Sharp claimed it was the 'natural propriety of women to be much seeing into that Art,' though nature should be augmented by 'a long and diligent practice, and be communicated to others of our own sex.'[36] The most vociferous proponent of women's distinctive capacity for midwifery was the English midwife Elizabeth Nihell. In her treatise of 1760, she professed the 'tender feelings it is so natural for me to have for the sufferings of my own sex,' and baldly stated 'I am myself a mother.'[37] Nihell went on to associate women with flesh and men with instruments, wondering 'where...is the person that would prefer iron and steel to a hand of flesh, tender, soft, duly supple, dextrous and trusting to its own feelings for what it is about.'[38] With this statement, she insisted men were notably lacking in both the necessary physical attributes and intrinsic understanding of birth possessed by women.

These accounts conflate the image of the ideal midwife with that of the ideal mother. In her extensive study of the representation of women in sixteenth-century French engravings, art historian Sara F. Matthews Grieco describes the image of the good mother. This maternal figure is invariably honest and gentle, obligated to care for and amuse her child for both biological and social reasons.[39] The roles of midwife as well as mother were considered natural for women, in part because of their bodily constitution and temperament, aspects commonly related during the early modern period. According to the Galenic doctrine that remained influential – especially in the feminist and anti-feminist writings associated with the *querelle des femmes* – cold and moist humours tended to dominate in women, making them more compassionate and possessed of patience, qualities thought necessary in mothering as well as midwifery.[40] Bourgeois certainly conflated these activities in her treatise. She not only stressed her embodied knowledge of childbirth, but also drew on her authority as a mother to offer advice to her daughter, evoking the traditional communication of 'women's secrets.'[41]

Despite the common association of female midwives with maternity, there were midwives such as Justine Siegemund who had never given birth. In her treatise of 1690, this German midwife admitted she had experienced neither pregnancy nor childbirth, but insisted she was nevertheless able to learn from the bodies of her female clients, as did male birthing assistants. All the same, Siegemund referred to her own menstrual disorders as if to counteract her childlessness. Her intimate and particularly feminine experience of reproductive problems was presented as a source of knowledge authorizing her to speak and write about childbirth.[42] Siegemund's own body therefore remained part of the physical evidence that established her abilities as a midwife. This emphasis on the first-hand knowledge of maternity continued into the eighteenth century. Although French midwife Angélique Marguerite Le Boursier du Coudray had never given birth, she compensated by adopting a 'niece' and training her in midwifery.[43]

The typical association of midwifery with maternity provided female midwives with a respectable image, sanctioning their public speaking, teaching, and writing as part of a traditionally feminine role.[44] Menstruation, pregnancy, childbirth, and maternity were part of an accumulated education, with bodily perception and pain providing paths to understanding.[45] Women's insistence on their natural abilities could justify their acquisition of 'male' knowledge, including anatomy. An anatomical understanding of the reproductive organs of women formed a necessary addition to the foundational knowledge women had already gained through first-hand experience. This elevation of practical over theoretical knowledge was also strategic, for it positioned men as perpetual outsiders in the birthing chamber. According to female midwives such as Bourgeois, men-midwives could only hope to attain a detached, theoretical understanding of women's bodies rather than an intimate appreciation of them.

How did male authors of early modern French obstetrical treatises respond to such arguments? Contrary to what might be expected, they did not shift attention away from the female midwife's physical qualities. Instead, they offered standardized descriptions of the ideal female midwife, considering her person, morals, and mind. Her physical characteristics often drew the most emphasis. In his *De l'heureux accouchement des femmes* of 1609, Jacques Guillemeau devoted several pages to the description of the female midwife.

> First, she must be of suitable age, neither too young, nor too old: well formed in her body, without being subject to any illnesses, and not deformed in any part, clean both in dress and person, having above all small, not coarse, clean hands, with rounded, short fingernails.[46]

The surgeon's insistence on the midwife's appropriate age, well-formed body, cleanliness, and delicate hands recurred in subsequent descriptions by French authors. In his treatise of 1623, surgeon man-midwife Jacques Bury similarly drew attention to the midwife's age, claiming that she should be between 35 and 50, past her prime childbearing years, but still young enough to possess bodily strength.[47] Age and endurance were likewise the primary concerns of surgeon man-midwife Paul Portal, who in 1685 claimed to have seen elderly midwives lacking the strength to pull children out in difficult cases, as well as youthful ones who endangered children through their negligence.[48]

In addition to endurance, a sound bodily structure was associated with the female midwife's ability to soothe clients. Bury contended that the midwife should not be hunchbacked, twisted or lame because badly formed people were both disagreeable and lacking in dexterity.[49] While Bury was uncustomarily specific about the appearance of a reassuring midwife – noting her 'gay eye' and 'smiling face' – other authors claimed the midwife's speech should encourage her suffering client to persevere during a lengthy labour.[50] In 1671, surgeon man-midwife Cosme Viardel insisted the midwife be both sober and chaste in her actions as well as sociable in her words, in order to divert the labouring woman and attendants gathered in the lying-in chamber.[51] A pleasant appearance and congenial demeanour went hand in hand. Yet according to surgeon man-midwife Pierre Dionis finding an agreeable-looking midwife who spoke modestly and with discretion could be difficult because women were naturally given to gossip.[52]

While education and intelligence were hardly undesirable in a female midwife, they were not considered crucial elements of her constitution. In fact, many male authors preferred personality traits that would render the female midwife easier to manage. In 1694, surgeon man-midwife Philippe Peu specified what kind of woman he would choose to assist him in the birthing chamber. Not only would she be gentle, silent, discreet, clever, strong, and agreeable to the suffering woman, she would also be 'prompt to obey' the surgeon.[53] Peu's account of the ideal female birth assistant resembled the moralizing descriptions of the model wife and mother offered by Claude Maillard; this Jesuit writer drew particular attention to the need for women to obey male authority figures, especially their husbands.[54]

A few male authors claimed female midwives should be equipped with anatomical knowledge in order to offer accurate reports to male practitioners when suffering women refused to expose themselves to men.[55] For the most part, however, men deviated from Soranus' model in the matter of the female midwife's education. When Guillemeau finally contemplated the mind of the ideal midwife, his account was rather cursory. She should be wise, discreet, witty, and able to devise flattering, even deceitful speeches to distract an apprehensive woman in labour.[56] In 1671, Viardel reiterated the necessity of these qualities, but also noted female midwives should be restrained in their prognoses, protecting their reputations by concealing their ignorance.[57] By 1718 Dionis argued that female midwives needed only as much theory as they were capable of acquiring – very little in his opinion.[58] Dionis' statement was unusual, however, for the midwife's theoretical education and literacy typically went unmentioned in obstetrical treatises penned by French men.[59]

French surgeon men-midwives suggested that assisting at natural births was a kind of bodily labour enhanced by practice. Most authors claimed the female midwife's primary obligation was to endure the birth physically and buoy the labouring woman's spirits. Declaring unnatural births their own more complicated domain, surgeon men-midwives argued that the role of the female midwife was simply to assist nature.[60] In cases of malpresentation, or where the child was weak, these men insisted the female midwife recognize her intellectual limitations and call on medical men to save both mother and child. The supposedly narrow capacities of female midwives were inscribed in the statutes of 1560, which directed midwives to call on the assistance of someone more experienced than them, either a doctor, surgeon, or older matron, if the child presented in a difficult birth posture.[61]

According to Lisa Forman Cody, eighteenth-century British men-midwives sought to rupture the natural connection between female midwives and maternity, rendering knowledge of childbirth attainable through rational-critical means rather than personal bodily experience.[62] In the earlier sources penned by French surgeon men-midwives, however, authors did not attempt to 'denaturalize' childbirth, distancing women from it. On the contrary, they reaffirmed women's natural affiliation with childbirth, stressing the midwife's bodily qualities in an effort to limit her traditional role. By insisting the female midwife primarily required physical strength and good-natured patience during a delivery, French surgeon men-midwives implied that her activity in the birthing room was both unskilled and utterly different from their own more learned interventions.

The female body was invoked in arguments for as well as against the constraint of the midwife's practice. These contradictory claims were possible because the female body was a slippery subject during the early modern period, imbued with conflicting values. Women's reproductive capacity was a site of authority and distinction, but was also considered potentially out of control.[63] Legal statutes in early modern France, for example, not only insisted that single pregnant women reveal the father's name, but made it illegal to hide a pregnancy or give birth clandestinely.[64] At the same time as the predominantly cold and moist humours in women encouraged certain positive qualities, they simultaneously gave rise to women's supposed inconstancy, fearfulness, and despair, making them prone to violent passions, while less capable of active virtue and intellectual pursuits.[65] These paradoxical understandings of women's nature explain why a good midwife could easily dissolve into a bad one. In male accounts, the midwife who knows her place during a normal delivery is labeled ignorant and presumptuous if she attempts a difficult delivery on her own.[66] But even in the treatise of Bourgeois, a generous midwife could unwittingly support sin by assisting at illegitimate births. Women's natural qualities and embodied knowledge ultimately provided an unstable foundation for female authors' arguments about midwifery skills. This situation should not be overstated, however, for men's claims about women's abilities were equally ambivalent. Reconfirming the link between women and natural childbirth may have distinguished the activities of surgeon men-midwives, but it also reestablished their own classification as outsiders summoned to the lying-in chamber only when birth deviated from its standard course.

Scrutinizing the Royal Midwife

Although Bourgeois stressed the embodied knowledge of the ideal female midwife, she did not follow the longstanding convention by mentioning her small, clean hands or sturdy frame. Nor did the royal midwife provide details about her own appearance, which the Queen apparently found so pleasing. An image of the royal midwife exists, however, in the form of the frontispiece author portrait in her treatise. This visual rendering of the midwife would seem to offer some concrete information about her appearance. During the early modern period author portraits typically functioned to represent the body from which the written text had issued. Often enhanced with an inscription of the author's name and rank, these images bound the text to a unique individual. Yet the portrait of Bourgeois is a complex and contradictory image providing far more than a likeness of the royal midwife.

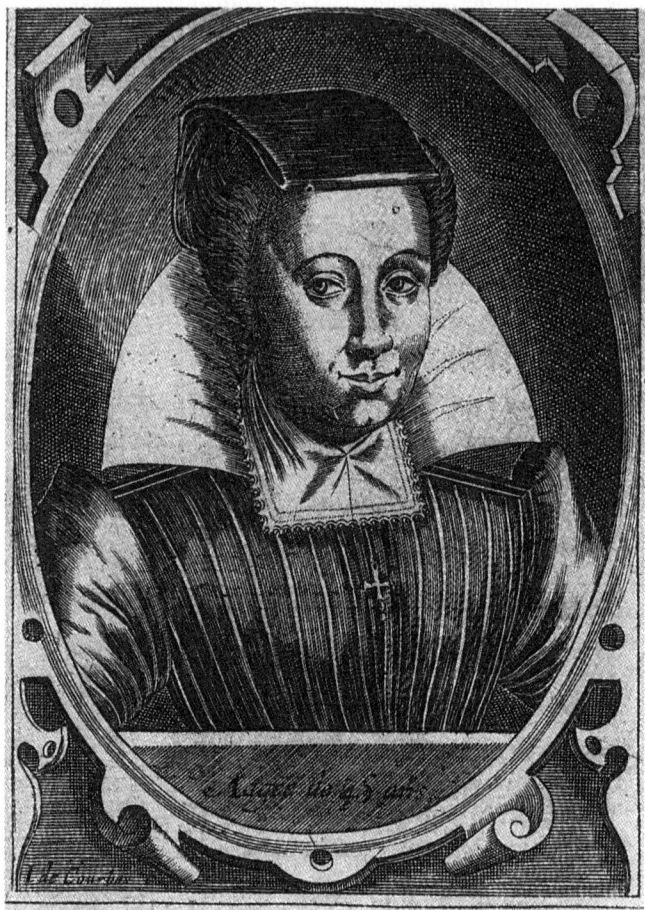

En ce parfait tableau le defaut de peinture,
Se congnoist auiourd'huy clairement à nos yeux;
Pource qu'on n'y peut veoir que du corps la figure;
Non l'esprit admiré pour chef d'œuure des Cieux.

Figure 3.1   Author portrait, from Louise Bourgeois' *Observations diverses sur la stérilité, perte de fruict, foecondité, accouchements et maladies des femmes et enfants nouveaux naiz*, 1626, Rouen. Courtesy of the Edward G. Miner Library, University of Rochester Medical Center, Rochester, NY

Bourgeois' portrait was engraved in 1608 by official French court artist Thomas de Leu, but to my knowledge no written records survive to document the complex web of negotiations leading to its production.[67] As indicated in Chapter 1, the manufacture of engravings was a group effort. In the case of an author portrait, a book's publisher would usually direct one artist to draw the image, and another to engrave it. The author in question also had a role to play. French historian Roger Chartier contends that early modern French writers took a vested interest in the construction of their books, specifying the language, type, paper, and plates to be used.[68] Engraved portraits would have received considerable attention, given the cost involved in commissioning them; during the seventeenth century they were more expensive than painted portraits.[69] An author may have had a voice in the selection of the engraver, especially since it was customary at the time for subjects to choose portrait painters. In any case, the author presumably did not remain mute during sittings, when important decisions about pose and costume were finalized.

Bourgeois' portrait appears near the front of her treatise, following the short dedication praising Queen Marie de Médicis' ability to recognize the midwife's skill.[70] Readers are thus asked to review the appearance found worthy by the Queen herself. They are offered an official image of the royal midwife, shown adorned with signs of royal favour. Bourgeois is portrayed wearing not only the high velvet collar and golden cross of the royal midwife, but also the velvet cap that formerly distinguished only the royal nurses. Recounting her promotion to the rank of royal midwife, Bourgeois insisted this headgear was first awarded to her by her royal patron, the Queen, and that no other midwife was allowed to wear it.[71] These references in the portrait point to both Bourgeois' elevated position as royal midwife and the importance of displaying that status during the early modern period.

The person of Bourgeois is characterized by her forthright countenance and broad shoulders. Her body is represented as well-formed and strong, qualities that Guillemeau and others emphasized as essential in a midwife. Bourgeois' rather stiff posture is itself a legible convention, and should not be mistaken for a natural inscription of her appearance in contrast to the more explicit visual signifiers of her rank. As historians Georges Vigarello and Herman Roodenburg have shown, a vertical carriage was increasingly linked with an upright social and moral status during the early modern period.[72] At the same time, a tranquil face signified a disciplined character.[73] Bourgeois underscored the quality of self-control in her open letter to her daughter, arguing that a midwife who 'lived within herself' was capable of remedying even the gravest situations.[74] The author furthermore insisted on her own ability to remain calm under stressful conditions, drawing attention to her absolute composure when she first realized the Queen had given birth to the much desired *Dauphin* in 1601, discussed below.

In addition to substantiating accounts of the ideal midwife, the portrait of Bourgeois conforms to early modern conventions of portraiture. Her image is more conventional than individualized, in keeping with the tradition of showing the sitter, according to art historian T. H. Thomas, 'not only as he [sic] looks but as he wants to look.'[75] The goal of French portraiture was not to capture a subject in an unguarded moment, but rather to configure a controlled, alert, and dignified figure aligned with social expectations. Numerous portraits by de Leu depict the stiffly upright heads and shoulders of noble subjects confined within an oval framework.[76] This commonplace format was not exclusive, however, to the court artist. De Leu's image of the royal midwife is standardized enough to be accredited to other artists. In his inventory of the plates held at the Bibliothèque Nationale in Paris, Roger-Armand Weigert names Jean de Courbes as the engraver of the portrait of Bourgeois.[77] This attribution is well-founded given that de Courbes signed the versions of the engraving he copied after de Leu, including one appearing in the 1626 edition of the midwife's treatise. The image of Bourgeois furthermore resembles other portraits produced by de Courbes. His depiction of the Spanish author Bernabé Moreno de Vargas in 1633, for example, similarly features the bust of a sitter with broad shoulders and a straightforward expression surrounded by an oval frame.[78] Bourgeois' portrait represents the midwife in a legible format regularly used to portray respectable writers and other notable figures, making it difficult to analyse exclusively in terms of the individual engraver or sitter involved.

At least one aspect of the author portrait of Bourgeois deviates from the norm. The frames surrounding most of the engraved portraits by de Leu, the author portrait of Moreno de Vargas by de Courbes, and various portraits of men who wrote obstetrical treatises – discussed in Chapter 4 – feature the names and official titles of their sitters. In contrast, the minute text directly beneath the representation of Bourgeois discloses only the date the image was made, 1608, and rather more prominently below this a statement identifying the subject as 45 years old. Although the age of a sitter was occasionally noted in portraits by de Leu, it did not replace but rather supplemented other textual information. The custom of noting the age of subjects waned during the seventeenth century, and no other portraits in French obstetrical treatises insist upon the author's life span in this fashion.[79] Bourgeois' age was therefore stressed as a significant element of her identity that surpassed in importance even her name and title.

Drawing attention to the age of Bourgeois may seem to accord with men's emphasis on the middle age of the ideal female midwife discussed above. Yet in her address to the Queen, Bourgeois indicated that certain people had judged her too young to merit the post of royal midwife. Only 38 years old when engaged by Marie de Médicis in 1601, Bourgeois had practised midwifery for a mere eight years and had held a license since 1598.[80] Moreover, Bourgeois was still in her childbearing years. When she first went to deliver the Queen at Fontainebleau, she left behind her third daughter, who was six months old. In contrast to Bourgeois' fertility and youth, written accounts of the ideal midwife both in France and throughout Europe favoured a midwife who was either widowed or no longer burdened with the care of young children, and able to respond to the call of a labouring woman any time of the day or night. Her maturity was made explicit in the Dutch ordinances that began to appear around the middle of the seventeenth century, specifying that the respectable female midwife had to be an older woman, either married or widowed, and equipped with a personal experience of childbirth.[81] Given the longstanding importance of the maturity of the ideal midwife, why did the portrait of Bourgeois emphasize her relative youth, especially when the royal midwife was defensive about it in her address to the Queen?

Even as noting the age of Bourgeois potentially drew attention to her purported lack of experience, it also highlighted her precocious accomplishments. By 1609 the royal midwife had already delivered all six of Marie de Médicis' children. Bourgeois' youth was in fact part of the reason the Queen selected her to replace the elderly Madame Dupuis.[82] The engraved reference to the midwife's age highlights her achievements in relation to her specific temporal and physical status. Insisting on the materiality of the female body that produced the text, it reinforces the traditional conflation of the female body with reproductive knowledge. By age 45, Bourgeois had given birth five times, in addition to delivering children for over a decade; it was in significant part these bodily experiences that empowered her to write an obstetrical treatise. Clearly, these experiences are not explicitly inscribed in Bourgeois' portrait, but age draws attention to her body in a way that name and rank could not have.

This emphasis on the material constitution of the midwife also accords with early modern theories of physiognomy, which held that a person's character was legible in his or her bodily appearance and facial features.[83] Such beliefs informed both the production and interpretation of portraiture, as already indicated by my association of Bourgeois' stiff posture in the image with the characteristic of self-control. The practice of physiognomy clearly influenced accounts of the ideal female midwife. Although the person, morals, and mind of the midwife were usually considered separately in obstetrical treatises, these categories were mutually informing. It may seem only obvious that bodily strength and cleanliness were considered desirable in a practising midwife, but in early modern France cleanliness was associated more with seemliness and good manners than with modern understandings of bodily hygiene.[84] The physical evaluation of character was standard procedure in a medical context. When Bourgeois gave advice about the selection of a wet nurse, for instance, she followed conventional wisdom by stressing the careful examination of a woman's appearance. Parents were to scrutinize not only for evidence of physical health – in white, well-ordered teeth – but also a suitable personality, which could be ascertained in a straightforward gaze, for a lowly or suspicious nature could be conveyed to the child by way of the nurse's breast milk.[85]

The predominance of physiognomy sheds light on the initial exchange between the Queen and Bourgeois. Marie de Médicis may have made a visual determination of the propriety and character of her potential servant, as much as Bourgeois' physical capacity to assist at the delivery. At the same time, by giving Bourgeois the royal 'once over,' the Queen performed her monarchical prerogatives. Philosopher Peter Harrison argues that the seventeenth-century desire to read the passions inscribed on the human countenance was associated with the ambition to master the language of nature in order to restore human dominion over nature (lost in the Fall); politically, such interpretive finesse could be used to maintain social hierarchies, including that of master over servant, husband over wife, and ruler over subject.[86] As her social superior, the Queen had the unquestioned right to evaluate the appearance of the potential royal midwife. Bourgeois presented herself, after all, as the woman who would not only enter the polite society of the court, but one who would be entitled to view as well as touch the body of the Queen. Bourgeois' strategic description of her elevation to the rank of royal midwife therefore included both a celebration of the Queen's recognition of her authority as a midwife, and her own submission to the conventions of the established order.

We too give Bourgeois the 'once over' when we examine her portrait, perhaps looking for evidence of her ability in the same way. Appropriately deferential, the eyes in the portrait of Bourgeois do not look back, confronting our gaze with her own. In the portrait, the royal midwife knows she is the one being looked at, not doing the looking herself. Although her eyes are shown to be open and clear, not squinting as they would be in a person with questionable morals, her pupils are slightly off-centre, aimed toward the left. This oblique gaze does not appear in de Leu's portraits of royal figures. In his image of Marie de Médicis in 1602, for example, the Queen addresses her viewer directly; she is equal or even superior to the subject who nevertheless evaluates her appearance.[87] In contrast, the carefully constructed portrait of Bourgeois presents her as perfectly suited to the role of royal servant. It provides evidence of the correspondence between her body, appearance, character, rank, and propriety.

The laudatory passage positioned beneath the portrait of Bourgeois, however, suggests a mismatch between her image and identity. Proclaiming 'In this perfect picture, the imperfection of the painting can be recognized clearly today because one can see there only the face of the subject and not the mind [or spirit] admired as a sublime masterpiece,' the quatrain by S. Hacquin implies that, although accurate as a record of Bourgeois' appearance, the portrait is unable to convey the intellectual or immaterial essence of the sitter.[88] Whether penned by Hacquin or another court poet, verses embellishing the portraits engraved by de Leu typically celebrate the sitter's beauty, courage, power, or wealth, often while associating him or her with an important historical event. The poems occasionally also express regret that the painter had not adequately represented the esteemed subject in question.[89] The quatrain written to accompany Bourgeois' portrait was therefore not entirely unique. It affirmed the sixteenth- and seventeenth-century conceit that visual reproduction could not fully capture the sitter's being, which readers were sometimes directed to locate in the text.[90]

Yet the differentiation of portrait and text, or material presence and essence, has particular significance within an obstetrical context. As we have already seen in descriptions of the ideal female midwife, it was typical for early modern Europeans to associate corporeality with women and intellectuality with men. This gendered distinction informed the association of female midwives with bodily knowledge and men with theory. The inscription beneath the portrait suggests that Bourgeois' intellectual abilities made her more than what her appearance – her female body – could convey. Hacquin's verse seems to act as a corrective to both the power of the image and inscription of the midwife's age, which draw attention to her body. The quatrain contends that Bourgeois' essential nature is to be found elsewhere, in the mind not commensurate with her body. In contrast to the midwife's account of her initial encounter with Queen Marie de Médicis, the verse implies that looking at Bourgeois' appearance and comprehending the full extent of her capacities are not equivalent.

Bourgeois' engraved author portrait sends several mixed messages. The royal midwife is both conflated with and distinguished from her body. Her image is presented as simultaneously accurate and inadequate. While these competing messages are potentially flattering, they could also be uncomplimentary to the midwife. On one hand, the exaltation of Bourgeois' mind implies she is an exceptional woman, whose intellect and ability surpass the confines of her womanly body and appearance. She is represented as a *femme forte*, a woman who outshines other women by excelling in activities usually associated with men, including intellectual endeavours such as writing.[91] Strong women were celebrated by feminist writers participating in the *querelle des femmes* as proof of women's considerable capacities. Bourgeois and other female midwives argued that women could excel in the masculine realm of medical theory. But on the other hand, learned women were considered unnatural in antifeminist literature. Boccaccio, for example, gave voice to a common sentiment when he wrote: 'what can we think except that it was an error of nature to give female sex to a body which had been endowed by God with a magnificent virile spirit.'[92] Women such as Bourgeois who went beyond the confines of their feminine nature could be considered monstrous mistakes. In the end, the author portrait supports both possibilities, associating Bourgeois with a hybrid identity that fluctuates between efficient female midwife and masculine writer.

The Midwife's Courtly Body

Bourgeois was subjected to a judgmental gaze both during her original encounter with Queen Marie de Médicis and as the character represented in her author portrait.

On the evening of 27 September 1601, however, the eyes of the royal court were on the midwife, watching her every move. She was at Fontainebleau, assisting the Queen of France with the delivery of her first child. The labour, which lasted over 22 hours, was nearing its end, and the large crowd gathered in the birthing chamber – including King Henri IV, the Princes of the Blood, and the Queen's ladies in waiting – eagerly awaited news of the child. Would the Queen produce the desired *Dauphin*, providing a male heir to continue the Bourbon dynasty? Or would she give birth to a girl, barred from succeeding to the throne? The royal child finally made its appearance, but the audience had to wait a little longer. According to the account written by Bourgeois herself, she quickly wrapped the newborn, so that those closest to the scene of birth could see only its face.[93] Although the royal midwife was the sole person in the room with knowledge of the child's sex, she did not betray this information. Her own face remained expressionless, and her demeanour calm. Bourgeois' inscrutable surface surprised the King and Queen, who thought the midwife would reveal the truth in her expression. In an earlier exchange, King Henri IV had insisted no woman in the world could keep quiet after recognizing the future King; Bourgeois would surely cry out with joy.[94]

Others also paid careful attention to the midwife's appearance. Mademoiselle de la Renoüilliere, the first *femme de chambre* [lady in waiting] of the Queen, had asked Bourgeois to provide her with a signal indicating the child's sex so that she could be the first to inform the King. Bourgeois agreed to perform a secret gesture, lowering her head if it was a boy, throwing it back if a girl arrived. Another attendant to the Queen, Mademoiselle Gratienne, had approached the royal midwife with a similar request. Although Mademoiselle Gratienne was beneath Mademoiselle de la Renoüilliere in age and rank, Bourgeois consented to appease both women. She would state 'Ma fille, chauffe-moi un linge' [My daughter, warm me a linen] to alert the younger lady that the child was male. When the time arrived, Bourgeois claimed to have performed her gestures and statements as promised. Both *femmes de chambre* conveyed their knowledge of the *Dauphin* to the King, but he scarcely believed them, pointing to Bourgeois' serious countenance as evidence of a female child. When Henri IV finally asked the midwife directly, she confirmed it was a boy, unwrapping the child to display him to the King. Overwhelmed with emotion, the King cried tears of delight, informed the Queen, and then allowed some two hundred people into the antechamber to celebrate the birth – arousing the anger of the royal midwife who feared for the Queen's delicate state. According to Bourgeois, a few days later the King jokingly renamed her *ma resoluë* [my resolute or resolved one], recognizing the midwife's exceptional composure at the royal birth.[95]

More than chronicling an important royal milestone, Bourgeois' story – part of the *Récit véritable* published in her obstetrical treatise – drew attention to how she had proved herself to be an accomplished royal midwife. At the birth of the *Dauphin*, the midwife's abilities were tested before a large and prestigious audience. But apart from describing how she revived the weak newborn by blowing wine into its mouth, Bourgeois included few details about the medical interventions she had undertaken. Instead, she emphasized her comportment at the birth, as well as her ability to manoeuvre within the complicated world of the French court, pleasing two *femmes de chambre* without abandoning her primary duty to the Queen. Bourgeois argued her regulated behaviour was designed to protect the health of Marie de Médicis as both elation and disappointment about the child could have had a deleterious effect on the Queen. In the end, however, it was not the midwife but rather the King who could not exercise self-control, putting his newly-delivered wife at risk.

Just as the author portrait does not simply reflect Bourgeois' appearance, this narrative of the royal birth does not necessarily record the event with accuracy. Other *raconteurs* offered strikingly different reports, ones less complimentary to the midwife. Jean Héroard, physician to Henri III, Henri IV and the *Dauphin*, described the same royal delivery in his *Journal sur l'enfance et la jeunesse de Louis XIII, 1601–1628* [Journal of the childhood and youth of Louis XIII, 1601–1628].[96] According to the physician, Bourgeois hesitated for some time before cutting the navel string because she was afraid to hurt the child. Héroard went on to cast even more doubt on the midwife's abilities. He implied that the weakened state of the *Dauphin* was caused, not by prolonged labour, but by the child's lengthy wait for the afterbirth to be delivered, a task traditionally assigned to the female midwife. Furthermore, the physician noted the newborn was revitalized by the royal surgeon Guillemeau, who used a spoon to administer wine to the *Dauphin*. Héroard favoured male medical practitioners by insisting that a man had stepped in to rectify the faults of an unnerved midwife barely capable of handling the extended labour.

In contrast to the physician, Bourgeois associated herself with the qualities of an ideal female midwife, including discretion and composure. At the same time, her controlled facial expressions and bodily movements correspond to the courtly body described by Norbert Elias and Norman Bryson, outlined in the previous chapter.[97] Both scholars emphasize the increasing value placed on self-control in early modern France, but pay little attention to distinctions of gender. The early modern French etiquette manuals studied by Elias nevertheless specified the bodily demeanour appropriate to individuals of varying sex, rank, and age. In *L'Honneste homme* [The honest man], a treatise first published in 1630 for male courtiers serving Louis XIII, for example, author Nicolas Faret argued that the man able to restrain his own passions, demonstrating self-mastery, would be able to govern others.[98] This ambition was not suited to women, who were naturally weaker, more passive, and more fearful than men, according to authors such as Marin Cureau de La Chambre in his *Art de connoistre les hommes* [The art of how to know men], published in 1660.[99] The physician to Louis XIV pointed out that such potentially negative qualities were not actually defects in women, but merely natural to their sex. The same etiquette manuals also urged women to avoid displaying any mastery they might possess. Even feminist writers encouraged them to be pleasant and agreeable, dissimulating rather than exposing their knowledge.[100] Cureau de La Chambre claimed that qualities desirable in men could only be deformities in women because 'those Women, who are born with that confidence and audacity, which are proper only to man, are commonly rash, impudent, unthrifty.'[101] According to this author and others who wrote about courtly behaviour before him, openly powerful or masculine women unsettled the natural order as well as, they implied, the political order of the absolutist court.[102]

Despite these descriptions of appropriately gendered behaviour, Bourgeois was not a modestly feminine figure in her account of the royal birth. The King's standard assumptions about women's vulnerability to expressing the passions in bodily form were thwarted by the royal midwife.[103] Acting more like a male courtier than a female servant, she presided over the birth in a lying-in room dominated by women. According to the royal midwife, she delivered her knowledge of the identity of the *Dauphin* to women first. Only two high-ranking female attendants to the Queen could interpret the midwife's body correctly, seeing the hidden truth. The King himself was duped, misreading Bourgeois' impassive visage as proof of a female child. All the same, the royal midwife argued that the King approved of her behaviour, rewarding her with an intimate nickname. His favour also assumed a more concrete form. Bourgeois maintained that during the lengthy labour, Henri IV instructed the royal physicians to confer with her about the Queen's treatment, as Marie de Médicis was suffering from colic.[104] The midwife's resolute demeanour within and control of the lying-in chamber resulted in the elevation of her rank within the courtly as well as medical hierarchy, at least according to Bourgeois; modern scholars find her claim that the King equalized the positions of the royal midwife and the royal physicians rather difficult to believe, doubting that male physicians would publicly defer to a young, relatively unknown midwife.[105]

The royal midwife drew additional attention to her power by describing an exchange she had with the young Duc de Vendôme, an illegitimate son born in 1594 to Henri IV and Gabrielle d'Estrées.[106] During the lengthy labour, Bourgeois reassured the five-year-old boy that the Queen would soon be delivered and that the newborn would be a boy. Implying her authority surpassed that of any monarch and even God, she playfully claimed she could make the child a boy or girl as she pleased. The story provided proof of Bourgeois' intimate contact with the royal family, but also enhanced her account of the carnivalesque atmosphere of the royal lying-in chamber, where hierarchies were overturned. Though the appearance of a legitimate male heir to the throne could only threaten the prestige of the Duc de Vendôme, it would dramatically increase that of Bourgeois.

Even in Bourgeois' treatise, however, the theme of the 'woman on top' is only temporary, ultimately reaffirming rather than undermining the status quo.[107] While maternity shifted the usual arrangement between the sexes – the King acted like a woman, while the midwife acted like a man – it finally reinforced the patriarchal structure of the state. The drama of the birth ultimately revolved around the desire for a male child who would become King. If a female child had been produced, Bourgeois' status would have suffered along with that of the Queen and her female entourage. At the same time, the royal midwife's demonstration of self-control was a sign, not simply of her powerful abilities, but also of her subjection. Only those of the highest rank were permitted to display openly their inner turmoil.[108] King Henri IV had not really made a social or political blunder with his emotional outburst. He had exercised his right to reject the rules of appropriate conduct. The Queen was also able to express herself, given her position as a birthing woman as well as monarch. When Bourgeois noticed Marie de Médicis was exercising self-restraint, the midwife urged her to moan in pain lest the Queen impede the birth or hurt herself.[109] Restrictions of behaviour did not apply equally to all; the royal midwife had to maintain her dignity within the court setting even if others did not.

Bourgeois was nevertheless conspicuously proud of having deceived the King with disingenuous behaviour apparently at odds with the conduct expected of an honest courtier and honourable midwife. Yet according to Castiglione's sixteenth-century Italian treatise, *Il Cortegiano,* as well as later French behaviour manuals, a kind of 'honourable dissimulation' was permitted in the complicated world of the court.[110] In addition, midwives were allowed to conceal the truth from those gathered in the lying-in chamber, if only for the good of their clients. Guillemeau argued, for example, that the practice of deceit and flattery was an essential part of the midwife's occupation.[111] This practice was only to be expected, given that duplicity was a trait frequently associated with women's natural inclinations. But anxieties about potential dishonesty suffused a court setting, and did not exclusively concern women. Bryson argues that the courtier was 'always deciphering and never experiencing without suspicion the influx of his sensations.'[112]

Bourgeois depicted a royal lying-in chamber rife with potential deception. King Henri IV, for example, did not trust the Queen's ladies in waiting when they informed him of the male child. In fact, the King believed the *Dauphin* existed only when he saw the child with his own eyes. In the end, it was Bourgeois who delivered the good news, usurping the status of both ladies in waiting. The royal midwife unwrapped the child that she herself had covered, presenting him to the King – as if she, and not the Queen, had produced him. Like the appearance of Bourgeois, the body of the newborn acted as a sign that conveyed meaning within the royal birthing chamber. In this case, however, the *Dauphin's* delicate body communicated the 'naked truth,' rather than harbouring hidden messages or ulterior motives. The sight of his penis is at the crux of the midwife's tale, as all the courtly machinations she described hinged on the revelation of this appendage. According to Bourgeois, once the child was uncovered, the drama was complete. The King perceived not only the sex of the royal child, but also the manly nature of the royal midwife.

Bourgeois' narrative is ultimately structured around the theme of the body as a site that both conceals and reveals the truth. This motif is not unique to her treatise, but can be related to a larger cultural paradox concerning the body during the early modern period. On one hand, the practice of physiognomy supported the contention that one could see the body and know the truth. Physiognomical theories were invoked not only to interpret portraiture, but also to assist royal servants at court. In his *Traité de la cour, ou instruction des courtisans* [Treatise of the court, or lessons for courtiers] of 1617, for example, Eustache de Refuge advised courtiers to ingratiate themselves with the Prince by determining his character. The inclinations and habits of the Prince, de Refuge argued, would be inscribed on his countenance, clearly visible to those who knew how to read them.[113] On the other hand, physiognomy was meant to help courtiers discover the secret designs of others, given that the court was a treacherous place where appearances did not always correspond with reality.[114] Literary critic Harry Berger contends that the sheer fiction of the self-representation promoted in etiquette manuals – urging readers to draw attention to the artful representation of natural virtues – eventually led to what he calls 'physiognomic scepticism' or apprehensions about the inevitable lack of authenticity in performance.[115] The early modern body was thus a means of both communication and miscommunication, truth and deceit. The courtly body (and, by extension, the body of the royal midwife) was a contradictory sign, at once legible, but also apt to dissemble.

In contrast to the initial meeting with Queen Marie de Médicis, during the royal delivery the relationship between looking at the midwife's body and seeing the truth was not obvious. Her carefully controlled body masked as well as exposed information about the royal birth. The disjunction between Bourgeois' appearance and the truth about the child's sex recalls the mismatch noted in her author portrait, which according to the inscription both accurately portrayed and yet potentially misconstrued her essential identity. In the royal lying-in chamber, the body of the female midwife was equally changeable, linked with power, duplicity, and submission. Bourgeois' representation of her courtly body is nevertheless distinct from the portrayal of her body in other parts of her treatise. Her account of the royal birth does not foreground her own personal experience of childbirth; nor does it relate her intellect to her feminine corporeality. Instead, Bourgeois emphasized how she had embodied masculine qualities in a way that enabled her to control the royal lying-in chamber, a feminine space sustaining the patriarchal order.

Conclusions

The three representations of Bourgeois analysed above indicate that visual display was an important aspect of midwifery practice in early modern France. In each case, the royal midwife was scrutinized for signs of appropriate physical qualities, demeanour, and appearance. As the primary means of communication, her body was a crucial element of her authority. The cases nevertheless provide three distinct images of Bourgeois, presenting her female body as a site of maternal knowledge, a form of materiality at odds with masculine intellect, and a carefully managed vector of (mis)information about childbirth. These different visions of the midwife can be at least partly explained in relation to the various conventions of representation with which they intersect. Bourgeois' description of the ideal female midwife both reaffirms and alters the standard accounts proffered in medical literature since Soranus, her frontispiece corresponds with contemporary conventions of portraiture, and her account of the royal birth presents the legible body required albeit mistrusted in a courtly setting. Yet the differences between these representations cannot be resolved with reference to stylistic variety or even the 'development' of Bourgeois' ideas. After all, both her letter to her daughter and narrative of the birth of the *Dauphin* were published in 1617. Considered together, the three cases foreground a lack of unity in arguments about the identity of the female midwife, despite their location in the same treatise. Bourgeois emerges from this study as an inconsistent figure with multiple voices. She shifts between the roles of mother, writer, and courtier, transforming from a defender of women's prerogative in the lying-in chamber to a masculine character serving the monarchy and back again.

This chapter demonstrates that the female body did not provide a stable ground for the identity of the female midwife. For even as maternal experience was valued, women's bodies were endowed with ambivalent qualities. At several points in Bourgeois' treatise, her body is differentiated from prevailing beliefs about women's nature, not just conflated with them. Midwifery emerges from her texts as a practice that required both feminine and masculine qualities.[116] Bourgeois consistently portrayed the lying-in chamber as a womanly realm, but she also argued that masculine abilities were sometimes required within it, indicating they could advance a female midwife's career. Overall, her treatise offers a complex view of the ideal midwife, while contesting the notion that men-midwives introduced 'male values' into the lying-in chamber to the overwhelming detriment of women.

Notes

1. Bourgeois's account is most accessible in the republication of François Rouget and Colette H. Winn, eds, *Récit véritable de la naissance de messeigneurs et dames les enfans de France* (Geneva: Droz, 2000), 57–96, and I will refer to this version in my notes.
2. When King Henri IV asked Bourgeois for a list of a dozen ladies of quality whom she had delivered, she supplied him with 30 names. Bourgeois, *Récit véritable*, 67.

3.   Louise Bourgeois, *Observations diverses sur la stérilité, perte de fruict, foecondité, accouchements et maladies des femmes et enfants nouveaux naiz*, Françoise Olive, ed. (Paris: Côté-Femmes, 1992; orig. 1652), unpaginated address to the Queen:

> Votre Majesté m'ayant vue, dès la première fois, sut par sa prudence juger l'affection que j'avais de vous faire un fidèle service, et que je n'avais la façon si téméraire de m'oser présenter devant elle, pour m'offrir de cueillir un si précieux fruit, que je n'en eusse l'industrie, sans l'endommager, ni la branche dont il sortirait.

4.   Bourgeois, *Récit véritable*, 64: 'je fis la reverence à la Reyne.'
5.   *Ibid.*, 58, Bourgeois noted 'c'est la principale piece de l'accouchement, que la sage-femme agrée à la femme qui accouche.'
6.   For recent publications on Bourgeois, see Philip A. Kalisch, Margaret Scobey, and Beatrice J. Kalisch, 'Louyse Bourgeois and the Emergence of Modern Midwifery,' *Journal of Nurse-Midwifery* 26, 4 (1981), 3–17, Evelyne Berriot-Salvadore, *Les femmes dans la société française de la renaissance* (Geneva: Droz, 1990), 257–66, Wendy Perkins, *Midwifery and Medicine in Early Modern France: Louise Bourgeois* (Exeter: University of Exeter Press, 1996), Colette H. Winn, 'De sage (-) femme à sage (-) fille: Louise Boursier, *Instructions à ma Fille* [1626],' *Papers on French Seventeenth-Century Literature* 24, 46 (1997), 61–83, François Rouget, 'De la sage-femme à la femme sage: réflexion et réflexivité dans les *Observations* de Louise Boursier,' *Papers on French Seventeenth-Century Literature* 25, 49 (1998), 483–96, and Bridgette Sheridan, 'At Birth: The Modern State, Modern Medicine, and the Royal Midwife Louise Bourgeois in Seventeenth-Century France,' *Dynamis* 19 (1999), 145–66.
7.   Bourgeois, *Observations diverses*, 175. For a discussion of the morals expounded in Bourgeois' letter to her daughter and the relationship of this text with contemporary pedagogical literature for women see Winn, 'De sage (-) femme à sage (-) fille,' 61–83.
8.   Bourgeois, *Observations diverses*, 178, 177.
9.   *Ibid.*, 177.
10.   *Ibid.*, 176.
11.   *Ibid.*, unpaginated preface in which Bourgeois stresses her desire to serve others.
12.   Hilary Marland, '"Stately and Dignified, Kindly and God-fearing": Midwives, Age and Status in the Netherlands in the Eighteenth Century,' Hilary Marland and Margaret Pelling, eds, *The Task of Healing: Medicine, Religion and Gender in England and the Netherlands 1450–1800* (Rotterdam: Erasmus Publishing, 1996), 277–8, and Doreen Evenden, *The Midwives of Seventeenth-Century London* (Cambridge: Cambridge University Press, 2000), 24–49.
13.   *Statuts et reiglemens ordonnez pour toutes les matronnes, ou saiges femmes de la ville, faulxbourgs, prevosté, et vicomté de Paris* (Paris, n.d.). The first royal edict for the entire realm was issued in 1692. For other midwifery regulations see *Statuts pour la communauté des maistres chirurgiens jurez de Paris* (Paris, 1699 and 1701). See also Jacques Gélis, *La sage-femme ou le médecin: une nouvelle conception de la vie* (Paris: Fayard, 1988), 40–55, Richard L. Petrelli, 'The Regulation of French Midwifery during

the *Ancien Régime,*' *Journal of the History of Medicine* 27 (1971), 276–92, and Matthew Ramsey, *Professional and Popular Medicine in France, 1770–1830* (Cambridge: Cambridge University Press, 1988), 23–4.

14. Gélis, *La sage-femme ou le médecin*, 47. In her discussion of the family–state compact, historian Sarah Hanley describes midwives as mediators, rather than servants, of the increasing state regulation of pregnancy and birth, collaborating with women to hide clandestine pregnancies, among other things. See her 'Engendering the State: Family Formation and State Building in Early Modern France,' *French Historical Studies* 16 (1989), 4–27.

15. Petrelli, 'The Regulation of French Midwifery during the *Ancien Régime,*' 287.

16. Laurence Brockliss and Colin Jones, *The Medical World of Early Modern France* (Oxford: Clarendon, 1997), 264–5.

17. Gélis, *La sage-femme ou le médecin*, 40–42. For some later Parisian decrees see *Statuts et reiglemens ordonnez pour toutes les Matronnes ou Saiges femmes de la ville* (n.l., 1587), *Arrêt de parlement portant nouveau réglement pour les apprentissages et réceptions des sages-femmes* (Paris, 1675), *Sentence du prevôt de Paris concernant les sages-femmes* (Paris, 1678), *Déclaration...portant défenses à ceux de la religion prétendüe réformée de faire les fonctions de sages-femmes* (Saint-Germain-en-Laye, 1680), and *Arrêt de la cour de parlement concernant la réception et prestation de serment des sages-femmes* (Paris, 1726).

18. *Sentence rendue par le lieutenant criminel contre plusieurs sages-femmes qui n'ont point prêté serment au Châtelet* (Paris, 1730).

19. Marcel Fosseyeux, 'Sages-femmes et nourrices à Paris au XVIIIe siècle,' *Revue de Paris* 19 (October 1921), 536.

20. Henriette Carrier, *Origines de la maternité de Paris. Les maîtresses sages-femmes et l'office des accouchées de l'ancien Hôtel Dieu (1378–1796)* (Paris: Steinheil, 1888), 76 and 81.

21. Helen King, *Hippocrates' Woman: Reading the Female Body in Ancient Greece* (London: Routledge, 1998), 175–6.

22. Soranus, *Gynecology*, Owsei Temkin, trans. and intro. (Baltimore: The Johns Hopkins University Press, 1956), 5.

23. *Ibid.*, 6.

24. Bourgeois, *Observations diverses*, 104.

25. *Ibid.*, 106–7. Bourgeois, 44, nevertheless reported that she had seen several dead women opened. For Bourgeois' call to education within the context of the *querelle des femmes* see Madeleine Lazard, *Images littéraires de la femme à la Renaissance* (Paris: Presses universitaires de France, 1985), 111.

26. *Arrêt de la cour du parlement rendu en faveur des jurées sages femmes en titre d'office et leurs aspirantes, contre les prévots gardes et communauté des maîtres chirurgiens de Saint Cosme et tous démonstrateurs anatomiques* (Paris, 1732).

27. *Mémoire signifié pour les prévots et communauté des chirurgiens-jurez à Saint-Côme de la ville de Paris, demandeurs, contre Louise Blanchon femme Jaunet et Lamare, jurées-sages-femmes en titre d'office au Châtelet de Paris, defenderesses* (Paris, 1737).

28. Baudoin, 'Lettre sur les accouchements,' Paul-Émile Le Maguet, ed., *Le monde médical parisien sous le Grand Roi, suivi du portefeuille de Vallant* (Paris: Maloine,

1899), 301–2:

> Elle avoit toutes les belles qualités qu'une sage-femme doit avoir, le jugement, l'esprit, la mémoire, la résolution et fermeté pour entreprendre de grandes opérations quand elles se présentoient. Elle parloit fort bien de sa profession, scavoit bien l'anatomie, particulièrement du bas ventre; je luy ay veu ouvrir plusieurs fois des femmes avec bien de l'adresse et nous faisoit des leçons parfaitement belles sur tout ce que nous luy demandions.

29. Carrier, *Origines de la maternité de Paris*, 74.
30. Marguerite de La Marche [du Tertre], *Instruction familière et très utile aux sages-femmes pour bien pratiquer les accouchemens* (Paris, 1710; orig. 1677), 1–2.
31. *Ibid.*, captions on plates that precede her text.
32. Soranus, *Gynecology*, 6.
33. Bourgeois, *Observations diverses*, 119: 'je dirai avec vérité en avoir porté un tourné six semaines, faisant tous les jours ma vacation.' Bourgeois, 42, also described the sensation of the child moving in the womb as the 'beating of the wing of a small bird,' claiming these movements were easy to judge for those who understood them.
34. *Ibid.*, 197.
35. *Ibid.*, 143.
36. Jane Sharp, *The Midwives Book* (London, 1671), 3.
37. Elizabeth Nihell, *A Treatise on the Art of Midwifery* (London, 1760), viii.
38. *Ibid.*, 36.
39. Sara F. Matthews Grieco, *Ange ou diablesse: La représentation de la femme au XVIe siècle* (Paris: Flammarion, 1991), 194.
40. Ian Maclean, *Woman Triumphant: Feminism in French Literature 1610–1652* (Oxford: Clarendon, 1977), 11, and 46–50. For more about the *querelle des femmes* see Joan Kelly, 'Early Feminist Theory and the *Querelle des Femmes*, 1400–1789,' *Signs* 8, 1 (1982), 4–28.
41. For the maternal messages in Bourgeois' letter to her daughter see Winn, 'De sage (-) femme à sage (-) fille,' 68–77.
42. Lynne Tatlock, 'Speculum Feminarum: Gendered Perspectives on Obstetrics and Gynecology in Early Modern Germany,' *Signs* 17, 4 (1992), 746.
43. Nina Rattner Gelbart, *The King's Midwife: A History and Mystery of Madame du Coudray* (Berkeley: University of California Press, 1998), 58.
44. For other accounts of how early modern women would reshape traditional roles to their social and political advantage see Sheila ffolliott, 'Catherine de' Medici as Artemesia: Figuring the Powerful Widow,' Margaret W. Ferguson, Maureen Quilligan, and Nancy J. Vickers, eds, *Rewriting the Renaissance: The Discourses of Sexual Difference in Early Modern Europe* (Chicago: University of Chicago Press, 1986), 227–41, and Elizabeth McCartney, 'The King's Mother and Royal Prerogative in Early-Sixteenth-Century France,' John Carmi Parsons, ed., *Medieval Queenship* (New York: St. Martin's Press, 1993), 117–41.
45. Lisa Silverman, *Tortured Subjects: Pain, Truth, and the Body in Early Modern France* (Chicago: University of Chicago Press, 2001), examines how the bodily experience of

pain and revelation of truth were linked in discussions of the efficacy of torture within legal proceedings. Her arguments shed light on early modern women's claims about the value of experiencing labour and delivery, as well as the state's insistence that women ask labouring women to name the fathers of their illegitimate children. In keeping with contemporary theories of torture, the belief was that while suffering the pains of childbirth, these women could no longer disguise the truth about paternity.

46. Jacques Guillemeau, *De l'heureux accouchement des femmes* (Paris, 1609), 151: 'Premierement elle doit estre de bon aage, ny trop jeune, ny trop vieille: bien composee de son corps, sans estre subjecte à aucunes maladies, ny contrefaicte en aucunes parties de son corps, propre en ses habits & en sa personne, ayant sur tout les mains petites & non grossieres, nettes, & les ongles rongnez de prez.' For similar descriptions of the ideal midwife, see Jacques Bury, *Le propagatif de l'homme* (Paris, 1623), 67–74, Cosme Viardel, *Observations sur la pratique des accouchemens naturels, contre nature & monstrueux* (Paris, 1671), 273–7, Denis Fournier, *L'accoucheur méthodique* (Paris, 1677), 61–5, Jean Bernier, *Histoire chronologique de la médecine, et des médecins* (Paris, 1695), 27–33, and Pierre Dionis, *Traité général des accouchemens* (Paris, 1718), 416–21.

47. Bury, *Le propagatif de l'homme*, 70.

48. Paul Portal, *La pratique des accouchemens* (Paris, 1685), 9.

49. Bury, *Le propagatif de l'homme*, 70.

50. *Ibid.*, 69.

51. Viardel, *Observations sur la pratique des accouchemens naturels, contre nature & monstrueux*, 275–6.

52. Dionis, *Traité général des accouchemens*, 417.

53. Philippe Peu, *La pratique des accouchemens* (Paris, 1694), 135: 'Ils les choisira, s'il est possible, doux, paisibles, silentieux, discrets, intelligens, forts, prompt a lui obéir, & agréables à la malade.' Bernier, *Histoire chronologique*, 31, argues that midwives should obey physicians.

54. Claude Maillard, *Le bon mariage, ou le moyen d'estre heureux et faire son salut en estat de mariage* (Douay, 1643), 289–300.

55. See Chapter 1, especially note 96.

56. Guillemeau, *De l'heureux accouchement des femmes*, 152–3.

57. Viardel, *Observations sur la pratique des accouchemens naturels, contre nature & monstrueux*, 276.

58. Dionis, *Traité général des accouchemens*, 417.

59. Male writers in other parts of Europe sometimes stressed the education of the female midwife. See, for example, Hendrik van Deventer, 'Of the Qualifications which are requir'd, to make a woman fit for the practice of midwifery,' *The Art of Midwifery Improv'd*, 3rd edn (London, 1728), 1–12.

60. See Chapter 1, especially notes 91–3.

61. See clause 11 of *Statuts et reiglemens ordonnez pour toutes les matronnes, ou saiges femmes de la ville, faulxbourgs, prevosté, et vicomté de Paris*.

62. Lisa Forman Cody, 'The Politics of Reproduction: From Midwives' Alternative Public Sphere to the Public Spectacle of Man-Midwifery,' *Eighteenth-Century Studies* 32, 4 (1999), 479–80.

63.   For a thorough account of women's purportedly 'dual nature' during the early modern period in France see Matthews Grieco, *Ange ou diablesse.*

64.   For King Henry II's edict of 1556 see Gélis, *La sage-femme ou le médecin*, 25.

65.   The physiognomical treatise by Marin Cureau de La Chambre, *The art how to know men*, John Davies, trans. (London, 1665), 26, features the negative traits that follow from women's cold, moist nature. She is distrustful, crafty, apt to dissemble, unfaithful, impatient, easily persuaded, and talkative. See also Jeannette Geffriaud Rosso, *Études sur la féminité aux XVIIe et XVIIe siècles* (Pisa: Libreria Goliardica, 1984).

66.   For example, Peu, *La pratique des accouchemens*, 402, explains that a judicious midwife would call for help when faced with an arm presentation. In contrast, 541–2, describes a female midwife reacting with great fear to a difficult birth, and 604 delineates the actions of ignorant midwives.

67.   For Thomas de Leu see Andrée Jouan, 'Thomas de Leu et le portrait français de la fin du XVIe siècle,' *Gazette des beaux-arts* 58 (1961), 203–22. For a history of the early modern title page see Robert Brun, *Le livre français* (Paris: Larousse, 1948), 65–6, and Lucien Febvre and Henri-Jean Martin, *The Coming of the Book*, David Gerard, trans. (London: Verso, 1976), 85–6.

68.   Roger Chartier, *The Order of Books: Readers, Authors, and Libraries in Europe between the Fourteenth and Eighteenth Centuries*, Lydia G. Cochrane, trans. (Stanford: Stanford University Press, 1994), 54.

69.   Linda C. Hults, *The Print in the Western World: An Introductory History* (Madison: University of Wisconsin Press, 1996), 283. For a discussion of the change from woodcut to engraved prints see Henri-Jean Martin, *Livre, pouvoirs et société à Paris au XVIIe siècle (1598–1701)*, vol. 1 (Geneva: Droz, 1969), 381–6.

70.   Though the 1609 edition of Bourgeois' book contained only her portrait, in later editions it followed a portrait of the Queen, seemingly based on an engraving made by de Leu in 1602 after a painting by François Quesnel. For a reproduction of the engraved portrait of Marie de Médicis see Bourgeois' *Récit véritable*, 54. The Queen strikes a posture similar to that of Bourgeois, but is adorned more elaborately. Brun, *Le livre français*, 78, claims that by the middle of the seventeenth century, it was common for treatises to be illustrated with portraits of the author as well as the patron. See also Ruth Mortimer, *A Portrait of the Author in Sixteenth-Century France* (Chapel Hill: University of North Carolina Press, 1980).

71.   Bourgeois, *Récit véritable*, 88–9.

72.   Georges Vigarello, 'The Upward Training of the Body from the Age of Chivalry to Courtly Civility,' Michel Feher, ed., *Zone: Fragments for a History of the Human Body*, vol. 2 (New York: Urzone, 1989), 149–99, and Herman Roodenburg 'How to Sit, Stand, and Walk: Toward a Historical Anthropology of Dutch Paintings and Prints,' Wayne Franits, ed., *Looking at Seventeenth-Century Dutch Art: Realism Reconsidered* (Cambridge: Cambridge University Press, 1997), 175–86.

73.   Ann Jensen Adams, 'The Three-Quarter Length Life-Sized Portrait in Seventeenth-Century Holland: The Cultural Functions of *Tranquillitas*,' Wayne Franits, ed., *Looking at Seventeenth-Century Dutch Art*, 158–74.

74.   Bourgeois, *Observations diverses*, 186.

75.   T H. Thomas, *French Portrait Engraving of the XVIIth and XVIIIth Centuries* (London: G. Bell, 1910), 57.

76.   Jouan, 'Thomas de Leu et le portrait français,' 218.

77.   Roger-Armand Weigert, *Inventaire du fonds français: graveurs du XVIIe siècle*, vol. 3 (Paris: Bibliothèque nationale, 1954), 188–9.

78.   The portrait of Moreno de Vargas is reproduced in Philip Hofer, *Baroque Book Illustration: A Short Survey from the Collection in the Department of Graphic Arts, Harvard College Library* (Cambridge, MA: Harvard University Press, 1951), plate 83.

79.   One portrait of surgeon man-midwife Paul Portal, engraved by Matthieu Lefebvre in 1688, includes the inscription 'Paul Portal Aagé de LVII ans,' but the different portrait appearing in Portal's treatise of 1685 does not mention his age, stressing instead his status as a master surgeon (see Chapter 4).

80.   See the chronology of Bourgeois' life in Rouget and Winn's edition of her *Récit véritable*, 49.

81.   Marland, '"Stately and Dignified, Kindly and God-fearing,"' 277. For the average age of German midwives see Mary Lindemann, *Health and Healing in Eighteenth-Century Germany* (Baltimore: The Johns Hopkins University Press, 1996), 206: 'Most midwives were older women, with an average age of about fifty-eight; the oldest was seventy, the youngest forty-two.' Merry Weisner, 'Early Modern Midwifery: A Case Study,' *International Journal of Women's Studies* 6, 1 (1983), 30, argues that the typical German midwife was a widow, or an older, unmarried woman.

82.   Bourgeois, *Récit véritable*, 58, indicates that the royal physicians looked for a midwife younger than Madame Dupuis, and, 66, claims the Queen stated 'Je veux une femme encor assés jeune, grande, et allegre.'

83.   For a popular and much reproduced manual of physiognomy see Charles Le Brun, *Conférence de M. Le Brun sur l'expression générale et particulière* (Paris, 1698), and Jennifer Montagu, *The Expression of the Passions: The Origin and Influence of Charles Le Brun's 'Conférence sur l'expression générale et particulière'* (New Haven: Yale University Press, 1994). According to Iain Pears, *The Discovery of Painting: The Growth of Interest in the Arts in England, 1680–1768* (New Haven: Yale University Press, 1988), 110–11, the observation of the human face and body linked the practices of medicine and art during the early modern period.

84.   Georges Vigarello, *Concepts of Cleanliness: Changing Attitudes in France since the Middle Ages*, Jean Birrell, trans. (Cambridge: Cambridge University Press, 1988), 78–89.

85.   Bourgeois, *Observations diverses*, 98–100.

86.   Peter Harrison, 'Reading the Passions: The Fall, the Passions, and Dominion Over Nature,' Stephen Gaukroger, ed., *The Soft Underbelly of Reason: The Passions in the Seventeenth Century* (London: Routledge, 1998), 49–78.

87.   For the 1602 portrait by de Leu see Jouan, 'Thomas de Leu et le portrait français,' 218. In the original engraving the Queen looks directly out at the viewer, though the image of the Queen eventually included in Bourgeois' treatise – perhaps another copy after de Leu by de Courbes – shows her looking to the left.

88.   The inscription beneath the portrait, which was very difficult to translate, reads:

En ce parfait tableau le defaut de peinture
Se congnoist aujourdhuy clairement a nos yeux
Pource qu'on n'y peut veoir que du corps la figure
Non l'esprit admiré pour chef d'oeuvre des cieux.

89.   Jouan, 'Thomas de Leu et le portrait français,' 206–15.

90.   W. McAllister Johnson, *French Royal Academy of Painting and Sculpture Engraved Reception Pieces: 1672–1798* (Kingston: Agnes Etherington Art Centre, Queen's University, 1982), 16.

91.   For a discussion of the *femme forte* or exceptional woman during the early modern period see Maclean, *Woman Triumphant*, 64–87, and Mary D. Sheriff, *The Exceptional Woman: Elisabeth Vigée-Lebrun and the Cultural Politics of Art* (Chicago: University of Chicago Press, 1996). See also Madeleine Lazard, 'Femmes, littérature, culture au XVIe siècle en France,' Danielle Haase-Dubosc and Eliane Viennot, eds, *Femmes et pouvoirs sous l'Ancien Régime* (Paris: Rivages, 1991), 101–19.

92.   Cited in Kelly, 'Early Feminist Theory and the *Querelle des Femmes, 1400–1789*,' 8.

93.   Bourgeois, *Récit véritable*, 78.

94.   *Ibid.*, 72.

95.   *Ibid.*, 78–82

96.   Madeleine Foisil, ed., *Journal de Jean Héroard*, vol. 1 (Paris: Fayard, 1989), 370–72. For another contemporary account of the birth that reinforces Bourgeois' narrative see Pierre Matthieu, *Histoire de France soubs les règnes de François I. Henry II. François II. Charles IX. Henry III. Henri IV*, vol. 2 (Paris, 1631), 442.

97.   Norman Bryson, 'The Legible Body: LeBrun,' *Word and Image: French Painting of the Ancien Régime* (Cambridge: Cambridge University Press, 1981), 41–2, Norbert Elias, *The Court Society*, Edmund Jephcott, trans. (Oxford: Blackwell, 1983), and Norbert Elias, *The Civilizing Process, I, The History of Manners*, Edmund Jephcott, trans. (New York: Urizen Books, 1978).

98.   Nicolas Faret, *L'honneste homme ou l'art de plaire à la court*, M. Magendie, ed. (Paris: Les presses universitaires de France, 1925), 68–9.

99.   Marin Cureau de La Chambre, *The art how to know men*, 11.

100. Maclean, *Woman Triumphant*, 55, notes that women could be mocked for writing. Winn, 'De sage (-) femme à sage (-) fille,' 68, argues that while women of quality were advised to dissimulate their knowledge and speak naturally about all things, Bourgeois encouraged her daughter to be ambitious.

101. Cureau de La Chambre, *The art how to know men*, 31.

102. For discussions of the political implications of the representation of women in Castiglione's influential advice book, *Cortegiano* (1527), for example, see Dain A. Trafton, 'Politics and the Praise of Women: Political Doctrine in the *Courtier*'s Third Book,' Robert W. Hanning and David Rosand, eds, *Castiglione: The Ideal and the Real in Renaissance Culture* (New Haven: Yale University Press, 1983), 29–44, and Carla Freccero, 'Politics and Aesthetics in Castiglione's *Il Cortegiano*: Book III and the Discourse on Women,' David Quint et al., eds, *Creative Imitation: New Essays on*

Renaissance Literature in Honor of Thomas M. Greene (Binghamton: Medieval and Renaissance Texts and Studies, 1992), 259–79.

103. Maclean, *Woman Triumphant*, 49.

104. Bourgeois, *Récit véritable*, 76.

105. Kalisch, Scobey and Kalisch, 'Louyse Bourgeois and the Emergence of Modern Midwifery,' 8–9.

106. Bourgeois, *Récit véritable*, 77. For another interpretation of this exchange see Caroline Bicks, *Midwiving Subjects in Shakespeare's England* (Aldershot: Ashgate, 2003), 1–5.

107. Natalie Zemon Davis, 'Women on Top: Symbolic Sexual Inversion and Political Disorder in Early Modern Europe,' Barbara A. Babcock, ed., *The Reversible World: Symbolic Inversion in Art and Society* (Ithaca: Cornell University Press, 1978), 147–90.

108. Bryson, 'The Legible Body: LeBrun,' 41.

109. Bourgeois, *Récit véritable*, 78.

110. Emmanuel Bury, 'Civiliser la "personne" ou instituer le "personnage"? Les deux versants de la politesse selon les théoriciens français du XVIIe siècle,' Alain Montandon, ed., *Etiquette et politesse* (Clermont-Ferrand: Association des publications de la Faculté des lettres et sciences humaines de Clermont-Ferrand, 1992), 127–8.

111. Guillemeau, *De l'heureux accouchement des femmes*, 153.

112. Bryson, 'The Legible Body: LeBrun,' 40.

113. Eustache de Refuge, *The accomplish'd courtier*, H. W. Gent, trans. (London, 1660), 7–10. See also Cureau de La Chambre, 'That the figure of the parts denotes the inclinations,' *The art how to know men*, 23–4.

114. De Refuge, *The accomplish'd courtier*, 39–41, and Cureau de La Chambre, *The art how to know men*, unpaginated preface, claims that physiognomy 'teaches the way to discover secret designs, private actions, and the unknown Authors of known actions.'

115. Harry Berger, Jr., *Fictions of the Pose: Rembrandt Against the Italian Renaissance* (Stanford: Stanford University Press, 2000), 137–52. For another account of the paradoxical nature of physiognomy see Jean-Jacques Courtine and Claudine Haroche, *Histoire du visage: exprimer et taire ses émotions XVIe–début XIXe siècle* (Paris: Rivages, 1988).

116. Marland, '"Stately and Dignified, Kindly and God-fearing,"' 273, notes that masculine qualities were often desired in early modern midwives, including Dutch midwife Catharina Schrader who combined the roles of midwife and man-midwife in one person.

Chapter 4

Looking the Part:
Men-midwives on Display

How could the male midwife put his best face forward in the lying-in chamber? François Mauriceau pondered this question in his obstetrical treatise of 1668, *Des maladies des femmes grosses et accouchées*, noting:

> There are some who say that a surgeon who wishes to practice midwifery ought...to be slovenly, or at least very careless, growing a long dirty beard, so as not to afford any occasion for jealousy to the husbands of the women who send for him to help them.[1]

In the end, however, the French practitioner disapproved of the dishevelled surgeon, claiming he would only look like a butcher. He argued that men-midwives should display an agreeable appearance, being healthy, strong, robust, and sober in order to avoid frightening those 'poor women' who required surgical intervention in childbirth.[2] Mauriceau was clearly more concerned with appealing to women than reassuring their husbands. At the same time, his discussion reveals the anomalous requirement of the male midwife to look dependable to his clients without evoking a sense of seductive allure in the female realm of the birthing room.

By considering the surgeon man-midwife's beard, Mauriceau raised the thorny issue of the appropriate display of masculinity in the lying-in chamber. The beard was, after all, a potent male signifier. A long tradition linked it with virility, from Augustine of Hippo who argued that a beard was a proper manly adornment, to the sixteenth-century physiognomist Jean Indagine, who remarked on the manliness of bearded women.[3] While hirsute women transgressed the laws of sexual difference by infringing on a male prerogative, men who lacked beards could find their virility in question. Part of the evidence in an impotence trial brought before the High Court of Paris in 1687 was that the accused man had only one testicle and no beard.[4] This penultimate sign of male sexuality was not necessarily welcomed, however, in the intimate realm of the birthing room, where women's chastity could be at stake and female midwives were the traditional assistants.[5] According to Mauriceau, some people advised the *chirurgien accoucheur* to cultivate masculinity in excess, growing a lengthy beard that would present him disguised as an elderly, unhygienic man. But Mauriceau favoured a clean-shaven, gentle male midwife able to comfort his female clients. He described a surgeon man-midwife who adapted to the feminine nature of his occupation by assuming womanly qualities.

Mauriceau's comments on the appropriate appearance of the male birthing assistant participated in a broader debate about the gendered identity of men-midwives in early modern Europe. The frontispiece of John Blunt's English treatise, *Man-Midwifery Dissected*, published in 1793, is among the most famous representations of how male midwives could challenge gendered categories. Entitled 'A Man-Mid-Wife,' the hand-coloured etching shows a figure sharply divided in half; on one side a young *accoucheur* in trousers is surrounded by the tools of his trade, while on the other an attractive female midwife attired in a long skirt is associated with a domestic setting (Figure 4.1). According to Ludmilla Jordanova, Blunt 'elaborates the idea that a man-midwife is and ought to be a contradiction in terms, an inappropriate, unnatural mixture of incompatible elements.'[6] The depiction of the man-midwife as a monster, neither man nor woman, but something in between, recurred well into the eighteenth century. Whereas female midwives were authorized to assist at births by their personal experiences of maternity as well as their ability to protect feminine modesty, men-midwives were affiliated with both sexual impropriety and danger. Yet male practitioners slowly produced a more positive image of themselves, and were increasingly called to serve wealthy, urban clients.[7]

In this chapter, I consider various arguments about the physical presentation of the French surgeon man-midwife, including what he should look like and how he should behave. This attention to the bodily display of *chirurgiens accoucheurs* extends my discussion of female midwives in the previous chapter. There I drew on descriptions of the ideal female midwife, considering how the relationship between her body and obstetrical abilities was represented. Here I analyse corresponding accounts of the ideal man-midwife. Although there are fewer written delineations of the model male midwife in obstetrical treatises, when they do appear they are usually positioned before or after discussions of the qualities desirable in a female midwife, inviting comparison. For the most part, the characteristics demanded in a female midwife were also those required of a male practitioner. His physical composition was described similarly; he was urged to dress modestly, have small, slender hands with short, rounded nails, and be of an age that would suggest accumulated experience without compromising bodily strength. According to these accounts, the consummate man-midwife would be like the ideal female midwife, but would surpass her in knowledge, skill, and status.

In addition to written descriptions, I examine visual articulations of the ideal man-midwife. Engraved author portraits regularly appear as the first plate in French obstetrical treatises, either prior to, or as part of, the official title page; I have been able to discover nine of these which date from the seventeenth and early eighteenth centuries. In contrast to the singular author portrait of royal midwife Louise

Bourgeois, this number is substantial. I contend that images of surgeon men-midwives constitute a form of strategic display in keeping with the wider goals of obstetrical treatises to present their authors as cultivated, skilled, and vastly experienced experts in childbirth. The portraits invite readers of obstetrical treatises to evaluate the appearance of male midwives, considering visual evidence that could influence their assessment of the men's written statements.

Jordanova argues that portraiture contributed to the construction of the identities of early modern British medical practitioners. There are relatively few author portraits of men-midwives in British treatises, and she analyses painted portraits such as Allan Ramsay's depiction of Scottish-born William Hunter, from around 1764, noting it precludes any suggestion of the sitter's contentious practice of midwifery.[8] In contrast, French obstetrical frontispieces became both increasingly prominent and more visually elaborate during the seventeenth century. A relatively early example inaugurates the treatise written by Jacques Duval in 1612, entitled *Traité des hermaphrodits, parties génitales, accouchemens des femmes* (Figure 4.2). The verse beneath the small bust of the author praises the 'rare Apollo' for his learned account of hermaphrodites. By 1671, the half-length portrait of Cosme Viardel dominates the frontispiece of his obstetrical treatise and depicts him touching a child, directly referring to his hands-on practice of midwifery (Figure 4.3). All the same, no straightforward story of chronological development can be told about these engravings. My interpretations of various French author portraits will refer to a number of different visual strategies. This diversity should not be surprising during a period when the *chirurgien accoucheur* lacked a stable professional identity. We will see that some images of surgeon men-midwives associate male practitioners with theoretical knowledge, while others relate them more directly with traditional maternal qualities. Almost all of the portraits, however, exhibit a desire to resignify the hands of the obstetrical surgeon, and to downplay his use of dangerous instruments.

Attention to the physical presentation and behaviour of practitioners was not exclusive to the lying-in chamber. Mary Lindemann argues that eighteenth-century German doctors received posts based on considerations of their personality and life-style as well as competence.[9] Nevertheless, such issues were especially crucial to men-midwives, given the controversial status of their occupation. To an even greater degree than other medical practitioners, men-midwives had to appeal to clients, principally women. They could not simply march into the lying-in chamber, brandishing instruments. According to Adrian Wilson, the man-midwife Hunter understood very well the need to attract clients. In the 1760s, he advised young male students that 'it is not the mere safe delivery of the woman will recommend an accoucheur, but a sagacious, well-conducted behaviour of tenderness, assiduity, and delicacy.'[10] In their obstetrical treatises, French *chirurgiens accoucheurs* likewise described the ideal male practitioner as having an agreeable manner and appearance,

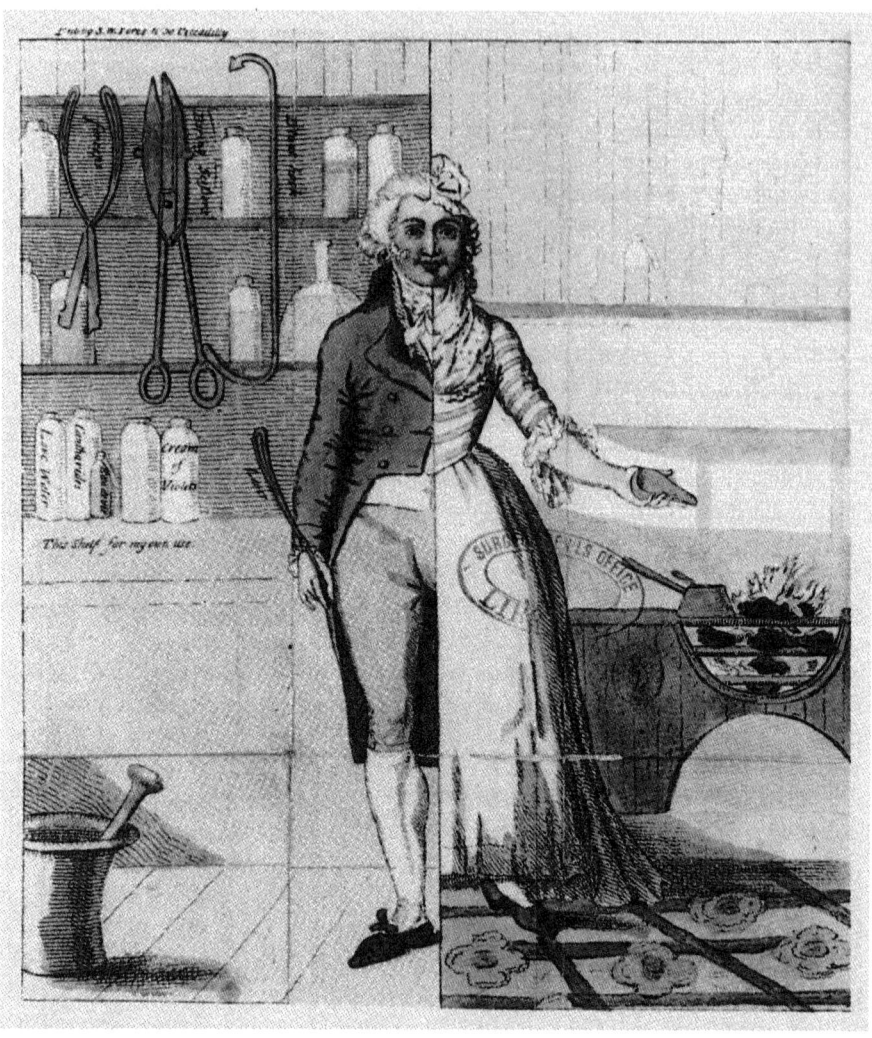

Figure 4.1   **A Man-Mid-Wife, from John Blunt's [Samuel Fores'] *Man-Midwifery Dissected*, 1793, London. Courtesy of the National Library of Medicine, Bethesda, MD**

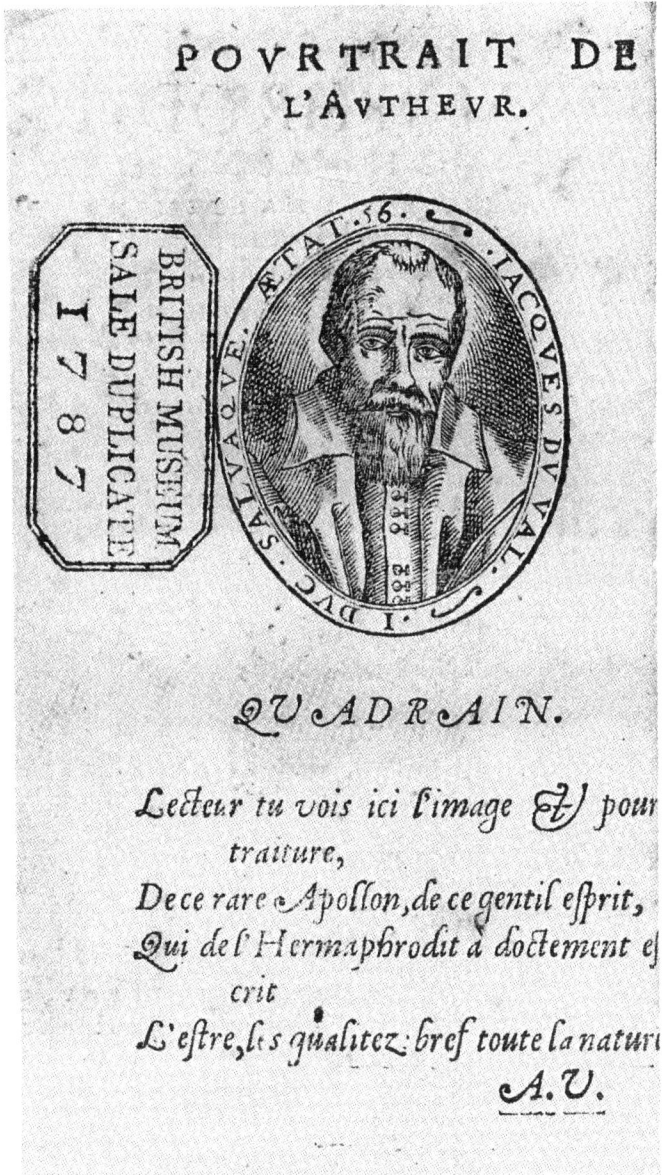

Figure 4.2   Author portrait, from Jacques Duval's *Traité des hermaphrodits, parties génitales, accouchemens des femmes*, 1612, Paris. Courtesy of the National Library of Medicine, Bethesda, MD

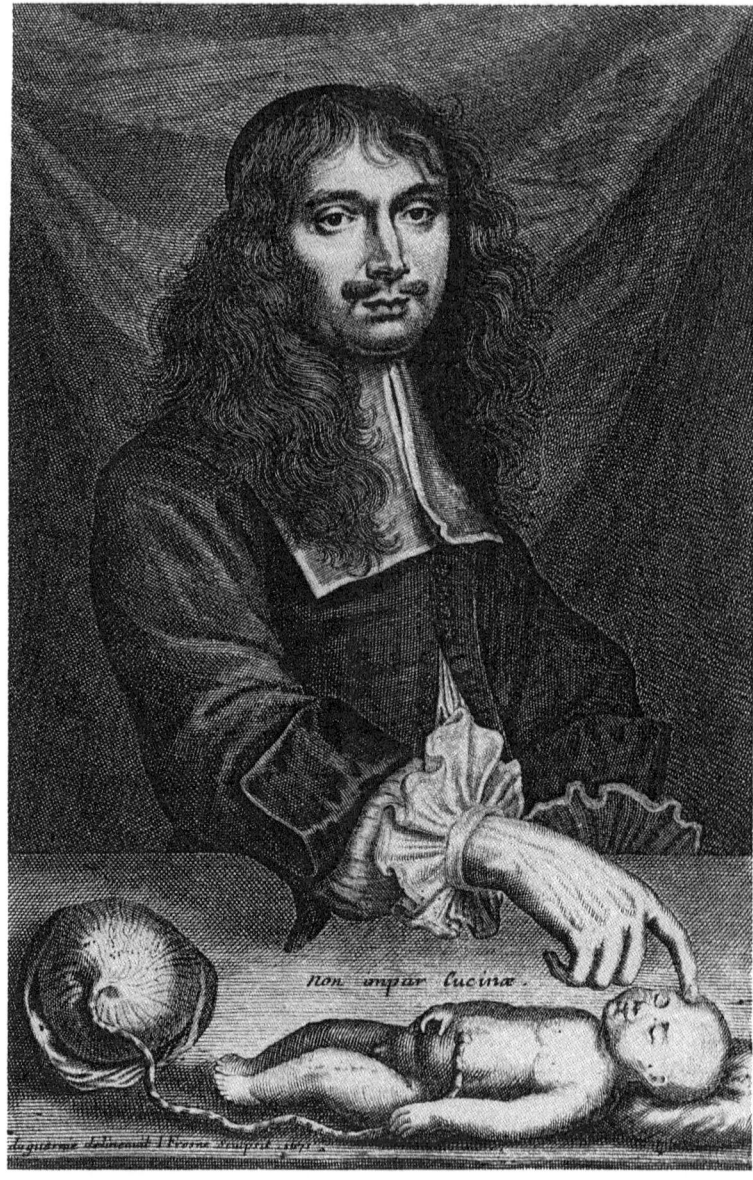

Figure 4.3   Author portrait, from Cosme Viardel's *Observations sur la pratique des accouchemens naturels, contre nature & monstrueux*, 1671, Paris. Courtesy of the National Library of Medicine, Bethesda, MD

free of any bodily defect that might cause the repugnance of female clients.[11] Their accounts lend support to arguments that women both scrutinized and appraised male birthing assistants, participating in their selection.[12]

Of course, depictions of the ideal practitioner do not necessarily correspond with what transpired in early modern French birthing chambers. The ephemeral performance of social graces – making polite conversation, lending a sympathetic ear, or having the proper dress and bodily comportment – is notoriously difficult to trace historically. Representations of the surgeon man-midwife nonetheless reveal the complex arguments made about him. Like the portrait of Bourgeois, written and visual descriptions of the ideal man-midwife portray a hybrid creature who challenges gendered boundaries. This image is not entirely at odds with the amalgamated figure pictured by Blunt. The ideal male birthing assistant delineated in French obstetrical treatises also fluctuates between masculine and feminine characteristics. In contrast to Blunt, however, the objective of French surgeon men-midwives was to garner respect for, rather than ridicule of, their occupation.

Writing the Man-midwife

If early modern descriptions of the ideal female midwife were ultimately inspired by the ancient precedent of Soranus, was there a similar model for the male midwife? The answer is two-fold. On one hand, there was no longstanding account of the exemplary man-midwife which outlined his appropriate age, bodily comportment, and behaviour. On the other hand, there was an antecedent – the same one informing early modern delineations of the female midwife. In fact, discussions of the ideal surgeon man-midwife in early modern France echo Soranus' text with more accuracy than do concurrent descriptions of the female midwife. Like Soranus' female birthing assistant, the accomplished surgeon man-midwife was expected to be intelligent, robust, experienced, and learned in several branches of medicine.[13] In contrast, outlines of the qualities desired in the female practitioner – especially those written by male surgeons – often paid little attention to her intellect, emphasizing bodily strength as opposed to theoretical training.[14] Obstetrical treatises produced by *chirurgiens accoucheurs* implied that by the seventeenth and early eighteenth centuries, Soranus' vision of the well-rounded female midwife could be realized only by male surgeons such as themselves.

In keeping with descriptions of the exemplary female midwife, surgeon men-midwives including Mauriceau, Viardel, and Pierre Dionis advised male colleagues to dress modestly – *sans fanfaron* [without boastfulness] – and be equipped with well-formed bodies able to withstand lengthy labours.[15] The surgeon man-midwife's bodily fortitude was related to his age: like the female midwife, he should be old enough to have acquired the requisite experience but young enough to retain strength. Authors often expressed doubts about the abilities of unseasoned and immature *chirurgiens accoucheurs*.[16] The physical characteristic receiving the most attention from male authors was, however, the hand of the male practitioner. According to Dionis in 1718 'a large, short hand is an essential defect in an accoucheur.'[17] While both male and female practitioners were ideally blessed with small, slender hands, they were deemed especially crucial to men. Mauriceau specified that the surgeon man-midwife's hand should be equipped with a long index finger able to touch the 'internal orifice' [cervix], and Viardel insisted that male practitioners be ambidextrous.[18] Guillaume Mauquest de La Motte was unique in disagreeing with the amount of attention given to the hand of the male practitioner. In the English translation of his 1721 treatise, he asserted: 'as for the smallness of the hand and length of the fingers, I am far from looking on them as necessary, having been intimately acquainted with the late Mr. Mingot, of the city of Caen, who was an excellent artist, notwithstanding his large thick hand.'[19]

Not only were surgeon men-midwives advised to have bodily qualities similar to those of the ideal female midwife, they were expected to behave in much the same way. Like the female birthing assistant, men working in the lying-in chamber were urged to be virtuous, prudent, honest, compassionate, modest, patient, charitable, religious, and able to keep secrets.[20] Many of these characteristics were typically associated with femininity, especially modesty, patience, and charity; indeed the latter attribute was often conflated with maternity itself.[21] Given the sensitive nature of their practices, a delicate demeanour was deemed indispensable to male midwives. Dionis explicitly recognized the unique position of the surgeon man-midwife, insisting he had to display politeness far exceeding that of the army or hospital surgeon.[22] Viardel similarly stressed the surgeon man-midwife's sensitivity, asserting he 'should be gentle in his words and agreeable in his conversation in order to cheer the sick woman.'[23] These French authors were not alone in claiming that male practitioners should demonstrate feminine qualities in the lying-in chamber. In his treatise originally published in 1701, Dutch man-midwife Hendrik van Deventer affirmed that like female midwives, male practitioners should be adorned with chastity, bashfulness, and modesty.[24]

Despite being described similarly, the behaviour of surgeon men-midwives was deemed more significant than that of female practitioners. After briefly outlining the demeanour of the ideal female midwife, Viardel expounded at greater length on that of the male midwife, claiming he was obligated to do so because life or death often rested on the surgeon's behaviour.[25] The English physician and man-midwife John Maubray also gave voice to the idea that more was demanded of the male midwife. In his treatise of 1724, he wrote that the man-midwife had to be especially compassionate toward his female client: 'He ought to *handle* her *decently*, and treat her *gently*; considering Her as the *weaker Vessel*, whose elegant tender Body, will admit of no *rough Usage*.'[26] While Maubray invoked the trope of the weaker vessel to support the man-midwife's indulgent treatment of female clients, Dionis highlighted the feminine weaknesses of female midwives. In his obstetrical treatise, the surgeon man-midwife adopted an approach at odds with that of Viardel by outlining the qualities desired in male practitioners before turning to a consideration of the ideal female midwife. The author argued that female practitioners should have all the positive characteristics demanded of the surgeon man-midwife, but needed to rid themselves of several defaults attached to their sex, including a propensity to gossip and to imagine themselves more knowledgeable than they really were.[27] With this statement, Dionis implied that good behaviour came more easily to male midwives; their masculine natures made it easier for them to display feminine qualities including compassion and charity while avoiding the negative aspects of femininity, such as indiscretion, vanity, and presumptuousness.

Even those male authors who did not delineate the appropriate physical and moral qualities of the ideal *chirurgien accoucheur* offered themselves as models of the behaviour required in the lying-in chamber. Their instruction often took the form of case studies, which included details about how the surgeon man-midwife in question had interacted with those gathered in the birthing room. In his obstetrical treatise of 1694, Peu, for example, described his ability to remain calm and collected when assisting at difficult deliveries. In one case, he was taking a brief rest after struggling to remove a child whose belly and arms presented first, when a servant suddenly pulled on the small body, causing its head to detach and remain in the womb. According to Peu, he 'dissimulated [his] distress to avoid frightening anyone,' before going to work with his *crochet* and employing a *lavement*, which finally expelled the severed head.[28] Dionis similarly argued that a surgeon man-midwife should not display a long, sad face, as if to announce some misfortune, while Mauquest de La Motte urged his colleagues to maintain a steady countenance in the lying-in chamber.[29] The surgeon man-midwife from Valognes provided examples of how he had concealed his own fear in dire circumstances, noting he had seen younger surgeons flee from a client's bedside after being overcome with fear.[30] These authors insisted that the surgeon man-midwife maintain an impassive facade during deliveries, echoing Bourgeois' account of her controlled behaviour at the birth of the *Dauphin* in 1601.[31] At the same time, male midwives suggested that the character of the surgeon called to intervene in difficult deliveries was as important as, or perhaps even more important than, his medical knowledge.

Theoretical learning was not overlooked in accounts of the ideal surgeon man-midwife. In his treatise of 1623, Jacques Bury argued that the *chirurgien accoucheur* required an understanding of anatomy in order to recognize the good or bad conformation of the parts of the human body.[32] Mauquest de La Motte excluded anatomical information from his treatise, contending that surgeons planning to undertake midwifery should already possess a thorough understanding of women's genital parts.[33] Such explicit references to surgical expertise and anatomical knowledge did not usually appear in concurrent accounts of the female midwife – at least not in those written by men. Bourgeois certainly insisted that female midwives needed to be educated in anatomy.[34] In contrast, male authors argued that surgeon men-midwives' medical knowledge distinguished them from female midwives. Viardel emphasized this point, claiming that male practitioners merited more than the name 'wise' accorded to women.[35] Without offering a more appropriate appellation, Viardel implied the man-midwife was not simply the equal of the female midwife, but her superior.

Accounts of the ideal male midwife furthermore suggested he was superior to other kinds of medical men. Despite emphasizing the necessity of the man-midwife's surgical training, several authors made it clear that not just any surgeon could operate in the lying-in chamber. According to Mauriceau, man-midwifery was the most difficult branch of surgery, requiring specialized knowledge as well as an indefatigable constitution.[36] Dionis pointed out that traditional surgical training would not suffice because women's modesty prevented apprentices from accompanying master surgeons into the birthing room. He encouraged the aspiring surgeon man-midwife to make extra efforts to acquire practice in midwifery, perhaps by working in the public lying-in ward at the Hôtel-Dieu in Paris.[37] By admitting it was difficult for men-midwives to accumulate hands-on experience at deliveries, Dionis acknowledged the longstanding criticism that male practitioners lacked an extensive personal experience of childbirth.[38] His confession, however, simultaneously portrayed man-midwifery as an especially challenging form of surgery, requiring the ability to overcome women's resistance as well as the need for extensive training.

This emphasis on expertise portrayed man-midwifery as both a distinctive and legitimate part of surgery. Dionis was most specific on this issue, stipulating that men-midwives had to be members of the company of master surgeons in their village. The author claimed such membership would not only ensure men-midwives were learned in surgery, but also that they had the right to attend deliveries, 'this operation being the domain of surgery.'[39] Dionis thus reinforced the corporate nature of early modern French medicine, which separated healers into guilds simultaneously defining and defending the boundaries of authorized practice. Himself a member of Saint-Côme, the Parisian community of surgeons, Dionis was clearly concerned with excluding outsiders or 'charlatans' from the lying-in chamber.[40] Charlatans were resented by syndicated practitioners because they ignored distinctions between medical practices, treating the entire human body, both inside and out. Such healers were denounced during the early modern period primarily because they disrupted the professionalization of medicine and competed with local practitioners; little inquiry was made into whether or not their treatments actually worked.[41] Dionis' focus on the incorporated status of men-midwives demanded that even well-trained practitioners be prohibited from performing manual operations in the lying-in chamber if they lacked the appropriate corporate identity.

His claims did more, however, than distinguish between male practitioners. They also excluded female midwives from intervening in those difficult deliveries, such as malpresentations, which Dionis and other male authors identified as specifically surgical in nature.[42] Although guilds had traditionally admitted both female surgeons and barber-surgeons, they gradually came to exclude them. After 1484 all women in France except the widows of surgeons and barbers were banned from practising surgery.[43] Though female midwives were licensed by the surgical guild in Paris, they were never full members of it. Dionis' insistence on guild membership consequently placed female midwives beneath surgeons in the medical hierarchy, reinforcing a situation already encoded in the official midwifery statutes.[44]

Overall, written accounts of the ideal surgeon man-midwife present an impressive figure. Undertaking interventions more challenging than other kinds of surgery, he pleased female clients, while eclipsing female midwives in terms of both intellect and status. Yet male authors did not simply differentiate the surgeon man-midwife from the female midwife. Despite criticizing female midwives, their descriptions of the ideal man-midwife reshaped accounts of the exemplary female midwife to associate feminine qualities with male bodies. According to male authors, the consummate surgeon man-midwife embodied all the positive qualities of the traditional female midwife, while avoiding the negative ones. Such claims can be related to the controversial status of male midwifery during the early modern period. They countered accusations that men made unprecedented incursions into the lying-in chamber, offending women. Male authors claimed to comfort and care for labouring women, portraying their practice as an extension of traditional maternal values. At the same time, the ambivalent situation of the male practitioner remains apparent in the written accounts. For even as the ideal surgeon man-midwife was advised to overcompensate for his male body, being especially polite and deliberately unthreatening, he was also urged to project a distinctively masculine professional identity.

Picturing the Man-midwife

Although written accounts of the ideal male practitioner describe his dress and bodily comportment, they provide few details. In contrast, portraits of surgeon men-midwives are richly embellished documents contributing to arguments about his identity. The elaborate frontispiece author portrait of Mauriceau, for example, displays the notably clean-shaven and well-dressed surgeon enclosed within an oval frame and surrounded by allegorical figures (Figure 4.4). Records of the commissioning of this portrait have apparently not survived, but the image was

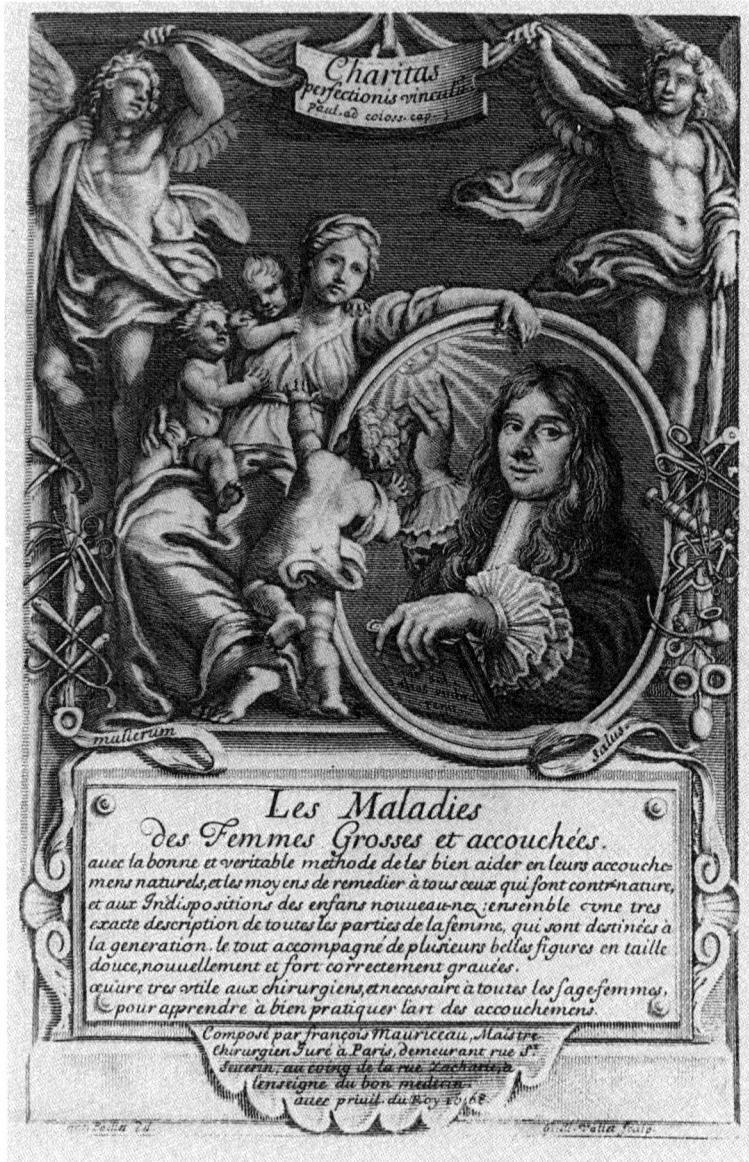

Figure 4.4   Author portrait, from François Mauriceau's *Des maladies des femmes grosses et accouchées*, 1668, Paris. Courtesy of the National Library of Medicine, Bethesda, MD

designed by artist Antoine Paillet and engraved by Guillaume Vallet, both members of the Académie royale de peinture et de sculpture, an artistic organization founded in Paris by royal decree in 1648.[45] By 1664 Paillet was a professor in the institution, an elevated post that recognized his artistic abilities, conferring additional prestige on his portrait of Mauriceau.[46] Producing the frontispiece in the Mannerist style for which he was known, Paillet created a complex composition that features a shallow, theatrical space containing multiple figures. To the left of the frame surrounding the surgeon, three children cling to a seated female figure dressed in a long robe. The upper edges of the engraving are demarcated by two winged and scantily clad male figures who reach upward to support a banner. Reading *Charitas perfectionis vinculum*, a quotation from Paul, Colossians, chapter 3, verse 14 – 'and above all these things, put on charity, which is the bond of perfection' – the religious ensign bestows a sense of overarching integrity to the image, binding the figures within a larger framework and counterbalancing the lengthy text inscribed below.

Writing is an important aspect of the intricate frontispiece. In fact, the image of Mauriceau is identified more closely with writing – considered an elevated, intellectual activity in early modern Europe – than with his practice as a surgeon man-midwife. His most important attribute is the book that he inclines toward the viewer. This bound volume bears an inscription reading *me sol, alios umbra regit* [me the sun rules, but others the shade]. The inscription not only proclaims Mauriceau's superior enlightenment but does so in Latin, the scholarly language primarily associated with university-educated physicians. At the same time, the oval portrait of the surgeon rests directly on a solid rectangular plinth covered in script announcing the long-winded title of Mauriceau's French treatise. This compositional arrangement implies that the reputation of the surgeon is firmly founded on his own text.

The portrait's emphasis on writing is in some ways at odds with the content of the treatise, which focuses on the surgeon man-midwife's manual interventions at difficult deliveries in addition to his theoretical education. The author portrait does not, however, simply efface all signs of the surgeon's manual activities. Although one of Mauriceau's hands touches a book, the other both reaches toward the sun and is positioned beside the head of a child that overlaps the oval frame around his image. This gesture, which could almost be read as a form of blessing, seems to invoke Mauriceau's delivery of children, displaying how he literally 'brings them into the light.'[47] It alludes to the hands-on, practical experience that allowed Mauriceau to write authoritatively about childbirth in the first place. As if echoing the surgeon's motion, the child reaches toward the seated female figure. She represents Charity, a traditional allegory of maternity often identified with female midwives.[48] The child acts to link the maternal realm with the masculine, theoretical domain of the surgeon.

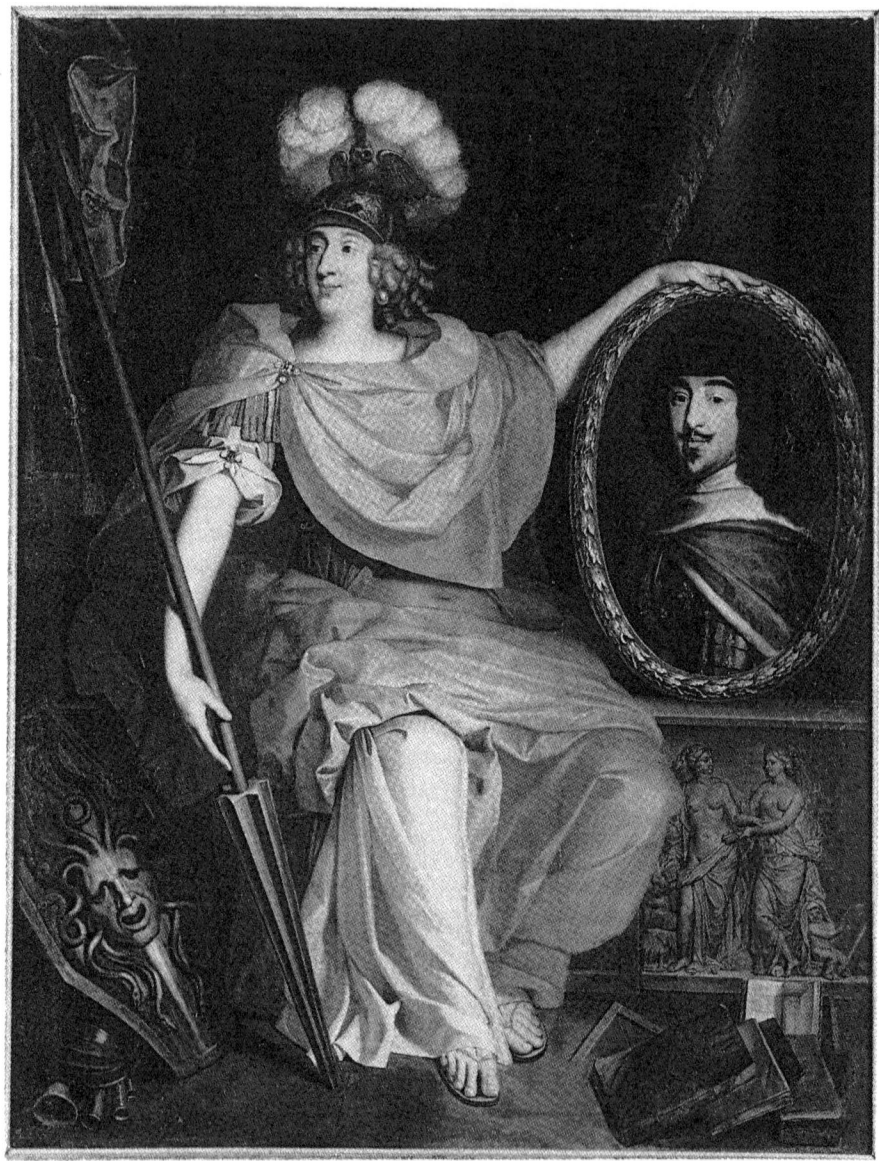

Figure 4.5   Pierre Bourguinon, *La Grande Mademoiselle*, 1671, Châteaux de
Versailles et de Trianon, Paris. Photo: Réunion des musées nationaux –
Gérard Blot

The composition of this frontispiece can be compared with that of the portrait of the Duchess of Montpensier, the wealthy cousin of Louis XIV, painted by Pierre Bourguignon in 1671[49] (Figure 4.5). Depicted allegorically as Minerva, La Grande Mademoiselle rests her delicate hand on an oval image of her father, Gaston d'Orléans. Although the noblewoman's identity is produced in relation to her father, who is portrayed as simultaneously present and absent, the patriarch is also potentially reduced to one of her ornamental attributes. Despite the similar configuration, however, the image of Mauriceau is not dwarfed by the maternal figure of Charity, but rather given prominence that draws the viewer's attention. Even so, his efforts do not trespass into the maternal sphere. The ponderous female body of Charity still bears most of the burden of child care, while the surgeon's eyes are discreetly directed away from her. Reference to the fleshliness of maternity needs, for reasons of professional status as well as sexual propriety, to be detached from the official identity of the surgeon.

Instead of looking at either the figure of Charity or the viewer, the surgeon gazes left, toward the instruments that simultaneously act as an ornamental border and intrude into his space. The surgical tools, including a syringe, a speculum, and several pessaries, are therefore given a certain importance. These tools provide another indication of Mauriceau's manual activities, but the surgeon man-midwife is shown with his back turned to the instruments, as if to deny a relationship with them. His most intimate attribute is the book he clutches; he does not actually touch a surgical tool. This rather ambivalent representation of surgical instruments can be related to the dubious reputation of men-midwives during the early modern period. Because surgeon men-midwives were initially identified with death and likened to butchers, it is not surprising that the instruments in Mauriceau's author portrait are portrayed as unthreatening decorative elements; they are acknowledged as signs of surgical expertise and yet distanced from the representation of the surgeon man-midwife.

The author portrait of Mauriceau displays even as it attempts to reconcile the fragmented identity and contested position of the *chirurgien accoucheur* in early modern France. The surgeon is shown rather literally in between the realms of maternity (on the left) and surgery (on the right). Like the instruments, the figure of Charity could also be considered an ornamental frame for the surgeon. Yet she is not as marginalized as the tools. The allegory of maternity occupies a significant amount of the visual plane, appearing to advocate his intervention in childbirth. Mauriceau points to the sun as the 'divine' source of knowledge that allows him to assist at deliveries, while the figure of Charity is inclined toward him. This circuit of gestures can be read as an argument for a beneficial exchange between the two gendered spheres, suggesting that male medical expertise keeps women and children safe and sound. At the same time, the muse of maternity is shown both to prop up and support herself on the image of Mauriceau. The frontispiece thereby represents interlocking masculine and feminine domains, each of which would collapse without the other. The rather precarious position of Mauriceau as a man-midwife is emphasized by the organizational structure of the engraving. In terms of composition, it looks as if the elements of the image have been selected from other works and pieced together to form a pastiche. This effect should not simply be attributed, however, to the working methods of the artist or his Mannerist tendencies. It can also be related to the fragmentation of Mauriceau's identity, as an intellectual man who touched women's bodies, and a dexterous surgeon who wrote books. The author portrait is divided up into various zones of signification, with the textual elements carefully delimited from the visual ones, and the representation of the surgeon separated from the maternal figure. Overall, the emphasis is on boundaries and the legitimate crossing of those boundaries. The rigid frame around the surgeon is traversed by both the unruly child and various surgical instruments. The female figure is depicted as approving of these border crossings; her own hand enters into the masculine sphere in order to guide the viewer's eye to him. This complex image could appeal to an equally fragmented audience, made up of men and women alike. Readers of both sexes could find points of identification, appreciating the traditional image of maternity, the framed picture of the surgeon, or the way in which the two representations have been combined to portray the uneasy position of the surgeon man-midwife.

While the elaborate portrait of Mauriceau represents a restrained surgeon blessed with intellectualized hands, the manual skills of the *chirurgien accoucheur* are foregrounded in the image that inaugurates Viardel's obstetrical treatise, *Observations sur la pratique des accouchemens naturels, contre nature & monstrueux*, first published in 1671 (Figure 4.3). Viardel was a royal surgeon to French Queen María Teresa, and not a member of Saint-Côme, the Parisian corporation of surgeons. Shown before a theatrical backdrop, the pose of the surgeon's left elbow is conventionally linked with self-confidence, and his dark coat alludes to intellectual learning.[50] Like Mauriceau's portrait, the image of Viardel was created by two members of the Académie royale, though they were less well-known. Pierre du Guernier, a miniaturist as well as portraitist, produced the design, while Jean Frosne engraved it.[51] The composition contains only two figures and is simpler than that of Mauriceau's frontispiece, but is more complex than the head and shoulders busts featured in the earlier author portraits of both Bourgeois and Duval.

In keeping with the image of Mauriceau, Viardel's portrait emphasizes the surgeon man-midwife's well-groomed appearance. It contains, however, fewer references to writing. For the most part, the authority of Viardel is displayed by his didactic gesture. Instead of indicating a book, the surgeon man-midwife points to the child arranged on a table before him. Although the child appears to be dead, it is whole, undamaged, and accompanied by an intact afterbirth. Viardel has managed, the portrait suggests, both to remove the infant from its mother's womb and to guarantee its eternal repose. The manual dexterity of Viardel is indicated by his gentle caress of its head. His long slender index figure corresponds with various written accounts of the ideal physical qualities of the man-midwife. At the same time, the gesture it performs, called the *dissidentiam noto* by John Bulwer in his seventeenth-century catalogue of the 'natural language of the hand,' traditionally conveyed the satisfaction of intellectual curiosity through the sense of touch.[52] An insistence upon the primacy of touch recurs throughout Viardel's treatise in both its written text and images. Numerous engravings depict the detached hand of the *chirurgien accoucheur* digitally examining the position of the infant in the womb. These fascinating images – discussed in Chapter 6 – reinforce Viardel's criticism of the potentially damaging *crochets* used to pull a dead child from the womb in pieces; he argued that the surgeon should use his hands alone to assist at deliveries.[53]

Although the pose of Viardel relates to his own practice of midwifery, it is also highly conventional. The same gesture appears in various early modern portraits, especially those of anatomists. In Jan van Neck's Dutch group portrait, *The Anatomy Lesson of Dr. Frederik Ruysch*, of 1683, for example, the anatomist gently lifts a portion of the intestine of the dissected stillborn baby between his thumb and forefinger, while the surgeon on the extreme left of the composition performs the *dissidentiam noto* gesture as he touches the afterbirth[54] (Figure 4.6). This delicate demonstration is a sign of the contact between fleshly beings. In the engraved image of Viardel, the surgeon's virtuosity is similarly shown to be based upon a physical comprehension of his subject matter. He looks directly out at the viewer as if making an observation based upon the evidence, namely the tiny corpse that is pushed into the viewer's space.

The perfectly preserved afterbirth in the lower left corner – elevated to receive the full attention of the spectator – not only illustrates Viardel's skill in removing it intact, but also emphasizes the child's detachment from the maternal body. The instructive tactile gesture of the surgeon links his own body with that of the child, implying a direct knowledge of the corporeal aspects of childbirth, one traditionally associated with women. This interpretation is supported by the Latin inscription, *Non impar Lucina*, positioned to the immediate left of the surgeon's outstretched hand. It insists he is not unequal to Lucina, the goddess of childbirth and muse of female midwives. Though the association of a surgeon man-midwife with Lucina was unusual, female midwives regularly invoked the goddess, linking their identities with her. In her obstetrical treatise, Bourgeois argued that Lucina provided her with divine instruction, guiding her during the royal deliveries of Marie de Médicis.[55] Viardel's portrait also affirms his relationship with Lucina, but he is not portrayed as her student or disciple. The text proclaiming *Non impar Lucina* is placed between the surgeon man-midwife's outstretched hand and the child, suggesting that his learned touch allows him to rival the goddess of childbirth. The implication is that he can replace Lucina and, by extension, the female midwives that follow her. Of course, only viewers possessing a knowledge of Latin could arrive at such an interpretation.

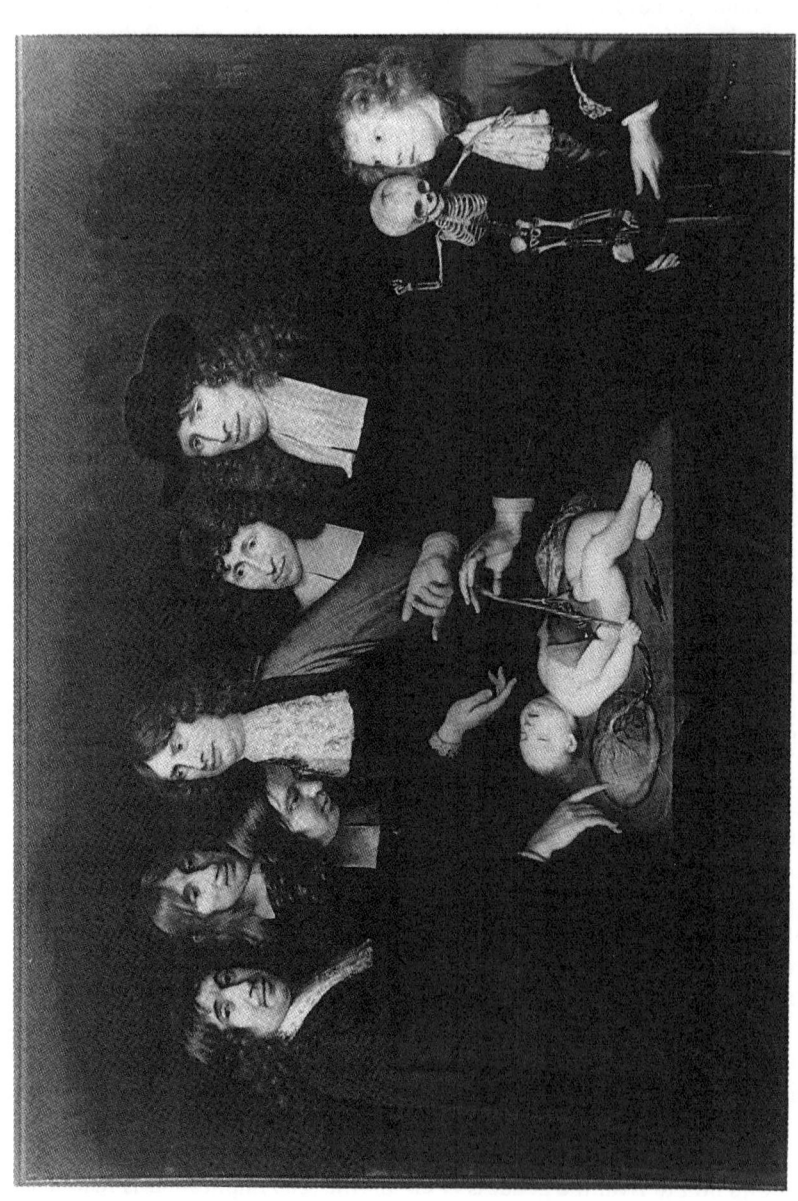

Figure 4.6   Jan van Neck, *The Anatomy Lesson of Dr Frederik Ruysch*, 1683, Amsterdam. Copyright Amsterdams Historisch Museum

Those women equipped with a strictly practical understanding of childbirth might attend to other aspects of the engraving, potentially appraising the condition of the afterbirth, a role expected of them in the lying-in chamber.[56]

Viardel's portrait contains no written text other than the short statement about Lucina and the minute signatures of the artists who made the image. In contrast to the frontispiece of Mauriceau's treatise, this portrait includes neither the title of Viardel's book, nor an inscription of the surgeon man-midwife's name and rank. Overall, Viardel is aligned less with his own writing and position as a royal surgeon than with his hands-on practices. These practices substitute for the maternal body, allowing him to succeed female midwives. Yet unlike the distinctly gendered spheres represented in the author portrait of Mauriceau, Viardel's portrait offers a vision of unity. Maternity is not simultaneously separated from and related to the surgeon; instead, Viardel's learned 'anatomical' touch is shown to embody both practical maternal and intellectual knowledge.

The author portrait inaugurating Paul Portal's treatise, *La pratique des accouchemens*, published in 1685, differs from the images of both Mauriceau and Viardel (Figure 4.7). Making no reference to either maternity or female midwives, the only attribute associated with the surgeon man-midwife is a copy of his own book, on which he places a small, steady hand. Like the portrait of Mauriceau, this juxtaposition identifies the surgeon's hand primarily with writing and theoretical knowledge. Portal's portrait is straightforward and while not as modest as that of Bourgeois, it functions to accentuate his reliable character. In fact, it recalls Jordanova's description of the portrait of Hunter as a 'masterpiece of denial' by excluding direct references to the surgeon's practice of midwifery.[57] The emphasis on respectability in the image of Portal counters characterizations of men-midwives as immoral and dangerous. Yet the restrained style of the engraving is at odds with other portraits by painter Gabriel Revel, a follower of Charles Le Brun. Joining the Académie royale in 1683, this established portraitist usually produced more elaborate images of aristocratic figures and fellow artists.[58]

Portal's understated portrait may inhibit the recognition of his specific social identity. The only indication of the surgeon man-midwife's expertise in childbirth is the spine of the book he holds, inscribed with both his name and a partial title 'Sur les accouchement.' Nothing indicates the treatise was based on the experiences of Portal, who as a *compagnon chirurgien ordinaire* at the Hôtel-Dieu in Paris from 1650 to 1663 was called to assist at obstetrical and other emergencies.[59] Instead, the large text encircling Portal's author portrait identifies him as a member of the Parisian corporation of surgeons, emphasizing his legitimate right to practise in the city, a value also favoured by Dionis. This script functions to link the role of master surgeon with the appearance of a well-groomed, and smartly attired gentleman. The visual and written aspects of Portal's frontispiece combine to represent the dignified appearance of an incorporated surgeon who produced a book about childbirth.

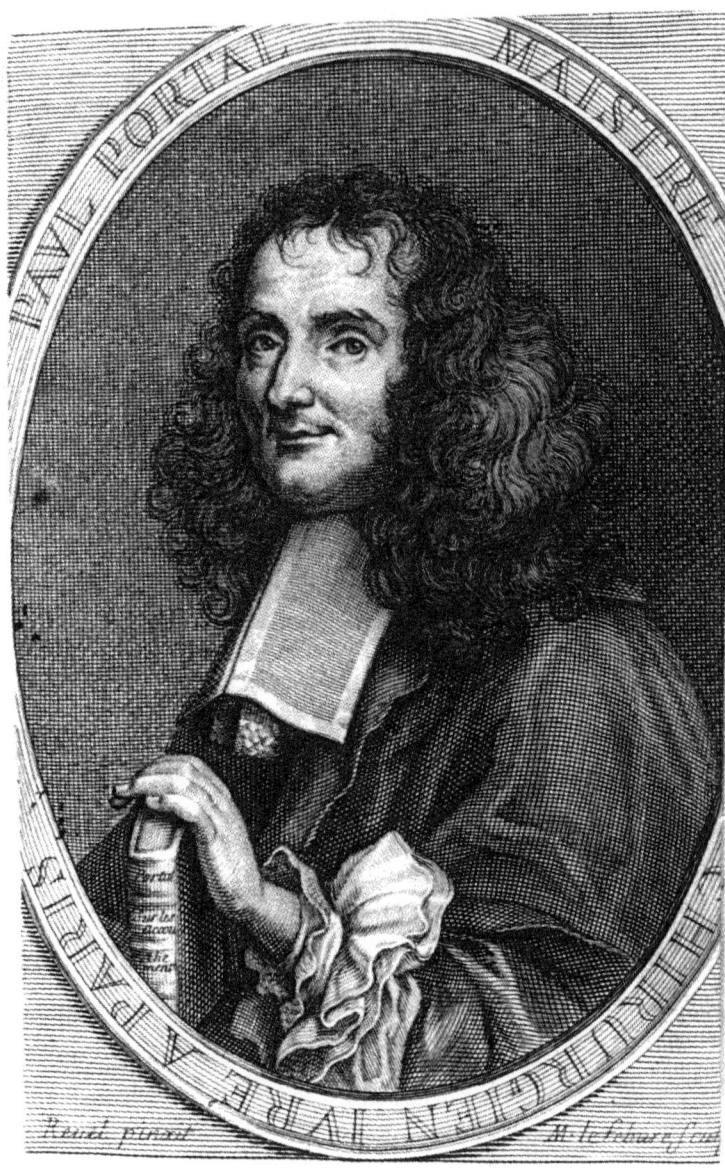

Figure 4.7   Author portrait, from Paul Portal's *La pratique des accouchemens*, 1685, Paris. Courtesy of the National Library of Medicine, Bethesda, MD

The reserved image offered by Portal's portrait corresponds with the austere style of the written text following it. In contrast to the loquacious texts by Mauriceau and Viardel, Portal's book is unassuming. The author rarely criticized male rivals, and was even sympathetic to female midwives, occasionally praising them.[60] Overall, his book is more serious than those of his predecessors, containing fewer embellishments and, as historian Emile-Jules-Alfred Maruitte points out, no witticisms.[61] In his study of Portal, historian François Duchatel claims the understated rhetorical style of the surgeon man-midwife may have contributed to the eclipse of his reputation, while Maruitte implies it hindered the republication of his treatise.[62] Though the singular edition of Portal's treatise was translated into English in 1705, the books produced by Mauriceau and Viardel enjoyed subsequent editions in French as well as other languages.[63]

Portal's age may provide one explanation for his restrained image. Age was highlighted in descriptions of the ideal qualities of both male and female midwives, which favoured middle-aged practitioners with an extensive understanding of childbirth. At the time his book was published, Portal was an established surgeon of about 55 years of age, with an indisputable amount of experience. In contrast, Mauriceau was only 31 years old when his more ornate and ambitious frontispiece was designed, a relatively young surgeon man-midwife striving to increase his practice. It is worth noting that a rather simple portrait of Mauriceau appeared in his obstetrical treatises after he had become more established.[64] A simple image of the head and shoulders of the *chirurgien accoucheur*, dated 1693, inaugurated both the fourth edition of *Des maladies des femmes grosses et accouchées,* and another book, *Aphorismes touchant la grossesse, l'accouchement, les maladies, et autres dispositions des femmes* [Aphorisms concerning pregnancy, childbirth, illnesses, and other dispositions of women], published in 1694[65] (Figure 4.8). Now aged 56 and sporting an elegant cravat and grandiose wig, Mauriceau looks directly out at the viewer. In an image more economical even than that of Portal, he is shorn of all props, and accompanied only by a small Latin text noting his official status as a master surgeon in Paris.

The conclusion that an older surgeon man-midwife would have had less need to insist on his obstetrical authority is challenged, however, by the elaborate image of Viardel. Although we have little information about his career, and no secure birth or death dates, historian Émile Placet convincingly argues that Viardel was of an advanced age when he wrote his treatise, despite looking rather young and dashing in the author portrait.[66] Questions about the abilities of Viardel were nevertheless raised by his peers. Even Portal disagreed with the teachings in Viardel's treatise. The respectable surgeon man-midwife argued, for example, that expelled *meconium* – the dark matter contained in the bowels of an unborn child – was not a sign of its death in the womb as Viardel contended.[67] Mauriceau was the most vociferous in his attacks on the Queen's royal surgeon, claiming the pages of Viardel's treatise were

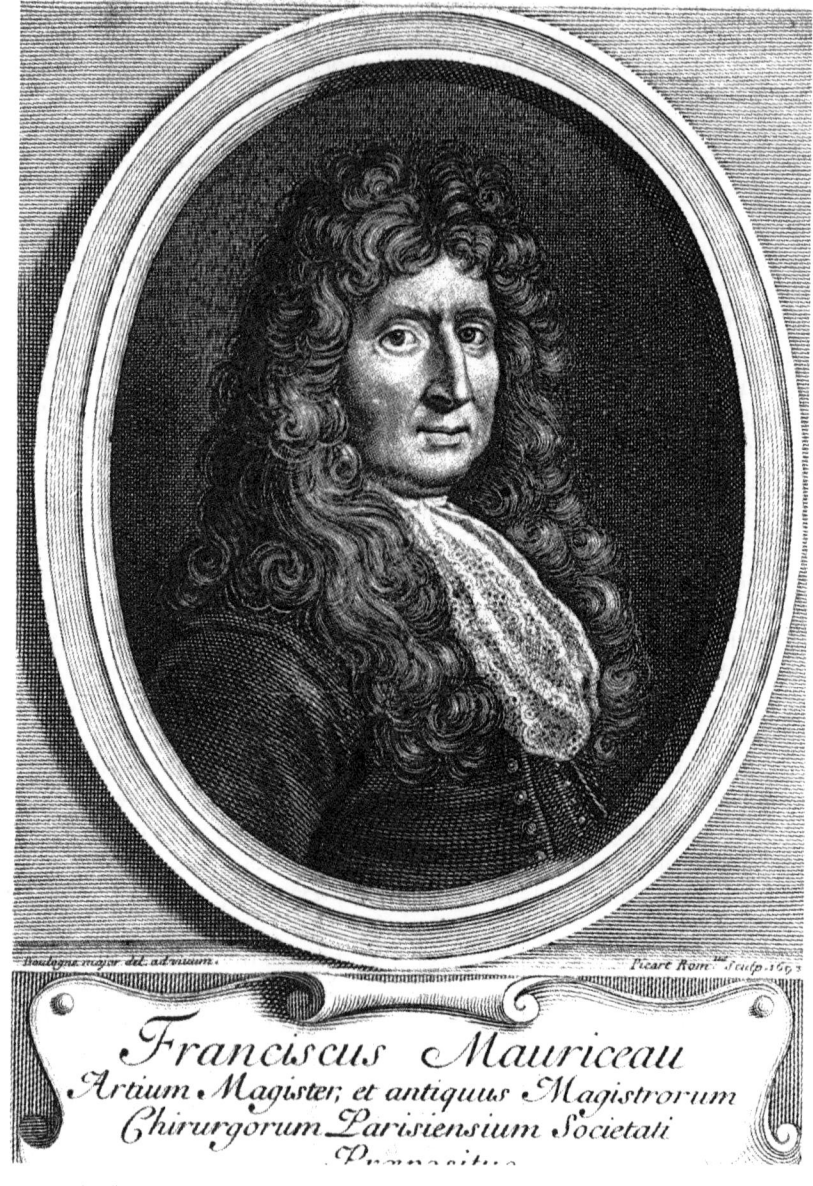

Figure 4.8   **Author portrait, from François Mauriceau's** *Des maladies des femmes grosses et accouchées*, **1694, Paris. Courtesy of the National Library of Medicine, Bethesda, MD**

fit only for wrapping cheese and butter at the market.[68] Although *chirurgiens accoucheurs* regularly denounced one another, the antagonism displayed toward Viardel was especially intense. Yet it is not difficult to explain. Unlike Mauriceau, Portal, and all of the other surgeon men-midwives who wrote obstetrical treatises, Viardel was not a member of an official corporation of surgeons. He was quite defensive about his lower status as a royal surgeon, located outside of the official medical hierarchy. In the preface to his treatise he assured readers that they should not doubt his book just because it was not written by a master surgeon; 'It is neither,' he insisted, 'the bonnet, nor the robe that makes a Doctor.'[69] Viardel associated official medical status with superficial ritual, questioning the link between appearance and ability. The members of Saint-Côme clearly resented Viardel's royal privilege, which enabled him to bypass their regulations as well as avoid demonstrating his skills for their adjudication. Consequently, Viardel had a greater need to prove his qualifications as a surgeon man-midwife, despite his claims of hands-on experience.

At 70 years of age, surgeon man-midwife Philippe Peu was even older than Viardel when he sat for the portrait in his treatise, *La pratique des accouchemens*, published in 1694 (Figure 4.9). Like the image of Portal and the later characterization of Mauriceau, Peu is depicted as a learned man in dark robes, solemnly addressing the viewer. Simon Thomassin the elder, an academic artist known for his engravings of religious subjects, both designed and inscribed the conventional image.[70] Peu's identity as a master surgeon is indicated only by the Latin script inscribed in the standard oval frame. The surgeon man-midwife is shown resting his idealized small and delicate hand not upon a book, but on his own chest, in a gesture typically associated with humility. The absolute denial of his hands-on practice and indeed of his undertaking work of any kind argues for the elevation of his status to that of an aristocrat or noble, an identity bolstered by his voluminous powdered wig. Instead of indicating his profession directly, Peu's gesture invokes the posture taken when swearing to tell the truth or taking an oath.[71] While this motion may refer to his status as sworn surgeon of Saint-Côme, it is also addressed to the viewer of the image as an act of pledging to serve his clients faithfully. At the same time, it can be read as a self-reflexive indication referring the viewer back to the body of the surgeon himself. Recalling Bourgeois' arguments about her presentation to Queen Marie de Médicis, the portrait suggests that Peu's appearance can stand as the ultimate evidence of both his character and his obstetrical abilities.

At least one of Peu's colleagues nevertheless found reason to criticize the surgeon man-midwife's appearance. Monsieur Simon, a fellow master surgeon of Saint-Côme, was angry at Peu for disparaging an operation he had undertaken in 1680 to open the calloused vagina of his client.[72] Although Peu referred only to the faulty methods of a 'young surgeon' in his treatise, Simon recognized himself and apparently feared other readers would as well. In 1695, Simon published a lengthy

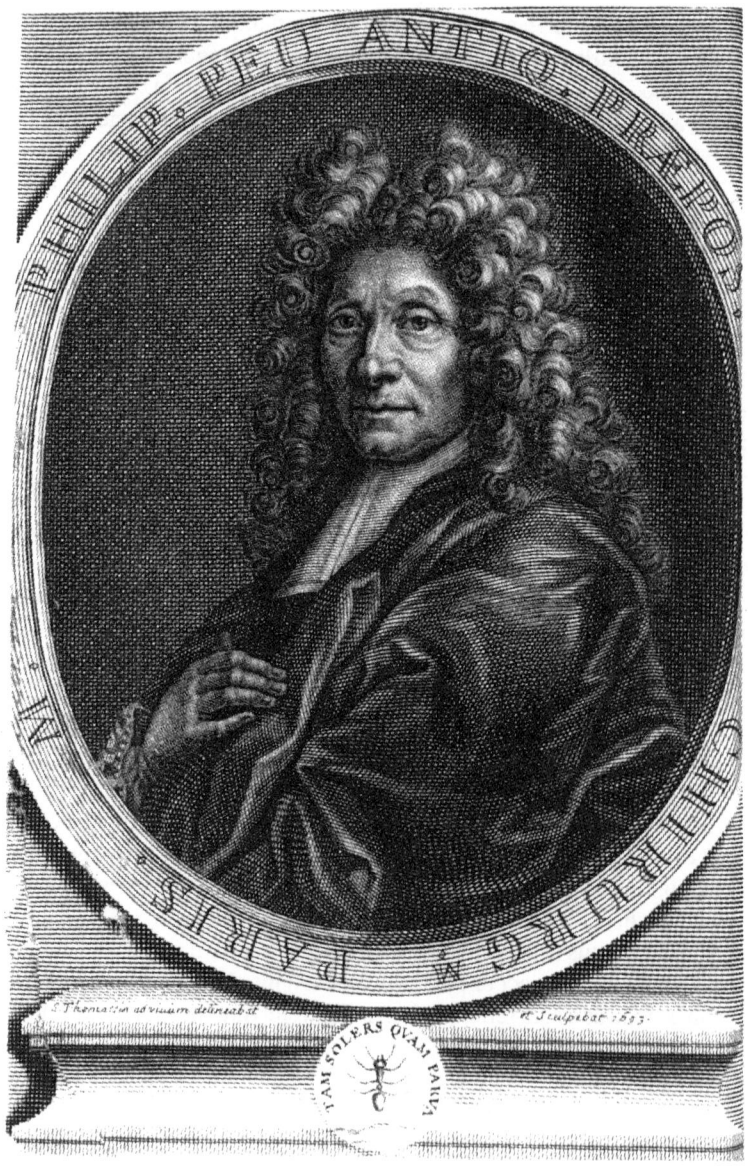

Figure 4.9   Author portrait, from Philippe Peu's *La pratique des accouchemens*,
1694, Paris. Courtesy of the National Library of Medicine, Bethesda,
MD

critique of Peu's account of the operation, but also took the opportunity to draw attention to Peu's preoccupation with his own appearance. According to Simon, Peu grew a great beard and moustache in his middle years, hoping to augment his *petite réputation* [small reputation] with flourishing facial hair. Realizing this strategy was not working, Simon continued, Peu suddenly shaved off his beard, and placed a blond wig over his scanty hair in an effort to conceal his advanced age 'which was making him a little decrepit.'[73] In a scathing appraisal of Peu, Simon correlated the surgeon man-midwife's balding head and increasing age with his diminishing abilities. Pointing out that Peu did not conform to the image of the ideal *chirurgien accoucheur* – middle-aged, strong, and pleasant to behold – Simon accused the older man of appearing to be something he was not. Simon's critique of Peu not only indicates that physical appearance and competence were closely linked, but also implies that the correspondence between the two could be manipulated to further career goals. In keeping with the 'physiognomic scepticism' rampant during the early modern period, Simon argued that appearances could be deceitful; the visual displays of surgeon men-midwives such as Peu required evaluation by a cautious and critical eye.[74]

Conclusions

This chapter showed that multiple strategies were used in the visual construction of the ideal image of the *chirurgien accoucheur*. Portraits of surgeon men-midwives vary according to the particular age, social status, and institutional affiliation of the subject. What links most of these images is an insistence on privileging hands, but even here there are differences. The hands of Mauriceau and Portal are primarily associated with the intellectual activity of writing, those of Viardel suggest an intimate knowledge of childbirth, and Peu's delicate hand is related to both loyalty and nobility. Given the moral questions that continued to surround the surgeon man-midwife's potentially illicit touching of women's bodies, and the overwhelming association of surgery with denigrated manual labour, resignifying the hands of the male practitioner was particularly important.

Visual and written descriptions of the ideal surgeon man-midwife provide insight into the unstable identity of *chirurgiens accoucheurs* in early modern France. During this period of shifting obstetrical practices, surgeon men-midwives were not a unified group. The case of Peu and Simon demonstrates that efforts to produce a positive image of the surgeon man-midwife could receive criticism even from fellow practitioners. Nor were surgeon men-midwives united in their opposition to female midwives. In fact, written accounts advise the men to adopt feminine qualities such as modesty, tenderness, and delicacy, without surrendering their masculine attributes of courage, self-control, and extensive medical knowledge. The elaborate author portraits of Viardel and Mauriceau (Figures 4.3 and 4.4) support the idea that male practitioners could be represented in relation to the maternal body, not exclusively in distinction from it. In the portrait of Viardel, the relational distance is collapsed altogether. Although the later images of Peu, Portal, and eventually Mauriceau erase all references to maternity, earlier portraits suggest that during the early and middle years of the seventeenth century *chirurgiens accoucheurs* did not, and perhaps could not – especially when attempting to expand and authenticate their practices – reject the continuing authority of the first-hand, subjective experience of childbirth. This evidence indicates that maternal experience was not disdained by French male midwives, a point explored further in the next chapter.

Notes

1. François Mauriceau, *Des maladies des femmes grosses et accouchées* (Paris, 1668), 267:

    Il y a des gens qui disent, qu'un Chirurgien qui veut pratiquer les accouchemens, doit...estre mal propre, ou à tout le moins fort negligé, se laissant venir une longue barbe sale, afin de ne pas donner aucune jalousie aux maris des femmes qui l'envoyent querir pour les secourir.

2. *Ibid.*, 267.
3. Cited in Barry Wind, *'A Foul and Pestilent Congregation': Images of 'Freaks' in Baroque Art* (Aldershot: Ashgate, 1998), 56. Jacques Duval, *Traité des hermaphrodits, parties génitales, accouchemens des femmes* (Rouen, 1612), 10, claimed that the hermaphrodite Marin de Marcis was demonstrably male because, among other things, he wore a beard on his chin. See also Will Fisher, 'The Renaissance Beard: Masculinity in Early Modern England,' *Renaissance Quarterly* 54 (2001), 155–87.
4. Pierre Darmon, *Le tribunal de l'impuissance: Virilité et défaillances conjugales dans l'ancienne France* (Paris: Seuil, 1979), 194.
5. For resistance to male midwives see Philippe Hecquet, *De l'indécence aux hommes d'accoucher les femmes* (Paris, 1708), and Roy Porter, 'A Touch of Danger: The Man-Midwife as Sexual Predator,' G. S. Rousseau and Roy Porter, eds, *Sexual Underworlds of the Enlightenment* (Chapel Hill: University of North Carolina Press, 1988), 206–32.
6. Ludmilla Jordanova, 'Feminine Figures: Nature Display'd,' *Nature Displayed: Gender, Science and Medicine 1760–1820* (London: Longman, 1999), 25. John Blunt was also known as Samuel Fores.
7. See my Introduction, especially notes 57–8.
8. Ludmilla Jordanova, 'Medical Men 1780–1820,' Joanna Woodall, ed., *Portraiture: Facing the Subject* (Manchester: Manchester University Press, 1997), 110.
9. Mary Lindemann, *Health and Healing in Eighteenth-Century Germany* (Baltimore: The Johns Hopkins University Press, 1996), 100.

10. Adrian Wilson, *The Making of Man-Midwifery: Childbirth in England 1660–1770* (London: UCL Press, 1995), 176.

11. See, for example, Mauriceau, *Des maladies des femmes grosses et accouchées*, 267, Pierre Dionis, *Traité général des accouchemens* (Paris, 1718), 413, and Jacques Mesnard, *Le guide des accoucheurs* (Paris, 1743), 5.

12. For this argument, see Chapter 2.

13. Soranus, *Gynecology*, Owsei Temkin, trans. and intro. (Baltimore: The Johns Hopkins University Press, 1956), 5–6. For the ideal physician in the Hippocratic corpus see Vivian Nutton, 'Beyond the Hippocratic Oath,' Andrew Wear et al., eds, *Doctors and Ethics: The Earlier Historical Setting of Professional Ethics* (Amsterdam: Rodopi, 1993), 10–37.

14. See Chapter 3, especially notes 46–59.

15. Mauriceau, *Des maladies des femmes grosses et accouchées*, 267, Cosme Viardel, *Observations sur la pratique des accouchemens naturels, contre nature & monstrueux* (Paris, 1671), 280, and Dionis, *Traité général des accouchemens*, 413.

16. Viardel, *Observations sur la pratique des accouchemens naturels, contre nature & monstrueux*, 279, Dionis, *Traité général des accouchemens*, 413, and Guillaume Mauquest de La Motte, *A General Treatise of Midwifry*, Thomas Tomkyns, trans. (London, 1746), 412.

17. Dionis, *Traité général des accouchemens*, 414: 'une main grosse & courte est un défaut essentiel dans un Accoucheur.' For an earlier account of the ideal surgical hand see Marie-Christine Pouchelle, *The Body and Surgery in the Middle Ages*, Rosemary Morris, trans. (New Brunswick: Rutgers University Press, 1990), 87.

18. Mauriceau, *Des maladies des femmes grosses et accouchées*, 267, and Viardel, *Observations sur la pratique des accouchemens naturels, contre nature & monstrueux*, 280.

19. Mauquest de La Motte, *A General Treatise of Midwifry*, 7.

20. Jacques Bury, *Le propagatif de l'homme* (Paris, 1623), 84, Philippe Peu, *La pratique des accouchemens* (Paris, 1694), 85, Dionis, *Traité général des accouchemens*, 416, and Mesnard, *Le guide des accoucheurs*, 4–5.

21. The allegorical figure of Charity was conventionally represented as a robed female figure breastfeeding a child, with older children standing on either side of her. The numerous editions and translations of Cesare Ripa's *Iconologia*, originally published in 1593, presented this image to artists and poets throughout Europe. See, for example, Caesar Ripa, *Iconologia*, P. Tempest, trans. (London, 1709), 12.

22. Dionis, *Traité général des accouchemens*, 413.

23. Viardel, *Observations sur la pratique des accouchemens naturels, contre nature & monstrueux*, 280: 'il doit...estre doux dans ses parolles, & agreable dans sa conversation afin de réjouir la malade.'

24. Hendrik van Deventer, *The Art of Midwifery Improv'd*, 3rd edn (London, 1728), 13–14.

25. Viardel, *Observations sur la pratique des accouchemens naturels, contre nature & monstrueux*, 278.

26. John Maubray, *The Female Physician* (London, 1724), 180, quoted in Robert A. Erickson, '"The Books of Generation": Some Observations on the Style of the British

Midwife Books, 1671–1764,' Paul-Gabriel Boucé, ed., *Sexuality in Eighteenth-Century Britain* (Manchester: Manchester University Press, 1982), 85.

27.   Dionis, *Traité général des accouchemens*, 417.

28.   Peu, *La pratique des accouchemens*, 312–13: 'Je dissumulai ma peine pour n'efraier personne.' On another occasion, 428, after an unnamed surgeon abandoned a suffering woman, Peu stepped in to remove the dismembered child from her womb without 'losing courage.'

29.   Dionis, *Traité général des accouchemens*, 415, and Guillaume Mauquest de La Motte, *Traité complet des accouchemens* (Paris, 1729; orig. 1721), 169.

30.   Mauquest de La Motte, *Traité complet des accouchemens*, 310, 421, and 424.

31.   Bourgeois, *Récit véritable de la naissance de messeigneurs et dames les enfans de France*, François Rouget and Colette H. Winn, eds (Geneva: Droz, 2000), 73–83, as discussed in Chapter 3.

32.   Bury, *Le propagatif de l'homme*, 83.

33.   Mauquest de La Motte, *Traité complet des accouchemens*, xi.

34.   Louise Bourgeois, *Observations diverses sur la stérilité, perte de fruict, foecondité, accouchemens et maladies des femmes et enfants nouveaux naiz*, Françoise Olive, ed. (Paris: Côté-Femmes, 1992; orig. 1652), 104–7.

35.   Viardel, *Observations sur la pratique des accouchemens naturels, contre nature & monstrueux*, 279.

36.   Mauriceau, *Des maladies des femmes grosses et accouchées*, 266–7.

37.   Dionis, *Traité général des accouchemens*, 414–15.

38.   See Chapter 3, especially notes 36–8 as well as Sarah Stone, *A Complete Practice of Midwifery* (London, 1737), vii, xi–xiii, and Elizabeth Nihell, *A Treatise on the Art of Midwifery* (London, 1760), xi.

39.   Dionis, *Traité général des accouchemens*, 414: 'cette operation étant du ressort de la Chirurgie.'

40.   For a history of Saint-Côme see Jeanne Rigal, *La communauté des maîtres-chirurgiens jurés de Paris au XVIIe et au XVIIIe siècle* (Paris: Vigot Frères, 1936), and E. Nicaise, 'Histoire abrégée du collège de chirurgie,' Pierre Franco, *Chirurgie*, E. Nicaise, ed. (Geneva: Slatkine Reprints, 1972; orig. 1561), cv–clii.

41.   Alison Klairmont Lingo, 'Empirics and Charlatans in Early Modern France: The Genesis of the Classification of the "Other" in Medical Practice,' *Journal of Social History* 19 (1986), 583–604. See also Roy Porter, *Quacks: Fakers and Charlatans in English Medicine* (Stroud, Gloucestershire: Tempus, 2000).

42.   See my discussion in Chapter 1, especially notes 91–3.

43.   Lingo, 'Empirics and Charlatans in Early Modern France,' 59.

44.   *Statuts et reiglemens ordonnez pour toutes les matronnes, ou saiges femmes de la ville, faulxbourgs, prevosté, et vicomté de Paris* (Paris, n.d.). See the discussion of these statutes as well as the licensing of female midwives in Chapter 3.

45.   For Paillet see Émile Bellier de la Chavignerie, *Dictionnaire général des artistes de l'école française* (Paris: Renouard, 1885), 191, and Emmanuel Bénézit, *Dictionnaire critique et documentaire des peintres, sculpteurs, dessinateurs et graveurs* (Paris: Gründ, 1966), vol. 6, 485. For Vallet see Bénézit, *Dictionnaire critique et documentaire*, vol. 8, 461.

46. The Académie royale was founded primarily to increase the social status of artists. For its history and hierarchical nature see Nathalie Heinich, *Du peintre à l'artiste: Artisans et académiciens à l'âge classique* (Paris: Minuit, 1993), Jacques Thuillier, 'Académie et classicisme en France: Les débuts de l'Académie royale de peinture et de sculpture (1648–63),' S. Bottari, ed., *Il Mito del Classicismo nel Seicento* (Messina/Florence: G. d'Anna, 1964), 181–209, and Louis Olivier, '"Curieux", Amateurs and Connoisseurs: Laymen and the Fine Arts in the Ancien Régime' (Ph.D. Diss., The Johns Hopkins University Press, 1976).

47. I thank Helen King for informing me of this longstanding way of describing childbirth. According to the eleventh- or twelfth-century book by Trotula, 'in the ninth month, it [the unborn child] proceeds from the darkness into the light.' See Monica H. Green, ed. and trans., *The Trotula: A Medieval Compendium of Women's Medicine* (Philadelphia: University of Pennsylvania Press, 2001), 107. Duval, *Traité des hermaphrodits, parties génitales, accouchemens des femmes*, 57, uses the same terminology.

48. The signs used by midwives are reported by Jacques Gélis, *La sage-femme ou le médecin: une nouvelle conception de la vie* (Paris: Fayard, 1988), 32, and Richard L. Petrelli, 'The Regulation of French Midwifery during the *Ancien Régime*,' *Journal of the History of Medicine* 27 (1971), 278.

49. For a discussion of Bourguignon's painting see Erica Harth, *Ideology and Culture in Seventeenth-Century France* (Ithaca: Cornell University Press, 1983), 109–10.

50. Joaneath Spicer, 'The Renaissance Elbow,' Jan Bremmer and Herman Roodenburg, eds, *A Cultural History of Gesture* (Ithaca: Cornell University Press, 1991), 84–128.

51. For Guernier see Bénézit, *Dictionnaire critique et documentaire*, vol. 4, 485, and for Frosne see vol. 4, 102–3, as well as Roger-Armand Weigert, *Inventaire du fonds français: graveurs du XVIIe siècle*, 4 (Paris: Bibliothèque nationale, 1961), 281–310.

52. John Bulwer, *Chirologia: Or the Naturall Language of the Hand* (London, 1644), 171–2.

53. Viardel, *Observations sur la pratique des accouchemens naturels, contre nature & monstrueux*, unpaginated preface.

54. For a discussion of this painting see Norbert E. Middelkoop, '"Large and Magnificent Paintings, all Pertaining to the Chirurgeon's Art". The Art Collection of the Amsterdam Surgeons' Guild,' Ben Broos et al., eds, *Rembrandt Under the Scalpel: The Anatomy Lesson of Dr Nicolaes Tulp Dissected* (Mauritshuis, The Hague: Six Art Promotion, 1998), 9–38.

55. Bourgeois, *Observations diverses*, 174.

56. For the visual appraisal of the afterbirth for appraisal see Chapter 2, especially notes 69–71.

57. Jordanova, 'Medical Men 1780–1820,' 110.

58. For Revel see Bénézit, *Dictionnaire critique et documentaire*, vol. 7, 195–6. Matthieu Lefebvre engraved the image. For him see Maxime Préaud, *Inventaire du fonds français: graveurs du XVIIe siècle*, vol. 10 (Paris: Bibliothèque nationale, 1989), 42–7. Most surgeon men-midwives hired academic artists to create their portraits, and I have already considered this issue in terms of the surgeons' desire for prestige, comparing the visual strategies used in portraits of both academic artists and aspiring surgeon

men-midwives in an unpublished paper given at the conference on Portraiture and Scientific Identity at the National Portrait Gallery in London in June 2000.

59. François Duchatel, 'Paul Portal (1630?–1er juillet 1703): Un accoucheur méconnu du XVIIe siècle,' *Histoire des sciences médicales* 14, 4 (1980), 407–18, and Émile-Jules-Alfred Maruitte, *Paul Portal. Sa vie. Son oeuvre* (Paris: Steinheil, 1900).

60. Paul Portal, *La pratique des accouchemens* (Paris, 1685), 59. He remarked on the skills of Mesdames Moreau and de France, sworn midwives who taught at the Hôtel-Dieu from 1660–1663.

61. Maruitte, *Paul Portal*, 41.

62. Duchatel, 'Paul Portal,' 410, and Maruitte, *Paul Portal*, 42.

63. Paul Portal, *The Compleat Practice of Men and Women Midwives* (London, 1705). Mauriceau's *Des maladies des femmes grosses et accouchées* appeared in four editions during the seventeenth century (1668, 1675, 1681, and 1694), numerous reprints during the eighteenth century, and translations into German, Dutch, Italian, Latin, Flemish, and English. Viardel's treatise of 1671 was republished in both 1673 and 1674, appearing in German in 1676.

64. This engraving is most likely based on the painted portrait of Mauriceau, currently in the collections of the Musée d'histoire de la médecine in Paris. I thank the Conservateur, Madame Marie Véronique Clin, for supplying me with a slide of this anonymous, undated work.

65. François Mauriceau, *Aphorismes touchant la grossesse, l'accouchement, les maladies, et autres dispositions des femmes* (Paris, 1694) is a very small book (about 5 by 12 cm.), which extracts the precepts outlined in the surgeon man-midwife's earlier books.

66. Émile Placet, *L'obstétrique aux XVIIe et XVIIIe siècles. Viardel, Portal, et Mauquest de La Motte* (Paris: Baillière, 1892), 46.

67. Portal, *La pratique des accouchemens*, 180, and 240.

68. Mauriceau, *Des maladies des femmes grosses et accouchées* (Paris, 1681), as cited in Joseph Lévy-Valensi, *La médecine et les médecins français au XVIIe siècle* (Paris: Baillière, 1933), 657.

69. Viardel, *Observations sur la pratique des accouchemens naturels, contre nature & monstrueux*, unpaginated preface: 'ce n'est pas le bonnet, n'y la robe qui fait un Docteur.'

70. For Thomassin see Bénézit, *Dictionnaire critique et documentaire*, vol. 8, 288. Author portraits of surgeon men-midwives not discussed in this chapter include those of Denis Fournier, Pierre Amand, and Pierre Dionis.

71. Bulwer, *Chirologia*, 88–9. A similar gesture is performed by Hendrik van Deventer in a painting by Thomas van der Wilt from 1700. See R.M.F. van der Weiden and W.J. Hoogsteder, 'A New Light Upon Hendrik van Deventer (1651–1724): Identification and Recovery of a Portrait,' *Journal of the Royal Society of Medicine* 90 (October 1997), 567–9.

72. Peu, *La pratique des accouchemens*, 252–6.

73. M. Simon, *Factum ou lettre écrite par Mr. Simon à Mr. Peu sur la falsification d'un fait qui se trouve à la fin du premier livre de sa Pratique des accouchemens* (n.l., n.d.), 15: 'qui commence à vous rendre un peu décrepite'.

74. For physiognomic scepticism see Chapter 3, note 115.

Chapter 5

Bodies in Labour:
Rhetoric, Rivalry, and Male Maternity

Although male authors of obstetrical treatises described the ideal surgeon man-midwife as modest, polite, and charitable, they also criticized rivals. Surgeon men-midwives regularly denounced other male practitioners, calling them unskilled, ignorant, and even killers of women and children. Producing an inverse image of the beneficial man-midwife, their written accounts outlined an injurious birthing assistant who lacked hands-on experience, overestimated his abilities, and flagrantly invented stories of the difficult deliveries he had remedied in an avaricious quest for fame. Castigating the negative qualities of fellow men-midwives allowed authors to construct a contrasting image of themselves. Many writers were not reticent about vaunting their own superior skills, more extensive training, and absolutely truthful descriptions of surgical interventions in childbirth. This discourse of rivalry portrays surgeon men-midwives as contenders in a competitive field, required both to display and defend their reputations.

Male authors criticized female midwives as well as male rivals. In addition to claiming that female midwives lacked a theoretical comprehension of childbirth, surgeon men-midwives referred to these women as ignorant meddlers whose arrogance prevented them from calling for male assistance when faced with dangerous deliveries.[1] Such assertions were initially accepted at face value by historians of childbirth. In 1966 Thomas Forbes, for example, agreed that early modern female midwives were both ignorant and incompetent.[2] More recent historical research has cast doubt on these claims. Archival evidence found by David Harley suggests that some English midwives were literate and relatively prosperous during the seventeenth and early eighteenth centuries.[3] Doreen Evenden's extensive research has similarly shown that seventeenth-century London female midwives were often from affluent families and well-trained after undergoing lengthy apprenticeships.[4] In terms of early modern French midwives, scholars Wendy Perkins and Nina Rattner Gelbart have challenged the myth of the incompetent matron by analysing the publications of influential midwives such as Louise Bourgeois and Angélique Marguerite Le Boursier du Coudray, women who were clearly capable of handling obstetrical emergencies.[5]

While male criticism of female midwives is increasingly viewed as part of men's strategic quest for advancement in the lying-in chamber, little attention has been paid to the ways in which these men portrayed each other. Maligning one's competitors was standard practice in early modern medical writing, and female midwives were not the only targets. Although men labelled these women untrained and crude, they said much the same thing about male practitioners, especially those unlicensed 'charlatans' who threatened to encroach upon an established clientele.[6] Highly educated medical men were not, however, immune from attack by both surgeons and physicians. The members of the Faculté de Médecine in Paris denounced physicians trained in other cities – including at the prestigious medical school in Montpellier – as unfit to practise in the capital.[7] Though surgeon men-midwives similarly criticized medical 'outsiders,' they often reserved particular animosity for fellow guild members. In 1694, *chirurgien accoucheur* François Mauriceau published a critique of the obstetrical treatise written by Philippe Peu, another sworn surgeon of Saint-Côme in Paris. Mauriceau claimed that Peu had never actually delivered a woman: the numerous complicated labours described in Peu's treatise were fabrications.[8] Peu responded in a lengthy polemical tract, accusing Mauriceau of having hastily produced a repetitive set of lewd and 'undigested observations' in his own treatise.[9]

In many ways, the accusations surgeon men-midwives launched at each other resemble the claims made against them by female midwives. English midwives Sarah Stone and Elizabeth Nihell complained that men-midwives lacked practical training, were too eager to intervene with instruments, and attacked female modesty.[10] In a similar vein, royal midwife Louise Bourgeois vaunted her intimate experience of pregnancy and childbirth, questioning the knowledge of male practitioners.[11] When criticizing a fellow surgeon man-midwife, male authors likewise emphasized his lack of sufficient practice, while drawing attention to their own extensive understanding of childbirth. Though surgeon men-midwives sometimes accused each other of publishing lascivious content – one of Peu's critiques of Mauriceau's treatise – such claims were relatively uncommon. Questions about the morality of men-midwives tended to come from non-surgeons concerned with upholding religious conventions and traditional understandings of female modesty. When physician Philippe Hecquet published his critique of man-midwifery in 1708, for example, he argued that the profession of *accoucheur* was both of recent invention and at odds with Christian morality because of its reliance on the dangerous touching of women's bodies.[12] Unlike Hecquet and various female midwives, surgeon men-midwives directed their comments toward specific individuals.

This chapter examines the written exchanges between *chirurgiens accoucheurs* published in both obstetrical treatises and shorter pamphlets during the seventeenth and early eighteenth centuries. To the best of my knowledge, these sources have not previously received extended scholarly attention, in contrast to recent examinations of the pamphlet war involving Bourgeois, also addressed below.[13] Disagreements among surgeon men-midwives are worth studying because they indicate these men were not a homogeneous group with identical approaches to childbirth. Such evidence challenges arguments insisting that increased male practice in the lying-in chamber resulted from a kind of 'gender war' in which medical men collaborated to oust female midwives.[14] While early modern surgeon men-midwives could cooperate with each other, there is much evidence of divisions among them. My efforts to understand the distinctions between male practitioners have been inspired by the work of Adrian Wilson. Examining the practices of early modern English men-midwives, Wilson has argued that these men were united neither by instrument use nor political belief.[15] French men-midwives similarly did not agree about which kinds of surgical instruments to employ or how frequently to use them (if at all). My focus on written disputes nevertheless departs from Wilson's approach. I am concerned with the kinds of arguments made in critical accounts of fellow surgeon men-midwives, as well as the rhetoric used and alliances represented in them. My goal is to examine the grounds on which obstetrical authority was both constructed and undermined, elaborating my larger thesis that obstetrical treatises were sites of contestation; they did not simply deliver medical instruction to readers.

In the first section of this chapter, I strive for an expansive vision of critical medical writing, examining disputes between surgeons and physicians, as well as between surgeon men-midwives. In addition to considering the conventional nature of the kinds of arguments made in published debates, I draw particular attention to pamphlets, including their format, and how they were distributed and read. Turning to specific debates between surgeon men-midwives, I explore the characteristic image of the 'bad' man-midwife emerging from them. Accounts of the unscrupulous male midwife echo the negative stereotype of the female midwife, with one notable difference. Whereas she was accused of wanting a theoretical understanding of medicine, the destructive man-midwife was primarily associated with a lack of hands-on practice in the birthing chamber.

In the second section, I focus on the criticism in obstetrical treatises to investigate how surgeon men-midwives exhibited their own practical knowledge of childbirth, while denouncing other male practitioners as inexperienced. Some of the strategies used in this effort are striking. Various male authors described the birthing experiences of their female relatives, including wives, sisters, and mothers. Such accounts associated surgeon men-midwives with a personal comprehension of childbirth, rather than an exclusively theoretical understanding of it. One author even referred to the circumstances of his own birth as evidence of his bodily encounter with both pregnancy and labour.[16] These remarkable passages provide additional evidence that surgeon men-midwives identified themselves with qualities traditionally valued in female midwives, including an intimate experience of childbirth. An important question, however, needs to be addressed: did men's association with maternity indicate a continued respect for maternal values, or was it based on a male appropriation of the maternal body? Finding evidence of both possibilities, this chapter explores a fundamental contradiction in tracts published by surgeon men-midwives. These authors celebrated male productivity and castigated the 'exclusively' corporeal knowledge of female midwives, but the female body remained a respected reference point in their assessments of obstetrical authority.

The Practices and Politics of Medical Criticism

One of the best-known medical disputes occurred in 1575. That year, Ambroise Paré, then royal surgeon to King Henri III, published a treatise entitled the *Oeuvres de M. Ambroise Paré*. A longtime military surgeon who had also trained for three years at the Hôtel-Dieu in Paris, Paré was famous for his treatment of gunshot wounds, replacing the previous method of painful cauterization with the application of ointment and dressings.[17] Paré's extensive treatise of 1575 included a book already published in 1573 as *Deux livres de chirurgie, de la génération de l'homme*. Among other things, it was devoted to the signs of conception, development of the embryo, and causes of miscarriage. Although Paré's book was protected by royal privilege, members of the Faculté de Médecine in Paris attempted to impede its diffusion.[18] Launching a legal case, the physicians insisted on the application of a decree created in 1535, which stated that no work of medicine could be sold before it was approved by the Faculté. The corporation of surgeons participated in the attack on Paré, arguing that his treatise was plagiarized and furthermore trespassed into the domain of surgery to reveal its secrets; although elevated to membership in Saint-Côme, Paré was trained as a 'mere' barber-surgeon. Paré's treatise was moreover accused of immorality. Filled with 'immodest' phrases, the text could, according to his accusers, negatively affect young girls and women.[19]

Paré responded by insisting his treatise was not lewd; he had discussed the causes of miscarriage in order to urge caution in women, not to assist them in procuring abortions, as charged.[20] His claims had little impact, for the real problem with the publication was not the accuracy or potential use of its contents, but rather the threat it posed to the established medical hierarchy. According to scholar Jean Céard, though the barber-surgeon's treatise of 1575 was similar to one he had published in 1573, it received negative attention because it was a weightier tome, written in French rather than Latin, which examined a number of questions pertaining to the medical domain.[21] Early modern physicians insisted that surgery involved a strictly manual labour, obliging surgeons to work under the direction of theoretically informed physicians. In publishing his significant treatise, Paré had effectively overstepped his rank and assumed the role of authoritative teacher.

In many ways, the debate occasioned by Paré's treatise epitomizes the disputes between Parisian surgeons and physicians recurring throughout the early modern period. As the position of surgeons gradually improved, conflicts between the Faculté de Médecine and Saint-Côme over medical status and privileges became both more numerous and more heated.[22] When the surgeons of Saint-Côme united with the barber-surgeons' guild in 1655, for example, physicians of the Faculté felt threatened, and undertook legal proceedings – not a surprising action during what has been called the litigious seventeenth century.[23] A court ruling in 1660 reaffirmed the subordinate status of surgeons, forbidding them to use titles, continue to refer to Saint-Côme as a College, and lecture publicly.[24] Despite this apparent decline in the situation of surgeons, historian Toby Gelfand has argued that the union of the two communities provided surgeons with a strong economic basis, allowing them to expand and ultimately secure increased prestige.[25] The amphitheatre of Saint-Côme was replaced with a larger building in 1691, for instance, to accommodate the surgical students seeking instruction in anatomy. The demand for such teaching continued even after the surgeons and barber-surgeons were divided in 1699, and a royal decree of 1725 established five surgical demonstrators to teach anatomy in the impressive new amphitheatre. The public lessons were implemented despite opposition from physicians who insisted surgeons were incapable of providing such theoretical instruction, and were furthermore forbidden to do so without the guidance of physicians.[26] All the same, surgeons did not attain complete independence from physicians until 1750.[27]

An extended written quarrel between a physician and a surgeon during the early seventeenth century indicates just how fierce these disputes could be as well as what was at stake in them. In 1613 Nicolas Habicot, a master surgeon of Saint-Côme, published *Gigantostéologie*, a work claiming that the curiously large bones exposed in Paris in July of that year were in fact the remains of the renowned giant, King Theutobochus.[28] Jean Riolan the younger, a professor of anatomy and member of the Faculté de Médecine, vehemently disagreed with Habicot. In his pamphlet of 1613, Riolan claimed that giants did not exist, suggesting the bones in question were those of an elephant.[29] Furious that a surgeon would assume authority in such an anatomical matter, and would furthermore presume to teach physicians as well as surgeons, Riolan wrote at least two other repudiations of Habicot's publication (in 1614 and 1618).[30] In 1614, the physician insisted Habicot understood nothing of the proportion of human bones, inviting the surgeon to attend anatomical lessons at the medical school, where they would speak French to ensure his comprehension – a jab at surgeons' purported lack of Latin. Reminding Habicot that surgeons and barbers were neither allowed to undertake anatomies without physicians present, nor to publish medical doctrine without their approval, he affirmed that physicians were the superiors of surgeons in all parts of medicine.[31]

Habicot did not respond directly to Riolan's allegations until 1618, when he accused the physician of jealousy, maliciousness, ambition, deception, slander, and a scanty knowledge of anatomy.[32] There were, however, earlier responses to the physician's critiques. In 1614 an anonymous author, identifying himself only as a 'compagnon chirurgien nouvelement arrivé de Montpellier' [journeyman surgeon recently arrived from Montpellier], reviled Riolan for writing such calumnious invectives against Habicot.[33] The author was offended by Riolan's claims that only physicians could truly understand anatomy, noting many surgeons, including Ambroise Paré, were well trained in the subject.[34] In 1615, another anonymous responder to Riolan asserted the physician had 'vomit[ed]' many insults against Saint-Côme. This author included passages in Latin in his pamphlet, arguing that surgeons such as Charles Guillemeau provided excellent anatomy lessons in that language.[35] Given that at least one scholar has identified the author of this pamphlet as royal surgeon Guillemeau himself, it seems the writer was concerned with protecting his own status rather than exclusively that of Habicot.[36]

This brief account simplifies a debate that spawned at least 15 publications between 1613 and 1618. It is nevertheless clear that the exchange went far beyond a disagreement over the proper identification of some marvelous bones. Riolan's multiple responses to Habicot's original publication, and the various replies the physician incurred, indicate that issues of institutional and professional identity were at stake. Even as Riolan put forward his own theories of the bones in order to discredit Habicot's ideas, the physician was especially eager to denounce all the surgeons of Saint-Côme as ignorant. Just as earlier physicians had attacked Paré for overstepping his position as a barber-surgeon blessed with royal privilege, so Riolan accused Habicot – also a former barber-surgeon – and his *confrères* of neglecting to defer to the superiority of the physicians of the Faculté de Médecine.

The lengthy debate involving Habicot and Riolan is particularly interesting because in addition to providing information about how critical publications were perceived during the early modern period, it reveals how such disputes developed. In the early stages of the quarrel, most authors did not sign their names to publications. Riolan endorsed his first response in 1613 'par un escholier en médecine' [by a novice in medicine], implying that even a young student of medicine could spot the errors in Habicot's arguments. The unknown *compagnon chirurgien* from Montpellier who responded to the physician's critique, however, explicitly identified Riolan the younger as Habicot's adversary. Guillemeau followed suit in 1615, naming Riolan as the offending author but neglecting to take credit for his own publication.[37] Apparently, the identities of all the primary characters were nevertheless common knowledge. The names of participants regularly appear in period script in the margins of surviving pamphlets.[38] The supposed anonymity of authors seems related less to the desire to conceal identity than to the conventions of such critical publications. Remaining anonymous was in any case unlikely, given the limited membership of both the Faculté and Saint-Côme; when not united with barber-surgeons the latter was particularly small.[39] By 1618, Riolan no longer maintained any pretense of anonymity, signing an extended attack on Habicot which essentially amalgamated the two earlier critiques of the surgeon.

The format of these publications suggests they were written for a limited, insider audience. They typically proceed by refuting the previously published argument point by point, assuming the reader is already familiar with the original tract. Although sections of the offending claims are often reproduced in order to be immediately disproved, sometimes only the page numbers of the earlier publication are noted. This organization implies the reader has both the first publication and the response to it in mind, and possibly even in hand, reading them side by side. Riolan claimed to have read a treatise and its rejoinder in this manner. The physician argued that when a copy of the first critique of Habicot – attributed to Riolan himself – 'fell into his hands' during the Christmas holidays, he carefully compared it with the surgeon's book on oversized bones. While finding the initial criticism of Habicot's text 'diligent,' Riolan argued he was obliged to write another assessment of it to refute even more of the surgeon's insupportable errors.[40]

Though ideally read as a series, it is less clear how the documents related to the dispute between Habicot and Riolan were distributed. Several pamphlets acknowledge neither the name of the author nor the publisher, but others give credit to publishers known to produce medical material. Although these publishers may have supplied readers with critical pamphlets, there is also evidence that such documents were circulated by individual authors. Another medical dispute refers directly to this method of dissemination. Monsieur Simon, a master surgeon of Saint-Côme, accused fellow master surgeon Philippe Peu of manually disbursing his written attack on François Mauriceau amongst their surgical colleagues.[41] While Simon meant to cast aspersions on Peu's action, he nevertheless alluded to the manufacture of published criticism as a personal quest presumably undertaken at personal expense and intended for a particular audience.

Members of the surgical audience who received a copy of such a pamphlet were likely not learning about the dispute for the first time. Simon narrated the circumstances of the production of his own critical publication of 1695, which denigrated Peu's obstetrical treatise, *La pratique des accouchemens*, published in 1694. Upset with a particular case study in Peu's book, Simon claimed to have confronted the surgeon with his accusations at an assembly of the members of Saint-Côme.[42] According to Simon, Peu challenged him to prove in writing that the case reported in the treatise was indeed false. If Simon did print such a critique, Peu threatened, he could certainly expect a response in turn. Simon's version of the dispute indicates both that it first erupted in the presence of fellow surgeons and that Peu considered a written composition to constitute an official accusation, one demanding a response from him.

Simon took up the challenge launched by Peu in order to defend his own reputation. The case study to which Simon so vehemently objected was based on an encounter in 1680. In his treatise, Peu criticized an operation undertaken by an unnamed 'young surgeon' who had attempted against the advice of Peu to remove the fleshy coherence obstructing a female client's vagina.[43] Recognizing himself as the overconfident and ultimately incompetent young surgeon in Peu's tale, Simon went on the defensive. He denounced the story as a fabulous work of Peu's imagination, and proceeded to contradict every one of the older surgeon's claims. When Peu declared himself the 'oldest and most learned' of the doctor and two other surgeons called to consult about the case, Simon insisted Peu was the most 'mal instruit' [badly instructed or unskilled].[44] Simon mocked not only Peu's scanty anatomical knowledge but also his 'mediocre reputation,' noting that the wealthy female client had first summoned Simon, a surgeon from her own neighbourhood, not Peu.[45]

Even as he was concerned to provide evidence that he was and always had been a competent surgeon, Simon attacked the character of his adversary. According to Simon, Peu was overcome with envy and ambition, inventing the case study in the hope of increasing his own reputation.[46] Peu was furthermore ignorant, imperious, and inexperienced in the practice of childbirth and delivery. When Peu worked at the Hôtel-Dieu, Simon continued, he delivered only those women infected with venereal disease. Peu never attended pregnant or newly-delivered women because the head midwife, Madame Le Vacher, preferred the assistance of Monsieur [Paul] Portal, a younger man. Peu thus blatantly lied when he claimed on page 38 of his treatise that he was called to the birthing room at the Hôtel-Dieu.[47] Linking Peu's failures with his advancing age at several points, Simon poked fun at Peu's balding head and increasingly decrepit appearance, as discussed in Chapter 4.[48]

In contrast to disputes involving members of different medical communities, Simon's attack on Peu did not question surgical training in general, but focused on that of his rival in particular. His critique nevertheless continued to emphasize issues of medical knowledge and experience, as had the disputes involving both Paré and Habicot. At the same time, questions of status remained at issue in Peu's case study as well as Simon's response to it. Whereas the written exchanges between members of Saint-Côme and the Faculté had invoked the hierarchy of their rival institutions, Simon and Peu articulated distinctions between members of the same community. Age emerged as a contested determinant of status among the surgeons. Peu's attention to Simon's youth, and Simon's disparagement of Peu's advanced age can be related to contemporary discussions about the ideal age of the male midwife; he should be neither so young as to lack appropriate training, nor so old as to want strength and energy.[49] Social status appeared as another factor dividing members of the same corporation. Simon alluded to Peu's mediocre rank and living conditions when he boasted that women of quality preferred to call the younger surgeon who inhabited their exclusive *quartier*.

Simon's published critique of Peu is conventional in many ways, quickly turning from a defence of his own actions to an attack on Peu's knowledge and character. It resembles other written disputes, including the one involving surgeon men-midwives

Peu and Mauriceau. Simon alluded to the earlier debate in his critique of Peu, allying himself with Mauriceau.[50] This apparently well-known altercation was sparked by another section of Peu's obstetrical treatise. The author devoted a chapter entitled 'Du tire-tête' [On the head-puller] to the condemnation of an instrument designed by Mauriceau to remove dead infants from the womb in cases of impacted head presentation[51] (Figure 5.1). Mauriceau quickly responded to Peu's criticisms in a brief admonitory *avertissement* appended to his own treatise, *Observations sur la grossesse et l'accouchement des femmes*, published in 1695.[52] When Peu reacted in turn by publishing his *Réponse à l'avertissement*, he received another critique from Mauriceau which outlined no less than 160 errors in Peu's obstetrical treatise. Although Mauriceau's second, longer critique of Peu's treatise has not survived, Peu's reply to these criticisms remains extant. Entitled *Réponse de M. Peu aux observations particulières de M. Mauriceau sur la grossesse et l'accouchement des femmes* [Response of M. Peu to the particular observations of M. Mauriceau on the pregnancy and delivery of women], and likely published in late 1694 or early 1695, Peu's 116-page-long publication refers in detail to Mauriceau's earlier pamphlet, providing a sense of the missing tract.[53]

In this debate, Peu and Mauriceau attempted to undermine each other's reputations as surgeon men-midwives, revealing what was considered essential to the dependable practice of that office. Both men argued that their rival lacked a longstanding, hands-on experience of childbirth. Like Simon, Mauriceau questioned the extent of Peu's practice at the Hôtel-Dieu, claiming that Peu had never delivered a single woman there.[54] In response, Peu provided certificates from administrators at the hospital, attesting to his extensive practice for over ten years at the institution. These official documents insisted that Peu's position as *compagnon chirurgien* and then *accoucheur* at the Hôtel-Dieu had enabled him to specialize in delivering women.[55] Peu then questioned the first-hand experience of Mauriceau, claiming the younger man had worked at the hospital for a mere four months in 1660 and yet professed to have delivered 300 women: 'You three hundred women in four months, and me not a single one in ten years!'[56] Attaching another certificate – from Jacques Petit, *chirurgien ordinaire* at the Hôtel-Dieu for some ten years – Peu supported his assertion that Mauriceau had delivered only four or five women during his stay at the hospital.[57] Peu was amazed that a man so much younger than he would pretend to have acquired more experience.

Surgical education and institutional identity were not at stake in the contest between Peu and Mauriceau. Instead, both men insisted on the sheer number of women they had delivered over the years, arguing that the lying-in chamber was the true school for surgeon men-midwives. This emphasis helps to explain why numerous case studies providing details of difficult deliveries were included in their pamphlets as well as obstetrical treatises. As these cases provided concrete evidence

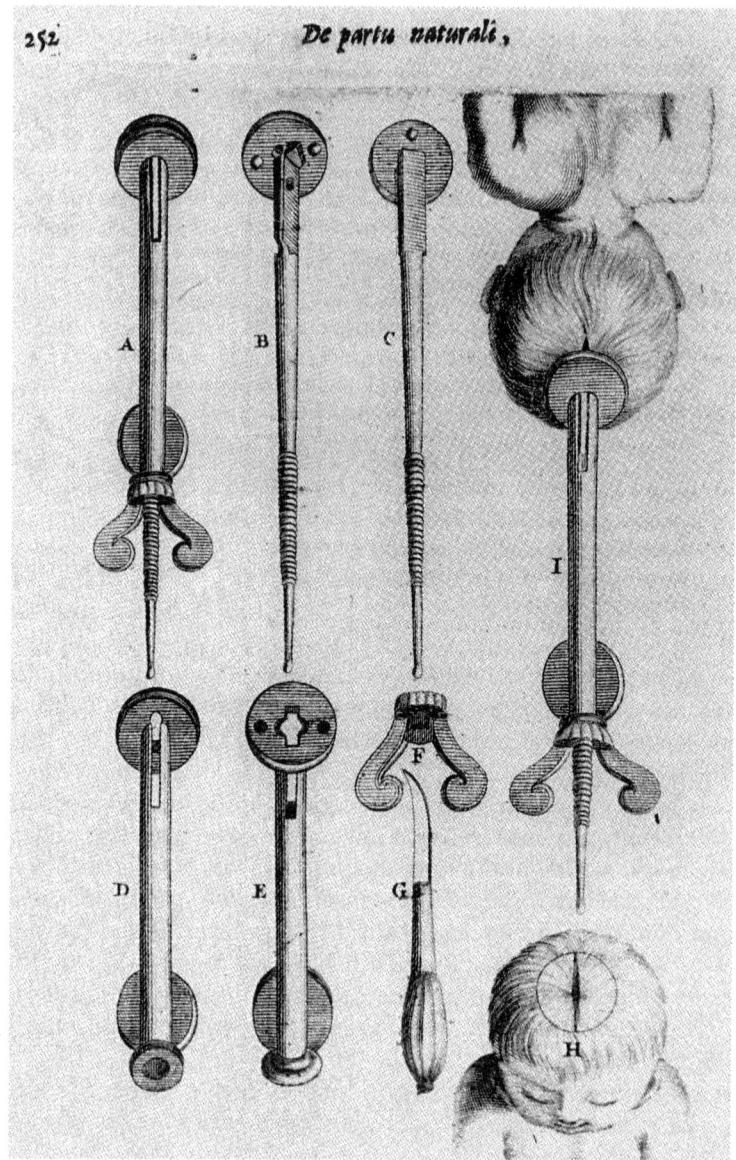

Figure 5.1 *Tire-tête*, from François Mauriceau's *De mulierum praegnantium*, 1681, Paris. Courtesy of the Edward G. Miner Library, University of Rochester Medical Center, Rochester, NY

of experience, they were both attacked and defended in critical publications. Mauriceau asserted that the observations in his own treatise were reliable, true, and based on personal experience, unlike the falsified accounts found in Peu's *La pratique des accouchemens*.[58] A better title for that treatise, Mauriceau affirmed, would be *La mauvaise pratique des accouchemens* [The bad practice of childbirth] in order to prevent young surgeons and midwives from falling into error.[59] Throughout his *Réponse*, Peu explained Mauriceau's scepticism about the case studies in his treatise as a simple lack of experience on the part of his rival.[60] According to Peu, Mauriceau did not accept the facts put forth in the treatise because he had not practised midwifery long enough to have had similar encounters.

Neither Peu nor Mauriceau was satisfied with declaring the other an inexperienced liar. Both men went even further, accusing his rival of being a dangerous murderer unfit to practise in the birthing chamber. In his treatise of 1694, Peu charged Mauriceau with killing children with his *tire-tête* because its use necessitated inserting the upper plate into the child's cranium before applying traction. According to Peu, the operator had to presuppose that the child was dead, or else believe it was permissible to destroy the child in order to save the mother when nothing else could be done. He insisted that such an approach was not only both criminal and barbarous, but also contrary to theological teaching.[61] In his angry response to Peu's accusations, Mauriceau maintained his head puller was never intended for use on live children. He argued that Peu posed the real threat to women and especially children through his use of *crochets*. Mauriceau directed readers to 11 different pages in Peu's treatise which described the 'horrible murders' Peu himself had committed.[62]

In their attempts to defame each other, Peu and Mauriceau reinforced the negative image of the man-midwife as an instrument-wielding butcher best avoided, even as they attempted to portray their own practices in a more positive light. A stereotype of the bad man-midwife emerges from these debates; he is impetuous, ignorant, bereft of an adequate experience of childbirth, and primarily interested in the vainglorious escalation of his reputation rather than the safety of his clients. This negative image of the man-midwife is at odds with representations of the beneficial male assistant as robust, dependable, in control of his emotions, and possessed of a reassuring appearance, analysed in the previous chapter. The injurious man-midwife was associated with qualities regularly identified with the unscrupulous female midwife. She too was described as vain, unskilled, overconfident in her abilities, emotionally unstable in the lying-in chamber, and prone to the ruthless treatment of women and children.[63] By displaying many of these same qualities, the bad man-midwife succumbed to feminine weaknesses, rather than distinguishing himself from them.

The defective male midwife was not portrayed, however, in exactly the same manner as the treacherous female midwife. Although the charges made against him echoed contemporary accounts of the ignorant and imprudent female midwife, she was repeatedly faulted for her lack of surgical training and theoretical knowledge, especially anatomy. Surgeon men-midwives likewise questioned their male rivals' knowledge of anatomy, issues also contested in earlier debates between physicians and surgeons. Both Simon and Mauriceau ridiculed Peu's anatomical learning, with the latter criticizing Peu's description of the structure of the umbilical cord.[64] Faulty surgeon men-midwives were nevertheless primarily accused of wanting an extensive hands-on experience of childbirth, the kind of practical knowledge typically associated with female midwives.

Negative accounts of male midwives should be approached carefully, just as the repeated criticisms of early modern female midwives are now questioned by scholars. Derisive descriptions of surgeon men-midwives do not confirm that these men were indeed inexperienced bunglers in the lying-in chamber, however unskilled and rash particular male midwives may have been. On the contrary, debates in which men attacked each other reveal the conventional nature of these critiques, which drew attention to deficient medical practices as well as dubious character traits. Furthermore, the debates reveal that early modern French men-midwives were not united in a common approach to intervening in childbirth. After all, Peu criticized Mauriceau's use of the *tire-tête,* advocating the more traditional *crochet* instead.[65] Other male midwives condemned the use of instruments altogether. In 1611, physician Jacques Fontaine accused men-midwives who used instruments of acting ruthlessly to achieve results at the expense of women and children.[66] Surgeon man-midwife Cosme Viardel echoed Fontaine in 1671 by arguing that surgeons should never use instruments in the lying-in chamber, relying instead on their skilled and supple hands.[67] Even those surgeon men-midwives who used instruments urged their fellow practitioners to be cautious, employing tools only when it was absolutely necessary, and doing so with the utmost discretion so as not to frighten clients.[68] Yet instrument use was not the only nor even the most important issue in evaluations of early modern French male midwives. Texts written by surgeon men-midwives predominately distinguish between practitioners on the basis of their social status, age, reputation, character, and degree of personal experience in the lying-in chamber.

Relative Maternity and the Labour of Men-midwives

Although the previous discussion focused on pamphlet wars between medical men, surgeon men-midwives also launched criticism at fellow practitioners in their obstetrical treatises. When authors recounted a difficult delivery to which they had been called, they often condemned the shoddy practices of the female midwife who had initially assisted the labouring woman. Surgeon men-midwives additionally referred, however, to any inadequate male practitioner called to assist the client before their own arrival. Noting that incompetent predecessors were either too young, too old, or simply baffled by the medical situation confronting them, male authors described themselves as heroes who entered the lying-in chamber in order to rectify the situation.[69] Surgeon men-midwives thereby extolled their own abilities by differentiating themselves from less capable colleagues.

Mauriceau regularly employed this strategy in the treatise he first published in 1668. In one case, he described the difficult labour and eventual death of his own sister both to cast aspersions on the surgeon man-midwife first called to deliver her and portray himself in a sympathetic light. To support his argument that pregnant women should be delivered promptly if they suffered a continual loss of blood, Mauriceau offered a lengthy account of the demise of his sister.[70] He recounted how the young woman, not yet 21 years of age, fell to her knees while approximately eight and a half months pregnant with her fifth child. Three days later, she experienced a great loss of blood and called a female midwife for assistance. According to Mauriceau, this midwife was not well informed and so recommended waiting for labour and delivery to proceed naturally, declaring that her feeble client had nothing to fear. After three or four more hours, however, the bleeding had not diminished, prompting the midwife to summon a surgeon. As Mauriceau was unavailable, a *chirurgien accoucheur* considered 'the most skilful man among all the surgeons' was invited instead.[71] Mauriceau related with disgust how, upon seeing his sister, the unnamed surgeon man-midwife simply declared she was a dead woman, recommended that the last rites be administered, and returned to his own home. When Mauriceau finally received news of his sister's plight, he ran to her bedside, only to be greeted with 'a spectacle so pitiful, that all the passions of [his] soul were agitated.'[72] In this distressed state, Mauriceau vacillated before attempting to deliver her, noting his hesitation was fuelled by the opinions of both the surgeon man-midwife and female midwife, who advised against delivery. After hours of delay, Mauriceau finally delivered his sister by *podalic* method, in time to baptize the child, but not to save the mother.

At first glance it is difficult to see how this story could reflect well on Mauriceau. After all, his emotional distress and lack of conviction contributed to his sister's decline. Why, then, did the author expound on the case at length? Mauriceau claimed that he told the sad tale to benefit the public, informing others who might be faced with a similar situation.[73] The author also strove, however, to shift the blame for his sister's death, directing it toward the female midwife and surgeon man-midwife called before him. Focusing on the failings of the male practitioner, Mauriceau accused him of malice, ignorance, and of having displayed 'false prudence' in order to safeguard his own reputation.[74] According to Mauriceau, this surgeon man-midwife had abandoned the young woman, failing to deliver her when there was still time to save her. Describing his own emotional distress in detail, Mauriceau argued that it had contributed to his bad judgment in trusting such a treacherous man.[75]

Yet in emphasizing his unstable emotions Mauriceau risked associating himself with the unruly passions of the dangerous man-midwife, rather than the qualities of the well governed male practitioner. Perhaps this risk was worth taking, for Mauriceau's impassioned descriptions of his affected state linked him with his sister, her labour, and her anguish. Before beginning his narrative, Mauriceau claimed the ink he used to transcribe the painful memory seemed to be made of blood: 'as much as in that pitiable and fatal occasion, [when] I saw to my great regret, pouring before me a part of my own.'[76] Mauriceau reaffirmed the blood tie between himself and his sister later in the story, describing 'the prodigious loss of this blood, which came from the same source as mine.'[77] With these statements, Mauriceau conflated his sister's blood, which flows unceasingly throughout the story, with his own. Just as the blood loss caused his sister to grow weak, so too did Mauriceau suffer during the course of her illness, losing control of his senses as well as his resolve as a surgeon man-midwife. Whereas her ordeal ended with death, however, his continued unabated. In a subsequent chapter of his treatise, Mauriceau referred again to the dangers of blood loss during pregnancy but refused to repeat the story of his sister's demise, claiming to be 'too sadly affected with it.'[78] In the end, the author had recounted his sister's suffering to produce a story about what he called his 'own experiences.'[79]

Mauriceau's extended account of his sister's labour linked him with a female family member, displaying his intimate understanding of childbirth as well as the losses that could be associated with it. This case study differs from the others in Mauriceau's treatise; they tend to be briefer, reporting a female client's symptoms along with the interventions performed by the stoic surgeon man-midwife. Mauriceau's description of his sister's dangerous condition was not, however, entirely unique. Accounts of the pregnancies and labours of female relatives recur not only in his obstetrical treatise, but also in publications by other surgeon men-midwives. In an earlier section of Mauriceau's treatise, for example, the author described the pregnancy and labour of his own mother. He did so to dispute the theory of the maternal imagination, which held that a pregnant woman's desires could affect her unborn children, causing birthmarks as well as deformities.[80] According to Mauriceau, a woman's imagination could influence her child only at the beginning of the pregnancy, especially the moment of conception. He referred to his own gestation – that is, to his mother's gestation of him – to prove that once a child was formed in the womb, the maternal imagination could have no influence on it.[81] Mauriceau explained that while his mother was pregnant with him, his six-year-old brother contracted small pox and eventually died. When Mauriceau was born the next day, he sported five or six red spots. It would not be correct to think, Mauriceau continued, that these marks stemmed from his mother's imagination. They were more likely caused by the contagious air she breathed while caring for her eldest son.

This air infected her blood, which in turn nourished the unborn Mauriceau and produced the red marks on his body.

In keeping with the story of his sister's death, Mauriceau emphasized the blood ties between him and his childbearing relative. He argued that his mother's contaminated blood was transferred to him, leaving visible but harmless traces. In both narratives, the author conflated male and female blood, identifying himself with the materiality of the maternal body. Mauriceau's physical experience of the pregnant female body is most conspicuous, however, in the description of him as an unborn child in the womb. While limiting the power of the maternal imagination by drawing attention to the fleshly nature of the connection between a mother and her unborn child, Mauriceau's tale also related his own experience.[82] It effectively portrayed the author's personal encounter with pregnancy, albeit as a child about to be born rather than a gestating mother. Like the case study of his suffering sister, Mauriceau's account of his mother's delivery of him displayed his bodily encounter with childbirth – the kind of encounter usually associated with female midwives. At the same time, Mauriceau indicated that he was familiar with the story of his own birth because his mother and father had recounted it on several occasions.[83] He thus demonstrated knowledge of the kind of orally transmitted childbirth lore traditionally identified with birthing women and their female relatives.

While Mauriceau elaborated on the labours of his sister and mother, other male authors drew attention to the reproductive experiences of their wives. Surgeon man-midwife Pierre Dionis criticized his cousin Mauriceau's lack of personal encounters with childbirth by contrasting the fertility of their respective wives. In his obstetrical treatise, *Traité général des accouchemens*, published in 1718, Dionis ridiculed Mauriceau's claim that women should not engage in intercourse while pregnant, pointing out that his cousin's 46-year-long marriage was childless; significantly, he backed up his argument for the safety of such sexual relations by referring to his own wife, who had been pregnant and successfully given birth some 20 times.[84] This argument not only vaunted Dionis' virility, but simultaneously displayed that he had a much more direct and abundant knowledge of pregnancy than Mauriceau. Although the force of his claims relied heavily on reference to his wife, this example indicates how Dionis tried to associate himself with a personal experience of childbirth rather than exclusively with its theoretical construction.

Dionis stressed Mauriceau's childlessness in another passage in his treatise, which praised fecundity for both its perpetuation and fortification of families; a husband's love increased if his wife was fruitful.[85] Furthermore, a desire for children was only natural. Mauriceau might pretend to disdain the pursuit of successors, Dionis argued, but 'all those who have never had children, and who have lost the hope of having them, speak like Mauriceau.'[86] Dionis claimed that Mauriceau clearly longed for children of his own. By repeatedly insisting on the sterility of the disillusioned Mauriceau, Dionis strove to undermine the authority of his famous cousin. He questioned Mauriceau's personal experience of childbirth and child rearing, implying that a childless man could have little authentic knowledge of pregnant women and the love of children.

Like Dionis, Guillaume Mauquest de La Motte referred to a husband's experience of his wife's parturient body, in this case to support his claims about the activity of the child in the womb. In the treatise he first published in 1721, Mauquest de La Motte argued that the unborn child often moved very vigorously within the maternal body, noting any man could make such an observation 'when he is in bed with his wife.'[87] In this instance addressing a male audience, the surgeon man-midwife invoked a commonsense understanding of pregnancy – one held by men rather than exclusively by women. The author implied that men's knowledge of childbirth, including his own, was in some part based on an intimate experience of it within the family. Pregnant wives provided one of the means by which men attained a first-hand comprehension of gestation and birth.

Although surgeon man-midwife Philippe Peu also referred to his personal experiences with childbearing women in his obstetrical treatise of 1694, he did not describe the deliveries of his sister, mother, or wife. Instead, he recounted how he had avoided marrying a deformed woman bound to have problems giving birth. Peu explained that when he was first established as a surgeon, it was suggested that he marry a young, wealthy, and religious woman, whose father he admired.[88] The young surgeon avoided the marriage, however, because the potential bride was rickety on one side of her body. Peu reported that when another man married her, she soon became pregnant, but because of her physical impediment was often subject to falls and died before giving birth. In contrast to the stories of other surgeon men-midwives, Peu argued that his medical training provided him with a superior understanding of women's fecundity, affecting his personal life rather than the other way around. However, like other authors, Peu drew attention to the connection between medical knowledge and family life, indicating that the two were closely aligned. The woman he almost married was another 'case study' used to illustrate the perception and learning of the authoritative surgeon man-midwife.

When early modern French surgeon men-midwives recounted stories of their female relatives or potential relatives, they provided evidence of their intimate understanding of childbirth. In some ways, these passages echo the writings of female midwives, who also referred to their personal experiences of pregnancy and birth in order to defend particular beliefs. As indicated in Chapter 3, Louise Bourgeois invoked her own maternity when insisting that a child in the womb could perform its somersault long before the actual delivery. She also mocked women who had given birth only a few times, and thus lacked a substantial comprehension of reproduction.[89] Dionis similarly criticized those men-midwives with a deficient experience of paternity, targeting the childless Mauriceau. Even as French surgeon men-midwives argued that they surpassed female midwives in their understanding of medical theory, the value of a bodily comprehension of childbirth was not simply renounced.

In fact, surgeon men-midwives regularly referred to the physical labour they undertook while assisting at difficult births. Mauriceau, for example, insisted the work was so taxing that even in the middle of winter surgeon men-midwives could find themselves covered in drops of sweat.[90] Fellow practitioners Portal, Peu, and Amand similarly described the physical pain and exhaustion they endured while performing their roles as male midwives.[91] Mauquest de La Motte was the most explicit, claiming one of the women he delivered in 1686 was out of her bed quickly, but 'the fatigue was so great that [he] was not well for several days.'[92] In another case he argued that after a particularly trying delivery the birthing woman's friends had to lay him down on a mattress before the fire, as if he was an *accouchée* [newly-delivered woman] recovering from labour.[93] Surgeon men-midwives implied that their own bodily labour substituted for and even surpassed that of the ill mother, suggesting the men had themselves given birth and suffered while doing it. Though Sarah Stone claimed to have endured physical pain for a full week after assisting at a particularly gruelling delivery, female midwives made such assertions less frequently.[94]

For the most part there is an important difference between the personal accounts of childbirth published by men and women. Female midwives could make reference to their own bodily experiences of maternity, but male practitioners were obliged to invoke their roles as brothers, sons, fathers, husbands, suitors, or birthing assistants. A childless female midwife such as Justine Siegemund alluded to her physical experiences of menstruation in order to reinforce her ability to serve parturient women.[95] The infertile Mauriceau, however, compensated by referring to the corporeal experiences of his sister and mother as well as the bodily exhaustion he suffered in the lying-in chamber. Even if surgeon men-midwives had fathered children, their experiences of maternity were less direct, necessarily mediated through the bodies of their wives. Yet some men claimed women's maternal experiences as their own.

How should surgeon men-midwives' accounts of their 'own' bodily experiences of maternity be understood? First of all, these narratives can be placed within a wider context, as they were not entirely unique. The image of male midwife who 'lies in' after assisting at a delivery resonates with, for example, accounts of the ritual of the *couvade* apparently practised into the nineteenth century in northern France as well as the Basque regions of Spain.[96] This custom required the husband of a pregnant woman to take to his bed, simulating the pains of labour and recovery from childbirth. The male's performance as mother has been variously interpreted by scholars, especially anthropologists. Some of them understand the 'labouring' man as asserting his patriarchal right to the child, while others see his actions in a more positive light, as an incorporation of maternal perceptions in preparation for fatherhood.[97]

In addition to folk tradition, literary texts could associate men with a bodily experience of maternity. Scholar Kirk Read argues that the representation of breastfeeding men was commonplace in sixteenth-century French literature. The poet Pierre de Ronsard, for example, figured his male teacher as a nursing mother.[98] According to Read, it was possible to praise the concept of the breastfeeding man during the early modern period because of the 'quasi hermaphroditic' conception of the body, described by literary critic Thomas Laqueur.[99] Laqueur argues that from antiquity through the early modern period a 'one-sex model' of the human body posited a kind of anatomical sameness between women and men.[100] Although similar in structure, women's genitals were less perfect than men's because they were turned inside out and lodged within the body. While exceptional women could attain bodily perfection if increased heat forced their genitals outside, men had the innate capacity to perform female as well as male functions. Apparently, men's maternal potential did not threaten their masculinity. On the contrary, Read concludes that the 'masculinized maternity' produced in the theme of the breastfeeding man empowered men's writing, with femininity providing the basis on which men related to each other.[101]

Men who gave birth surpassed even those male mothers who nursed. Childbearing men were regularly featured in both literary and medical texts during the early modern period.[102] In *Le progrès de la médecine* [The progress of medicine], 1697, for example, editor Claude Brunet collected the medical reports of various practitioners, including one concerning male pregnancy. The story, related by a 'reliable' but anonymous source, described the secret encounters of a Cistercian monk and a nun in June of 1696.[103] While the couple engaged in the 'lively caressing' of each other's 'lower parts,' they apparently did not have intercourse. Nevertheless, the monk's passions fermented his semen, causing the painful enlargement of his right testicle. When surgeons and physicians first amputated and then dissected this testicle, they discovered it contained more than the tumour they expected to find. Evidence of a fleshy mass complete with solid bones and a cranium surrounded by an afterbirth convinced the medical practitioners that the monk's testicle incorporated a child. The report concluded that this phenomenon favoured the views of animaculists who believed male semen was replete with 'very tiny animals' able to reproduce independently of women.[104]

The narrator went on to recount a male birth that supposedly took place in 1330 in a Flemish village. In this case, a man became pregnant after mocking his wife while she was in labour, imitating her grimaces and postures.[105] Later on, a painful tumour developed in his right buttock, and continued to grow for nine months. The living child finally pulled from this swelling was a boy awarded the name of his father, Louis Roossel. According to the author, the father's impassioned imitation of his wife had caused the semen circulating through his body to ferment, rendering him fertile. The story ended with a consideration of why men did not become pregnant more often, given their obvious ability to reproduce. The author asserted that men were greatly inconvenienced by birth, suffering more pain than women. Women's organs were thus more disposed to childbirth, despite men's capacity for it.

Accounts of men giving birth as well as breastfeeding feature male fecundity. References to nursing affirm men's ability to nourish other men, binding them together while removing women from the picture. In a similar way, tales of male childbirth secure the paternal connection – the Flemish man gives birth to his own son – while celebrating maternity without women. Both accounts of male childbirth noted by Brunet drew attention to the potency of male semen, insisting that it alone was capable of engendering children. This emphasis was in keeping with ongoing fantasies about the possibility of male generation. Male semen had long been considered the productive element in childbirth. According to Aristotle, women exclusively contributed matter to the developing child, but even the 'two semen' theory propounded in the Hippocratic and Galenic corpuses asserted that male seed was more powerful than the seed produced by women.[106] The act of insemination, even self-insemination, was thus identified with manliness, not femininity or hermaphroditism, during the early modern period.

Male fecundity was also featured in obstetrical treatises, though without surgeon men-midwives describing either themselves or other men actually giving birth. Dionis drew attention to his own virility most directly, asserting that he had impregnated his wife some 20 times. The productivity of surgeon men-midwives, however, was more often displayed in accounts of the number of deliveries they had attended, as well as their heroic efforts within the lying-in chamber, physically intervening to save women and children. Male fruitfulness was furthermore linked with the texts they published. Authors of obstetrical treatises occasionally referred to the generation of their books. Both Mauriceau and Peu called their books the 'fruit' of their labours, a striking expression given that unborn children were often described as unripe fruit during the early modern period.[107] Peu nevertheless accused Mauriceau of having given birth to his second treatise – a 'monster' – prematurely, implying the younger man had published it before spending enough time labouring as a *chirurgien accoucheur*.[108] Peu's statement alluded to his view that treatises should encompass a life's work, with case studies spanning many years of practice.[109] Surgeon men-midwives Jacques Guillemeau, Barthélemy Saviard, and Mauquest de La Motte similarly indicated they had published treatises after a full career, drawing on a long experience with childbirth.[110] They portrayed their work in the lying-in chamber as a kind of gestation period that led to the production of books. Like Ronsard's depiction of his lactating male mentor, a masculine form of maternity both authorized surgeon men-midwives' writing and enriched their texts.

Did these surgeon men-midwives thereby appropriate maternity to increase their own power, establishing their reputations at the expense of the feminine? In their texts, male authors of obstetrical treatises frequently spoke for women, interpreted female bodies, and usurped the position of both labouring and newly-delivered women. Understanding these representations as appropriations of maternity might seem to be only too obvious, given that the men operated within the birthing chamber, traditionally a feminine domain supervised by female midwives. Yet narratives of birth penned by surgeon men-midwives also betray a continuing respect for the maternal body, its productive abilities, and the pain it endured. Even as pregnancy was often linked with illness and disease, maternity was not entirely medicalized in obstetrical treatises. Vivid tales of labouring sisters, mothers, and wives indicate that childbirth was also represented as a physical act of fleshly transformation bound up with emotions and impacting on a broader community – one that included men. In many ways, maternity was portrayed as desirable in the obstetrical treatises penned by surgeon men-midwives, even if particular births ended in disaster.

The work of historian Gianna Pomata offers an alternative method for understanding the ways in which surgeon men-midwives attempted to associate themselves with maternal embodiment. Analysing descriptions of male menstruation in early modern European texts, Pomata explains that certain men were thought to discharge excess blood periodically, from their genitals, noses, haemorrhoids, or other bodily openings.[111] Menstruating men were neither stigmatized nor feminized. Instead, their courses were often depicted in glowing terms, associated with longevity, fertility, and the maintenance of general well-being, just as regular flows signified health in women. According to Pomata, this longstanding phenomenon challenges Laqueur's assertion that the male body was always considered the paradigm for human physiology during the early modern period, the theory informing Read's interpretation of breastfeeding men.[112] Pomata argues that male menstruation offers one instance in which the male body was understood through the model provided by female physiology. Accounts of bleeding men reveal a 'deep curiosity and respect' for the female body, one which endured throughout the early modern period.[113]

Surgeon men-midwives' attempts to associate themselves with childbirth could provide another case in which the female body set the standard for men. Critical pamphlets as well as obstetrical treatises indicate that an immediate, physical experience of childbirth continued to be valued, and that many male practitioners attempted to identify themselves with it. This evidence suggests that the experienced female body remained the norm in the lying-in chamber throughout the early modern period, a norm to which men had to adapt or else risk having questions raised about their authority. The point should not be overstated; surgeon men-midwives certainly criticized female midwives, viewing their bodies as limits to theoretical knowledge.

Yet it offers an important corrective to interpretations that understand obstetrical treatises to have imposed male knowledge on women, with no regard for the practical understanding of maternity traditionally associated with female midwives.

Conclusions

Early modern French obstetrical treatises contain more contradictions than have previously been realized. The physical experience of maternity remained a powerful ideal in these sources, an ideal that would seem to favour the continued practice of female midwives. It was therefore one which surgeon men-midwives had simultaneously to downplay and work hard to display. Even as male authors disdained the purely empirical understanding of childbirth supposedly held by female midwives, they also condemned fellow male practitioners if these men lacked practical experience. Surgeon men-midwives argued that men with an extensive hands-on experience in the lying-in chamber – especially those with wives and children of their own – could incorporate the physical qualities of female midwives, while surpassing the women in terms of theoretical knowledge. All the same, obstetrical treatises convey an ongoing anxiety about surgeon men-midwives' potential lack of a sufficiently personal and physical comprehension of childbirth, particularly when male authors defended themselves against accusations of inexperience in the lying-in chamber and ignorance of the parturient body.

In addition to highlighting the contested status of maternal experience, this chapter offered a fuller appreciation of medical criticism. Male attacks on female midwives have often been considered in isolation from the broader spectrum of early modern medical criticism, implying that women alone were accused of ignorance and incompetence. Attending to the conventional nature of such complaints reveals how they both converged and diverged from those directed at male practitioners. The well-known pamphlet war involving Louise Bourgeois provides a case in point. In 1627, Marie de Bourbon-Montpensier, sister-in-law to Louis XIII, died after being delivered by Bourgeois, and Queen Marie de Médicis ordered an autopsy. The report, published by ten royal physicians and surgeons, did not state a precise cause of death, but significantly noted that a piece of the placenta remained in the Princess' gangrenous womb.[114] As removal of the afterbirth was traditionally the responsibility of the female midwife, Bourgeois understood herself to be blamed for the death. She quickly launched a rebuttal attacking the authors of the report as both ignorant and malicious, referring to her longstanding practice of midwifery as the basis for her superior understanding of the anatomy of the womb.[115] Bourgeois' denunciation of the autopsy report in turn received a reply – attributed to Charles Guillemeau though perhaps written by more than one medical man – which directly implicated her in the death of Madame de Bourbon-Montpensier. Guillemeau criticized her presumption in challenging the medical opinions of her male superiors, arguing she had failed to perform well that which was in fact her duty – the gentle delivery of both child and afterbirth, as well as the subsequent care of the newly-delivered woman.[116]

In her comprehensive analysis of this pamphlet war, literary scholar Wendy Perkins frames it as a gender conflict between male and female midwives, as well as theory and practice.[117] Further nuances are revealed, however, when the dispute is compared with other exchanges, especially the earlier one involving Habicot and Riolan. Like the men involved in this pamphlet war, Bourgeois accused her adversaries of lacking adequate anatomical learning as well as vicious behaviour. Claiming the men had less experience than she had, she offered them an anatomy lesson to display her superior knowledge of the womb. By doing so, the royal midwife challenged the medical hierarchy. At the same time, she exhibited her comprehension of the practice of medical criticism, as well as her facility in producing the kinds of arguments typically associated with men. The printed rebuttal of her attack was equally standard. Guillemeau charged Bourgeois with impertinence in daring to offer those more knowledgeable than her a lesson in anatomy. He defended the medical hierarchy more than the individuals involved, just as he had done in his denunciation of Riolan's critique of Habicot twelve years earlier. Distinguishing Bourgeois from a good midwife, Guillemeau claimed she was the kind of unscrupulous woman capable of causing the death of a Princess. By responding to Bourgeois as a type of midwife rather than an individual, the author (or authors) employed the same approach Riolan used when he criticized Habicot by arguing that all surgeons were uneducated manual labourers bereft of anatomical knowledge. Though the written attack on Bourgeois was clearly meant to undermine her, it employed a set of strategies that were not always directed at women.

The claims made against Bourgeois were in many ways commonplace, but the potential harm they could cause was not. Women were disadvantaged in such exchanges. In contrast to the often protracted disputes involving men, Bourgeois did not produce a subsequent rebuttal to the damning reply of her male adversaries, nor did anyone leap to her defence, providing her with the kind of support Habicot had received. While several royal physicians had helped Bourgeois attain her post as royal midwife in 1601, there is no evidence they continued to champion her after the publication of the autopsy report. Female midwives officially held a lowly status in the medical hierarchy, which meant they had more 'superiors' interested in maintaining that position, and fewer allies who could benefit from protecting the women. That is part of the reason the written denunciation of Bourgeois effectively ended her career at court. There is no indication that the careers of Riolan and Habicot – as well as Simon, Peu, and Mauriceau – suffered irreparable damage when the men were attacked in print. The hierarchical structure of early modern French medicine should not, however, be overstated. For Bourgeois' case makes it clear that women did respond to negative evaluations of them, and obstetrical treatises demonstrate that women had advantages, notably their ability to claim a personal experience of maternity.

Notes

1.   For a discussion of the continuing 'diatribe' against traditional midwives in the French literature see Madeleine Lazard, 'Médecins contre matrones au 16e siècle: La difficile naissance de l'obstétrique,' Marc Bertrand, ed., *Popular Tradition and Learned Culture in France* (Saratoga: Anma Libri, 1985), 25–41, and Evelyne Berriot-Salvadore, *Les femmes dans la société française de la renaissance* (Geneva: Droz, 1990), 267–75. While not exhaustive, the following references indicate the recurrence of male criticism of female midwives in medical publications: Pierre Franco, *Chirurgie*, E. Nicaise, ed. (Geneva: Slatkine Reprints, 1972; orig. 1561), 236, Laurent Joubert, *Erreurs populaires* (Bordeaux, 1578), 347–52, Jacques Guillemeau, *De l'heureux accouchement des femmes* (Paris, 1609), 169, Jacques Duval, *Traité des hermaphrodits, parties genitales, accouchemens des femmes* (Rouen, 1612), 11, 57, 177, 196, François Mauriceau, *Des maladies des femmes grosses et accouchées* (Paris, 1668), 243–4, 259, 278, 350–51, Philippe Peu, *La pratique des accouchemens* (Paris, 1694), 25, 145, 155, 260–62, 403, Pierre Amand, *Nouvelles observations sur la pratique des accouchemens* (Paris, 1715), 161, 182, 215, and Pierre Dionis, *Traité général des accouchemens* (Paris, 1718), 203, 228, 261. Though now well-known, the diatribe by Gervais de la Tousche, *La Tres haute et tres souveraine science de l'art et industrie naturelle d'enfanter, contre la maudicte et perverse impericie des femmes que l'on appelle saiges femmes ou belles meres, lesquelles par leur ignorance font journellement perir une infinité de femmes et d'enfans à l'enfantement* (Paris, 1587) was unusual. Written by a 'gentleman' rather than a doctor, it urged women to give birth with no assistance whatsoever.

2.   Thomas Rogers Forbes, *The Midwife and the Witch* (New Haven: Yale University Press, 1966), viii.

3.   David Harley, 'Ignorant Midwives – a Persistent Stereotype,' *Society for the Social History of Medicine Bulletin* 28 (1981), 6–9.

4.   Doreen Evenden, *The Midwives of Seventeenth-Century London* (Cambridge: Cambridge University Press, 2000).

5.   Wendy Perkins, *Midwifery and Medicine in Early Modern France: Louise Bourgeois* (Exeter: University of Exeter Press, 1996), and Nina Rattner Gelbart, *The King's Midwife: A History and Mystery of Madame du Coudray* (Berkeley: University of California Press, 1998).

6.   Alison Klairmont Lingo, 'Empirics and Charlatans in Early Modern France: The Genesis of the Classification of the "Other" in Medical Practice,' *Journal of Social History* 19 (1986), 583–604.

7.   Laurence Brockliss and Colin Jones, *The Medical World of Early Modern France* (Oxford: Clarendon Press, 1997), 16.

8.   Cited in Philippe Peu, *Réponse de M. Peu aux observations particulières de M. Mauriceau sur la grossesse et l'accouchement des femmes* (n.l., n.d.), 12, 16.

9.   *Ibid.*, 3.

10.   Sarah Stone, *A Complete Practice of Midwifery* (London, 1737), vii, xi–xiii, and Elizabeth Nihell, *A Treatise on the Art of Midwifery* (London, 1760), ii–vi. Female midwives also regularly accused other female practitioners of being untrained and inexperienced. See Louise Bourgeois, *Observations diverses sur la stérilité, perte de fruict, foecondité, accouchements et maladies des femmes et enfants nouveaux naiz*, Françoise Olive, ed. (Paris: Côté-Femmes, 1992; orig. 1652), 56, 104, Stone, vi, and German midwife Anna Elisabeth Horenburg, who asserted in 1700: 'Unfortunately, there are far too many known cases of various and often grave mistakes and neglect in working with women in labor, which are made partially by the women themselves, but mostly by the ignorant and clumsy midwives, who are not sufficiently trained for such dangerous undertakings.' See Agnes Risko, '"Gott Zu Ehren, Dem Neben=Christen Zu Nutz...": Anna Elisabeth Horenburg's Manual for Midwives' (Ph.D. Diss., The Ohio State University, 1998), 161.

11.   Bourgeois, *Observations diverses*, 119, 143, and 197. See also Louise Bourgeois, *Fidelle relation de l'accouchement, maladie et ouverture du corps de feu Madame* (1627), reprinted in François Rouget and Colette H. Winn, eds, *Récit véritable de la naissance de messeigneurs et dames les enfans de France* (Geneva: Droz, 2000), 99–109, a pamphlet discussed below.

12.   Philippe Hecquet, *De l'indécence aux hommes d'accoucher les femmes* (Paris, 1708). Hecquet was also concerned with the competition *chirurgiens accoucheurs* posed to physicians. See Laurence Brockliss, 'The Medico-Religious Universe of an Early Eighteenth-Century Parisian Doctor: The Case of Philippe Hecquet,' Roger French and Andrew Wear, eds, *The Medical Revolution of the Seventeenth Century* (Cambridge: Cambridge University Press, 1989), 206.

13.   Wendy Perkins, 'Midwives versus Doctors: The Case of Louise Bourgeois,' *Seventeenth Century* 3 (1988), 135–57. See also Achille Chéreau, ed. and intro., *Les six couches de Marie de Médicis* (Paris: Léon Willem and Paul Daffis, 1875), 12–18.

14.   See my discussion of this issue in the Introduction.

15.   Adrian Wilson, *The Making of Man-Midwifery: Childbirth in England 1660–1770* (London: UCL Press, 1995), 65–144.

16.   François Mauriceau, *Des maladies des femmes grosses et accouchées* (Paris, 1668), 58–60, discussed below.

17.   For Paré's biography and medical theories see Ambroise Paré, *Oeuvres complètes d'Ambroise Paré*, 3 vol., J.-F. Malgaigne, ed. (Paris: Baillière, 1840–41), and Paule Dumaitre, *Ambroise Paré, chirurgien de quatre rois de France* (Paris: Librairie Académique Perrin Fondation Singer-Polignac, 1986). For Paré's writings on childbirth see Henri Stofft, 'Ambroise Paré, accoucheur,' *Histoire des sciences médicales* 32, 4 (1998), 399–407, and Paule Dumaître, 'Autour d'Ambroise Paré, ses élèves, ses amis,' *Histoire des sciences médicales* 30, 3 (1996), 351–7.

18.   Wallace B. Hamby, *Ambroise Paré: Surgeon of the Renaissance* (St. Louis: Warren H. Green, 1967), 153–6.

19.   Alison Klairmont Lingo, 'Print's Role in the Politics of Women's Health Care in Early Modern France,' Barbara B. Diefendorf and Carla Hesse, eds, *Culture and Identity in Early Modern Europe (1500–1800): Essays in Honor of Natalie Zemon Davis* (Ann Arbor: The University of Michigan Press, 1993), 207–8.

20.   Ambroise Paré, *Responce de M. Ambroise Paré, premier chirurgien du Roy, aux calomnies d'aucuns médecins, et chirurgiens, touchant ses oeuvres* (n.l., n.d.), 8–9. Despite presenting his case, the 1535 edict supporting physicians was reinstated by the Parlement. The outcome of the trial nevertheless remains unclear. Paré's treatise was eventually distributed for sale, suggesting the intervention of his royal patron may have been a factor.

21.   Ambroise Paré, *Des monstres et prodiges*, Jean Céard, ed. (Geneva: Droz, 1971), xiv–xvi.

22.   Jeanne Rigal, *La communauté des maîtres-chirurgiens jurés de Paris au XVIIe et au XVIIIe siècle* (Paris: Vigot Frères, 1936), 25–72, François Millepierres, *La vie quotidienne des médecins au temps du Molière* (Paris: Hachette, 1964), 169–87, Toby Gelfand, *Professionalizing Modern Medicine: Paris Surgeons and Medical Science and Institutions in the 18th Century* (Westport: Greenwood Press, 1980), 21–57, and Brockliss and Jones, *The Medical World of Early Modern France*, 170–229, 553–621.

23.   Brockliss and Jones, *The Medical World of Early Modern France*, 215.

24.   Franco, *Chirurgie*, E. Nicaise, ed., cxliii–cxlv. See also Nicaise's entire chapter: 'Histoire abrégée du collège de chirurgie,' cv–clii.

25.   Gelfand, *Professionalizing Modern Medicine*, 29–30.

26.   *Ibid.*, 62–3.

27.   *Ibid.*, 76.

28.   Nicolas Habicot, *Gigantostéologie, ou discours des os d'un géant* (Paris, 1613).

29.   Jean Riolan, fils, attr., *Gigantomachie, pour respondre à la Gigantostologie* (n.l., 1613).

30.   Jean Riolan, fils, attr., *L'imposture descouverte des os humains supposés et faussement attribués au roy Theutobochus* (Paris, 1614) and *Gigantologie. Discours sur la grandeur des geants. Où il est demonstré, que de toute ancienneté les plus grands hommes, & geants, n'ont esté plus hauts que ceux de ce temps* (Paris, 1618).

31.   Riolan, *L'imposture descouverte*, 3, 72–6.

32.   Nicolas Habicot, *Antigigantologie, ou contrediscours de la grandeur des géans* (Paris, 1618), 2–3, 7–8.

33.   Anon., *Monomachie ou response d'un compagnon chirurgien nouvelement arrivé de Montpellier, aux calomnieuses invectives de la Gigantomachie de Riolan, docteur la en* [sic] *faculté d'ignorance, contre l'honneur du College des chirurgiens de Paris* (n.l., n.d.).

34.   *Ibid.*, 8.

35.   Charles Guillemeau, attr., *Discours apologétique touchant la verité des geants. Contre la Gigantomachie d'un soy disant escollier en Medecine* (Paris, 1615), 2, 35.

36.   Nicolas-François-Joseph Éloy, *Dictionnaire historique de la médecine* (Mons: Hoyois, 1778), vol. 2, 425.

37.   Guillemeau, attr., *Discours apologétique*, 37.

38.   This statement is based on my own research as well as the discussion of the debate in Éloy, *Dictionnaire historique de la médecine*, vol. 2, 425.

39.   Gelfand, *Professionalizing Modern Medicine*, 23.

40.   Riolan, *L'imposture descouverte*, 2–3.

41.   M. Simon, *Factum ou lettre écrite par Mr. Simon à Mr. Peu sur la falsification d'un fait qui se trouve à la fin du premier livre de sa Pratique des accouchemens* (n.l., n.d.), 2.

42.   *Ibid.*, 4.

43.   Peu, *La pratique des accouchemens*, 252–6.

44.   Simon, *Factum*, 9.

45.   *Ibid.*, 16.

46.   *Ibid.*, 19.

47.   *Ibid.*, 14.

48.   *Ibid.*, 15–16.

49.   See the discussion in Chapter 4, especially note 16.

50.   Simon, *Factum*, 1–2.

51.   Peu, 'Du tire-tête,' *La pratique des accouchemens*, 357–76. Mauriceau did not discuss the *tire-tête* until the third edition of his *Des maladies des femmes grosses et accouchées* (Paris, 1681), 325, 353–8.

52.   François Mauriceau, *Observations sur la grossesse et l'accouchement des femmes* (Paris, 1695), unpaginated preface.

53.   Philippe Peu, *Réponse à l'avertissement* (n.l., n.d.), and Peu, *Réponse de M. Peu*.

54.   Peu, *Réponse de M. Peu*, 12.

55.   *Ibid.*, 12–14.

56.   *Ibid.*, 16: 'Vous trois cens femmes en quatre mois: & moi pas une seule en dix années!'

57.   *Ibid.*, 17.

58.   Mauriceau, *Observations sur la grossesse et l'accouchement des femmes*, unpaginated preface.

59.   Mauriceau, *Observations sur la grossesse et l'accouchement des femmes*, unpaginated preface.

60.   Peu, *Réponse de M. Peu*, 91.

61.   *Ibid.*, 54, 80.

62.   *Ibid.*, 49. Mauriceau, *Observations sur la grossesse et l'accouchement des femmes*, unpaginated preface.

63.   See note 1 above.

64.   Simon, *Factum*, 8, and Mauriceau, *Observations sur la grossesse et l'accouchement des femmes*, unpaginated preface.

65.   Peu, *La pratique des accouchemens*, 373–6.

66.   Jacques Fontaine, *Deux paradoxes, appartenant à la chirurgie, le premier contient la façon de tirer les enfans du ventre de leur mère par la violence extraordinaire* (Paris, 1611), 18–19.

67.   Cosme Viardel, *Observations sur la pratique des accouchemens naturels, contre nature & monstrueux* (Paris, 1671), unpaginated preface.

68.   See Chapter 2, especially notes 63–5.

69.   For some examples of this narrative structure see Guillaume Mauquest de La Motte, *Traité complet des accouchemens* (Paris, 1729; orig. 1721), 267–8, 424, Paul Portal, *La pratique des accouchemens* (Paris, 1685), 103, and Amand, *Nouvelles observations sur la pratique des accouchemens*, 209–10. Nancy G. Siraisi, *Medieval and Early Renaissance Medicine: An Introduction to Knowledge and Practice* (Chicago: University of Chicago Press, 1990), 172, argues it had long been commonplace for surgeons to publish stories contrasting their successes with the failures of another.

70.   Mauriceau, *Des maladies des femmes grosses et accouchées*, 159–70.

71.   *Ibid.*, 160: 'le plus habile homme de tous les Chirurgiens.' Peu, *La pratique des accouchemens*, 273–6, and *Réponse de M. Peu*, 70–72, also referred to this incident, claiming a colleague had called him too late to help his sister. Peu said he found Mauriceau's sister already delivered and advised there was nothing to do but wait for her death, which quickly followed. According to Peu, the violent dilation of the mouth of the womb was never advisable in such cases; he thus cast blame on Mauriceau. According to Peu, he was not the unnamed surgeon originally called by Mauriceau. Dionis, *Traité général des accouchemens*, 170, also mentioned the tragic death of Mauriceau's sister, arguing that similar situations should not intimidate a surgeon with the probity and capacity to act.

72.   Mauriceau, *Des maladies des femmes grosses et accouchées*, 161: 'un si pitoyable spectacle, que toutes les passions de mon ame furent agitées.'

73.   *Ibid.*, 159.

74.   *Ibid.*, 167.

75.   *Ibid.*, 163.

76.   *Ibid.*, 159: 'd'autant qu'en cette pitoyable & fatale occasion, j'en vis à mon grand regret, épancher devant moy une partie du mien.'

77.   *Ibid.*, 163: 'la prodigieuse perte de ce sang, qui estoit sorti de la même source que le mien.'

78.   *Ibid.*, 341–2: 'que je ne repeteray point, parce que le ressouvenir m'en est trop sensible.'

79.   *Ibid.*, 159: 'par mes propres experiences.'

80.   *Ibid.*, 58–60. Mauriceau, 124, also reported a story about how he helped a kinswoman to recover after she stumbled while six months pregnant.

81.   For the theory of the maternal imagination see Herman Roodenburg, 'The Maternal Imagination: The Fears of Pregnant Women in Seventeenth-Century Holland,' *Journal of Social History* 21, 4 (1988), 701–16, Marie-Hélène Huet, *Monstrous Imagination* (Cambridge, MA: Harvard University Press, 1993), and Valeria Finucci, 'Maternal Imagination and Monstrous Birth: Tasso's *Gerusalemme liberata*,' Valeria Finucci and Kevin Brownlee, eds, *Generation and Degeneration: Tropes of Reproduction in Literature and History from Antiquity to Early Modern Europe* (Durham: Duke University Press, 2001), 41–77.

82.   In a similar vein, the deaths of relatives and friends were thought to affect the health of survivors during the early modern period. See Mary Lindemann, *Health and Healing in Eighteenth-Century Germany* (Baltimore: The Johns Hopkins University Press, 1996), 314.

83.   Mauriceau, *Des maladies des femmes grosses et accouchées*, 59.

84. Dionis, *Traité général des accouchemens*, 143.
85. *Ibid.*, 64.
86. *Ibid.*, 64: 'Tous ceux qui n'ont point d'enfans, & qui ont perdu l'esperance d'en avoir, parlent comme Mauriceau.'
87. Mauquest de La Motte, *Traité complet des accouchemens*, 94. See also Duval, *Traité des hermaphrodits, parties genitales, accouchemens des femmes*, 10, where the author referred to his long and happy marriage to counter suggestions that his book might be lascivious, and 197, to the death in childbirth of his first wife.
88. Peu, *La pratique des accouchemens*, 107.
89. See note 11 above.
90. Mauriceau, *Des maladies des femmes grosses et accouchées*, 266–7.
91. Portal, *La pratique des accouchemens*, 109, 113, Peu, *La pratique des accouchemens*, 395, and Amand, *Nouvelles observations sur la pratique des accouchemens*, 215.
92. Mauquest de La Motte, *Traité complet des accouchemens*, 348.
93. *Ibid.*, 381. For similar accounts see also 375, 392, 395, and 481.
94. Stone, *A Complete Practice of Midwifery*, 80.
95. Lynne Tatlock, 'Speculum Feminarum: Gendered Perspectives on Obstetrics and Gynecology in Early Modern Germany,' *Signs* 17, 4 (1992), 746.
96. See the classic text by Warren R. Dawson, *The Custom of Couvade* (Manchester: Manchester University Press, 1929), 9–15.
97. Nor Hall and Warren R. Dawson, *Broodmales: A Psychological Essay on Men in Childbirth* (Dallas: Spring Publications, 1989), 11–12, 17–19.
98. Kirk Read, 'Mother's Milk from Father's Breast: Maternity without Women in Male French Renaissance Lyric,' Kathleen P. Long, ed., *High Anxiety: Masculinity in Crisis in Early Modern France* (Kirksville: Truman State University Press, 2002), 72–3.
99. *Ibid.*, 76–7.
100. Thomas Laqueur, *Making Sex: Body and Gender from the Greeks to Freud* (Cambridge, MA: Harvard University Press, 1990).
101. Read, 'Mother's Milk from Father's Breast,' 76.
102. Roberto Zapperi, *The Pregnant Man* (Chur, Switzerland: Harwood Academic Publishers, 1991), and Elizabeth D. Harvey, 'Matrix as Metaphor: Midwifery and the Conception of the Voice,' *Ventriloquized Voices: Feminist Theory and English Renaissance Texts* (London: Routledge, 1992), 76–115.
103. Claude Brunet, 'D'une grossesse d'home [sic],' *Le progrès de la médecine* (Paris, 1697), 62–5.
104. *Ibid.*, 66.
105. *Ibid.*, 68–70.
106. For an overview of this commonplace belief see Finucci, 'Maternal Imagination and Monstrous Birth,' 48. Early modern theories of generation are covered in more detail in my Chapter 6.
107. Peu, *La pratique des accouchemens*, unpaginated preface: 'le fruit de mes travaux.' Mauriceau, *Des maladies des femmes grosses et accouchées*, unpaginated preface: 'ce premier fruit de mes veilles.' Peu, 156, also referred to an unborn child as an unripe fruit. For a discussion of the longstanding comparison of children with fruit see Jacques

Gélis, *L'arbre et le fruit: la naissance dans l'Occident moderne, XVIe–XIXe siècle* (Paris: Fayard, 1984).

108.   Peu, *Réponse de M. Peu*, 3: 'vous avez enfanté le monstre avant-terme.'

109.   Peu, *La pratique des accouchemens*, unpaginated *privilège du roi*, reaffirmed the surgeon had recorded his midwifery observations during more than forty years of practice.

110.   Guillemeau, *De l'heureux accouchement des femmes*, unpaginated preface, Barthélemy Saviard, *Nouveau recueil d'observations chirurgicales* (Paris, 1702), unpaginated *avertissement*, and Mauquest de La Motte, *Traité complet des accouchemens*, vii.

111.   Gianna Pomata, 'Menstruating Men: Similarity and Difference of the Sexes in Early Modern Medicine,' Valeria Finucci and Kevin Brownlee, eds, *Generation and Degeneration*, 109–52.

112.   *Ibid.*, 112–13. For other critiques of Laqueur's one-sex model see Katharine Park and Robert A. Nye, 'Destiny is Anatomy,' *The New Republic* (February 18, 1991), 53–7, and Michael Stolberg, 'A Woman Down to Her Bones: The Anatomy of Sexual Difference in the Sixteenth and Early Seventeenth Centuries,' *Isis* 94 (2003), 274–99. For Laqueur's response to the latter critique see Thomas Laqueur, 'Sex in the Flesh,' *Isis* 94 (2003), 300–306.

113.   Pomata, 'Menstruating Men,' 152.

114.   *Rapport de l'ouverture du corps de feu Madame* (1627), reprinted in François Rouget and Colette H. Winn, eds, *Récit véritable de la naissance de messeigneurs et dames les enfans de France*, 108–9.

115.   Bourgeois, *Fidelle relation de l'accouchement, maladie et ouverture du corps de feu Madame*, 108, 105.

116.   Charles Guillemeau, attr., *Remonstrance à Madame Bourcier, touchant son apologie* (1627), reprinted in François Rouget and Colette H. Winn, eds, *Récit véritable de la naissance de messeigneurs et dames les enfans de France*, 111–20.

117.   Perkins, 'Midwives versus Doctors,' 135–57.

Chapter 6

Handling the Unborn:
Men-midwives between Vision and
Blindness

Fourteen images of unborn figures enrich *La pratique des accouchemens*, the obstetrical treatise published by *chirurgien accoucheur* Philippe Peu in 1694 (Figure 6.1). Resembling playful toddlers, the figures float in spacious egg-shaped wombs. Delicate flaps of viscera have been peeled back to reveal their contorted postures. The unborn children are clearly at risk of strangulation, and one even pulls at the umbilical cord wrapped around its neck. At the same time, references to danger are belied by the blissful expressions on their faces. The engravings in Peu's treatise are remarkably beautiful, but they are not unique. Representations of child-like figures in perilous situations routinely appear in early modern French obstetrical treatises. Sometimes the normal birth position is pictured, and the figure's limbs are drawn in to its torso. Such representations provide, however, a point of contrast for the unnatural positions that prevail in the treatises. Unborn figures are usually shown with appendages flung in all directions, extending one hand toward the mouth of the womb (Figure 6.2), in a breech position with arms raised overhead (Figure 6.3), or with feet and hands presenting together (Figure 6.4).

In this chapter, I undertake careful visual analyses of these images, approaching them as signs that were interpreted within a specific historical context. Though my goal is to determine how depictions of unborn figures conveyed meaning during the early modern period, it is difficult to eschew present beliefs when looking at them. Images such as those in Peu's treatise may seem familiar to contemporary eyes because representations of fetuses detached from the maternal body proliferate in Western culture, appearing in television commercials, parades, and posters carried by protestors at women's health clinics.[1] Inscribed with various meanings, these fetuses are understood as signs of innocence, commodity consumption, politics, or religious belief. The sign status of fetal imagery is often disavowed altogether in medical contexts, with ultrasound and photographic representations offered as revelations of the contents of women's bodies.[2] In response, feminist scholars argue that by separating the fetus from the maternal body, modern representations discount women's crucial role in parturition. Visual depictions of the fetus as an autonomous

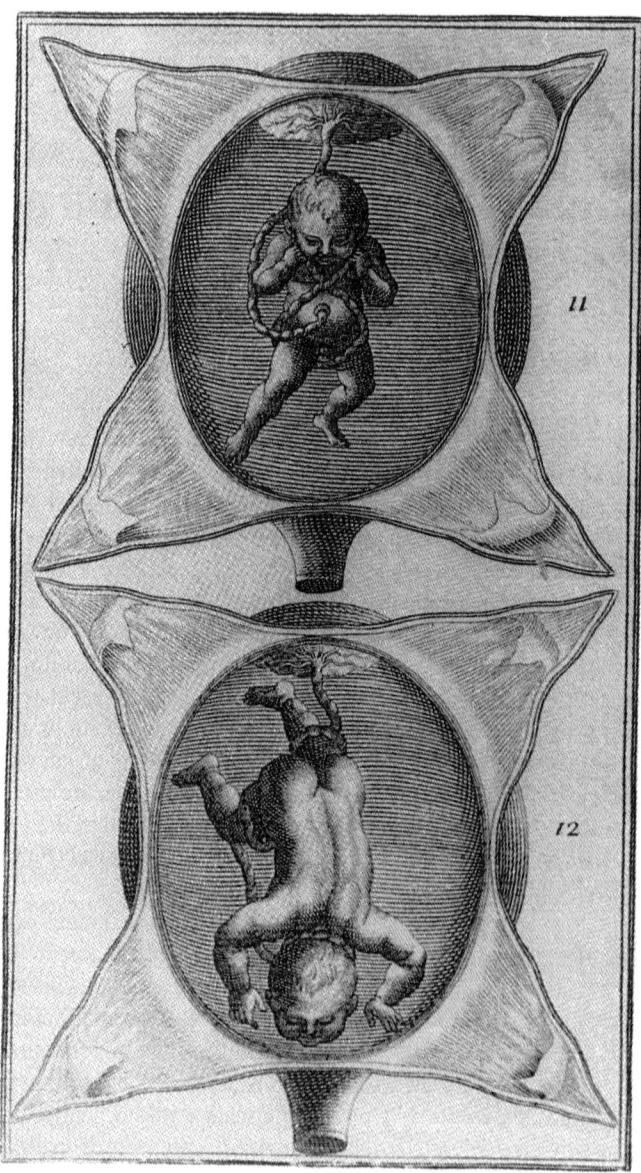

Figure 6.1   Unborn figures, from Philippe Peu's *La pratique des accouchemens*, 1694,
Paris. Courtesy of the Edward G. Miner Library, University of Rochester
Medical Center, Rochester, NY

312 De l'accouchement naturel, & de ceux

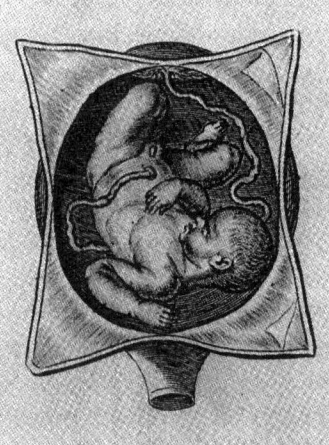

CHAPITRE XXI.

Le moyen d'accoucher la femme, quand l'enfant preſente une ou deux mains ſeules.

LORS que l'enfant preſente une ou deux mains ſeules, ou un bras qui ſort quelquefois juſques au coude, & parfois juſques à l'épaule, c'eſt une des plus mauvaiſes & des plus dangereuſes poſtures que puiſ-ſe tenir l'enfant, tant pour luy que pour ſa mere, à cau-ſe des violens efforts que le Chirurgien eſt toûjours obligé de faire à l'un & à l'autre, pour luy aller cher-
cher

Figure 6.2   Unborn figure, from François Mauriceau's *Des maladies des femmes grosses et accouchées*, 1668, Paris. Courtesy of the Edward G. Miner Library, University of Rochester Medical Center, Rochester, NY

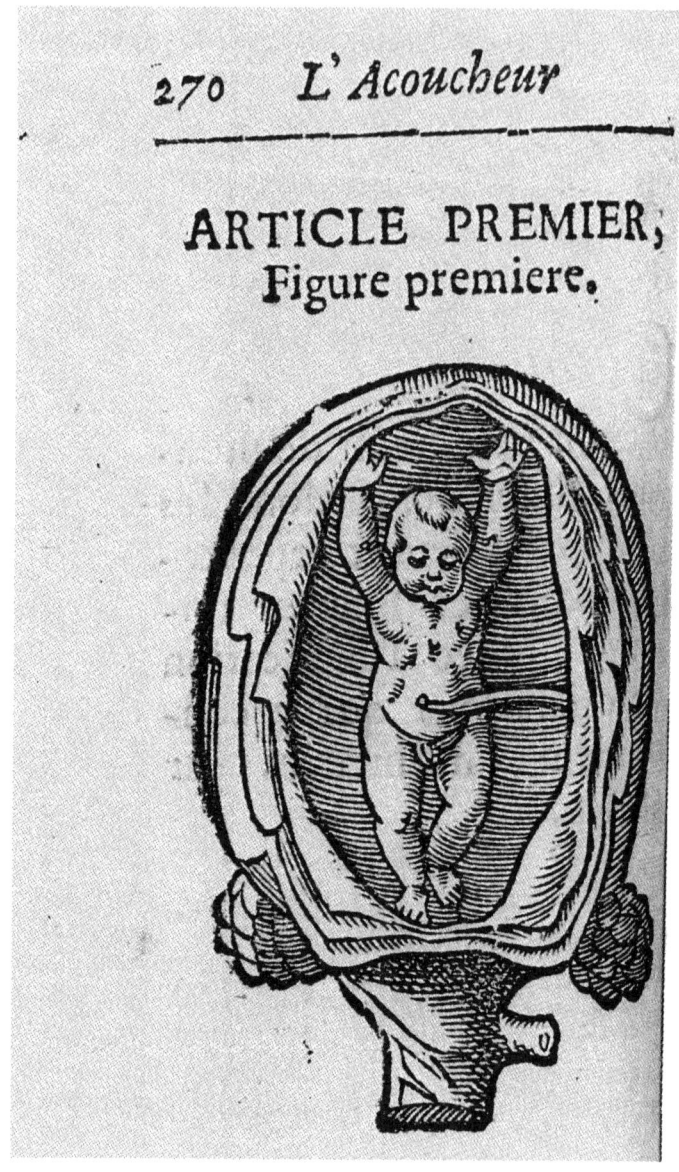

Figure 6.3 Unborn figure, from Denis Fournier's *L'accoucheur méthodique*, 1677, Paris. Courtesy of the National Library of Medicine, Bethesda, MD

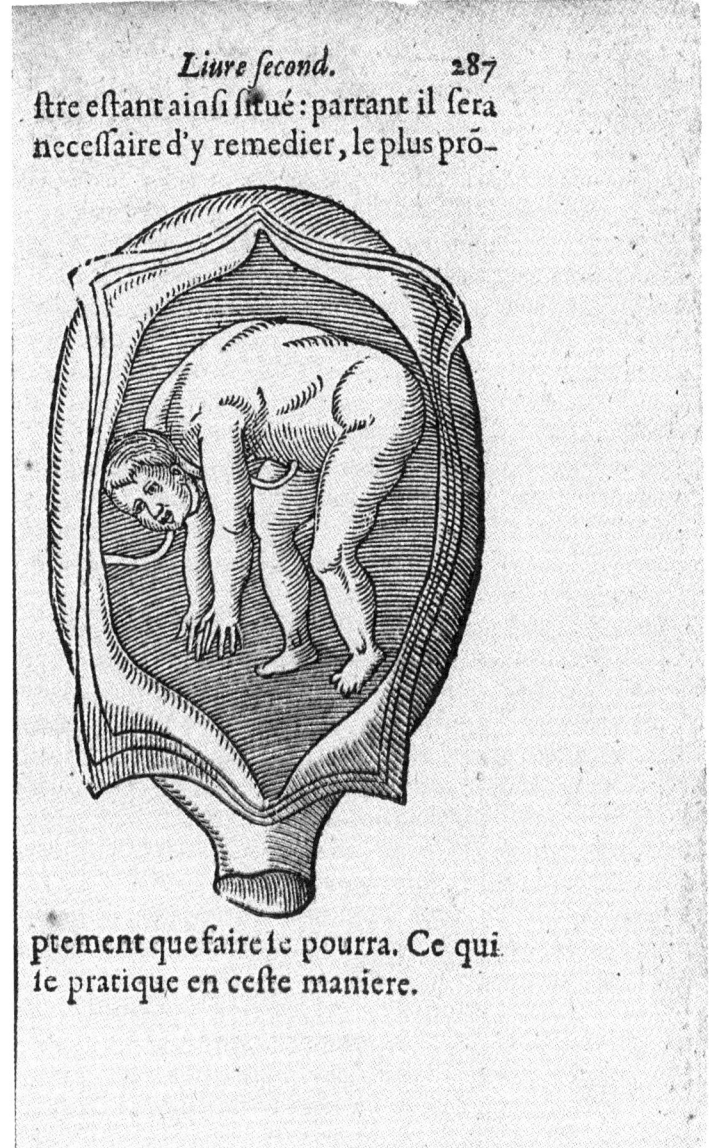

Figure 6.4   Unborn figure, from Jacques Guillemeau's *De l'heureux accouchement des femmes*, 1609, Paris. Copyright Bibliothèque nationale de France, Paris

being go hand in hand with constructions of it as a masculine figure in need of protection from an aggressive and dangerous female body.[3]

Is something similar happening in early modern images of the unborn? Literary scholar Karen Newman answers this question in the affirmative. Gathering an array of representations of the unborn from the ninth century to the present day, she postulates a long and persistent history of visualization which portrays the fetus as an inviolable, rights-bearing individual.[4] At first glance, Newman's observations seem convincing. After all, the images in early modern obstetrical treatises show male figures in wombs detached from the maternal body. Yet there are many problems with her analysis. Newman's argument recontextualizes diverse representations in different mediums – wax sculptures, obstetrical engravings, anatomical drawings – within a narrative of the longstanding depiction of fetal subjectivity. She undertakes little investigation of either individual images or the sources from which they have been excised. Instead, the literary scholar explains the erasure of the maternal body and insistence on the unborn child with reference to medical beliefs in maternal passivity and fetal activity. Newman assumes the images render in graphic form what people in the past thought about the fetus. This unsophisticated approach to the visual representations implies they simply reflect social and cultural precepts.

My analysis departs from Newman's to arrive at different conclusions. I focus on engravings of malpresenting birth figures within a single source – early modern French obstetrical treatises – to avoid offering a pan-European account that conflates distinct visual mediums and simplifies theories of conception and birth. I also examine the relationship between written and visual depictions of the unborn in these treatises. Contrary to Newman's claims, the images do not correspond to written descriptions of the womb, translating dominant medical belief into a visual format. Early modern representations of the unborn are often at odds with written accounts, which describe the maternal body in ways that can hardly be characterized as passive, and the unborn child as anything but a unique individual. Several authors of obstetrical treatises explicitly acknowledged that engravings of the unborn did not illustrate their understanding of the womb or its contents.

What, then, was the purpose of these images? At least one early modern writer argued they were intended to guide the intellectual activity of practitioners asked to intervene in difficult deliveries. He essentially described the engravings as diagrams that could be applied and reshaped in order to imagine the womb's interior. Exploring this suggestion, I draw on the theories of philosopher Charles Sanders Peirce. His systematic investigation of how visual signs communicate meaning distinguishes between icons, symbols, and indexes to counteract the supposition that all images are based on the principle of visual resemblance. According to Peirce, diagrams are one kind of iconic sign not based on visual similarity between the image and the object it portrays. Instead, diagrams offer an abstracted representation of the relationship between the parts of the object. These structures support the conceptual processes of those who use them and promote the creation of new ideas. Regarding images of the unborn as diagrams fosters a more historical understanding of them, while providing insight into how they actively produced meaning.

Attending to the specificity of the images furthermore demonstrates they were not the same over time. In contrast to ancient precursors, early modern depictions of the unborn refer to the hands-on interventions of medical practitioners. By the end of the seventeenth century, some engravings even include representations of detached hands reaching into the womb. My consideration of how and why these images changed emphasizes the broader goals of obstetrical treatises. Surgeon men-midwives described their hands as instruments of perception that discovered the womb, enabling them to undertake difficult deliveries with success when both labouring women and female midwives failed to do so. These men were expected to know the womb through the tactile sense, rather than through vision, and authors linked the images of malpresenting figures in their treatises to this haptic knowledge. Visual representations of the unborn contributed to arguments about the manual skills of surgeon men-midwives, supporting claims about when and why it was appropriate for these men to enter the lying-in chamber. They overwhelmingly portray the unborn child in an unnatural situation, not a 'state of nature' as Newman claims.[5] I contend that instead of referring exclusively to an unborn creature, the images invoke an 'other,' namely the skilled practitioner who would remove the child from the womb when it was in danger.

My close readings of early modern images of the unborn also consider what is excluded from them – the maternal body. The pregnant woman appears not as subject but as object, reduced to a womb portrayed for the most part as a hindrance to the unborn figure. It is this disappearance of women that seems to link early modern representations with those modern visions of independent fetuses. I argue, however, that the absence of the parturient body from early modern images emphasizes the unnaturalness of the difficult birth positions portrayed. Establishing that the unborn creatures are separated from maternal assistance and thus endangered, it creates an operative space for the medical expert. Pregnant women are certainly not missing from the written portions of obstetrical treatises. Numerous narratives of protracted or irregular labours describe women as a force to be reckoned with, making decisions, shrieking in pain, and refusing to be touched by men. Images of the unborn suppress this active maternal body in order to produce the subjectivity of the male practitioner.

The authority figure invoked by images of the unborn is not always male. Female midwives occasionally included comparable representations in their own treatises, portraying female rather than male hands assisting with malpresentations. In these cases, conventional representations of unborn figures have been reshaped to signify the medical expertise of women. They provide further evidence that images of the unborn did not have a single, fixed meaning over time. I contend these images were flexible sites of representation deployed in the strategic display of obstetrical authority. Studying them contributes to an increased understanding of how gender, status, and medical identity were portrayed in obstetrical treatises. At the same time, it establishes that images of the unborn were not associated with fetal subjectivity during the early modern period. This realization promotes a more historical understanding of current beliefs in an independent fetus able to transcend time and place.

Image Meets Text

Visual depictions of unborn figures in early modern French obstetrical treatises typically appear as part of a series. The publications feature ten, twelve, or even sixteen different malpresentations surrounded by written texts describing how to intervene in each difficult case to bring about a successful delivery. In François Mauriceau's *Des maladies des femmes grosses et accouchées* of 1668, for example, the first image of an unborn figure appears just over half way through the lengthy treatise, above the chapter heading: 'The means to deliver a woman, when the child presents one or two feet first.' A small engraving portrays a fully-formed male infant with his knees bent and feet oriented toward the mouth of a womb opened to admit the viewer's gaze (Figure 6.5). The text below this image admonishes the male surgeon not to attempt to correct the adversity by turning the child to a head-first position. Instead, the surgeon man-midwife should open the cervix, dilating it if necessary with fingers anointed with oil or fresh butter. He should place his hand in the womb to search for the child's feet and then gently pull both of them together while ensuring the child faced its mother's back lest its chin become lodged behind the pubic bone.[6] In the course of the next fifty pages of Mauriceau's treatise, fourteen comparable images accompany chapters that discuss the management of increasingly complicated birth presentations. Mauriceau recommended locating the child's feet to perform *podalic* version no matter which part of its body presented first: knee, chest, back, arm, or buttocks.[7]

The function of the images placed in relation to these texts would seem obvious. As illustrations of the womb, the engravings apparently portray every situation a surgeon man-midwife could encounter. Revealing the characteristics of various malpresentations, they indicate where practitioners could expect to find the legs and feet of unborn figures no matter what their situation. The images thus shed light on the womb in a pedagogical effort aimed at audiences equipped with varying levels of literacy. They represent a womb that would otherwise remain hidden, employing a visual format to educate but perhaps also to divert readers by providing them with something interesting to look at. In short, images of unborn figures in awkward poses *qui ſont contre nature. Liv. I I.*   *28ſ*

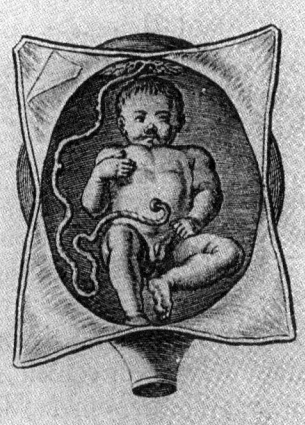

CHAPITRE XIV.

Le moyen d'accoucher la femme, quand l'en-
fant preſente un ou deux pieds les
premiers.

C'EST une verité tres-conſtante & connuë à tous
ceux qui pratiquent les accouchemens, que les
differentes poſtures contre nature auſquelles les enfans
ſe preſentent pour ſortir de la Matrice, ſont cauſe de
la plus grande partie des mauvais travaux, & des ac-
cidens qui s'y rencontrent, pour leſquels on a ordinai-
rement recours au Chirurgien.

N n iij

Figure 6.5   Unborn figure, from François Mauriceau's *Des maladies des femmes*
grosses et accouchées, 1668, Paris. Courtesy of the Edward G. Miner
Library, University of Rochester Medical Center, Rochester, NY

supplement and embellish written texts, extending the instructions offered by authors of obstetrical treatises.

This preliminary interpretation is unable, however, to withstand analysis. Visual and written representations of the unborn do not correspond to each other in any straightforward way. In fact, they often convey conflicting information. For instance, although engravings picture spacious wombs that house thoroughly visible unborn figures, textual accounts emphasize the cramped quarters of unborn children. Surgeon men-midwives described how difficult it was to manipulate a malpresenting child, wedging their hands into the constricted womb while attempting to differentiate between the tangled limbs enclosed there. Paul Portal was among those authors to remark on the pain caused by a uterus squeezing his hand.[8] Writers also drew attention to the containment of the unborn figure when explaining the nature of the membranes surrounding it. Distinguishing between two layers, they defined the tough exterior skin known as the *chorion* and the inner, transparent veil, called the *amnios*. While there was disagreement about the nature of the liquid enclosed within these membranes, many authors insisted they were filled with a mixture of the child's sweat and urine.[9] If still intact, these membranes could act as a barrier to practitioners, forcing them to wait until the waters broke before attempting to determine the child's position.[10] The written contents of obstetrical treatises repeatedly indicate that the limbs of the unborn were neither easily accessible nor legible.

Visual representations of the unborn furthermore depict acrobatic figures, evidently able to move freely within accommodating wombs. Yet written representations portray unborn creatures who do not move independently, assuming bizarre postures at will. Although the unborn figure was awarded some range of motion after it 'quickened' around the third or fourth month of gestation (depending on its sex), its movements were limited.[11] Authors of obstetrical treatises described the tiny creature confined to a standard position – curled up in a ball with heels touching buttocks, hands resting on bent knees, and head bowed – during the better part of the pregnancy. The only major movement of the unborn child was its performance of a somersault sometime after the seventh month.[12] At this point, the child turned itself from an upright to a natural head-first position in anticipation of its departure from the womb. Guillaume Mauquest de La Motte was one of the few writers to argue that unborn figures did not always assume this posture. He wrote: 'I judge that the child's situation in the uterus is without any rule, and that it alters upon anything extraordinary happening to the mother or child.'[13] But even as the surgeon man-midwife maintained the unborn child could change position, he did not believe it did so independently. The practitioner argued that situations departing from the natural one resulted from the application of an external force. Like other surgeon men-midwives, he searched for the causes of malpresentations, ascribing them to any number of events, including a perilous fall experienced by the pregnant woman, or a beating she had received.[14]

This suggestion of interaction between the unborn figure and the maternal body contradicts another aspect of the visual images. Engravings of the child in the womb remove the maternal body from the picture. Newman explains this erasure with reference to early modern beliefs in preformation and the passive role of women during labour, but authors of French obstetrical treatises did not adhere to such theories.[15] The vast majority of authors advanced the Galenic explanation of conception, which was informed by Hippocratic texts maintaining that a mixture of male and female semen was required to form a child. In her publication of 1677, midwife Marguerite de La Marche summarized what she called the 'common opinion' that 'conception is an enlivening of the [two] semens procured by the power of the womb.'[16] While La Marche drew attention to the action of the womb – it stimulated the seed with its heat – the Hippocratic/Galenic theory did not necessarily promote a vision of sexual equality. Although contributed by both men and women, semen was thought to be produced in various strengths, with powerful seed issuing from men, and thinner seed from women. All the same, physician Charles de Saint-Germain explained in his treatise of 1650 that the potency of semen varied in both men and women.[17] A masculine woman could secrete strong seed to create a male child, whereas a feminine man might contribute weak semen to the formation of a less perfect female child.[18] Though gendered, the two seed theory awarded women an active role in conception, one that surpassed Aristotle's identification of women's contribution with the inert menstrual blood acted upon by male seed.[19]

The enduring influence of the two seed theory of conception might seem surprising, however, given that by 1651 English physician William Harvey had declared 'all animals are in some part produced out of an egg.'[20] According to historian Jacques Roger, most anatomists working on the reproductive organs were persuaded that eggs existed in viviparous females by 1680 if not earlier; the proof largely consisted of analogies made with animals, as the human egg was not actually discovered until 1827.[21] Yet the *ovum* theory was not defended in French obstetrical treatises until the eighteenth century, with surgeon man-midwife Pierre Amand among the earliest in 1714.[22] All the same, in the 1729 edition of his treatise Mauquest de La Motte reaffirmed the two seed theory, arguing that embryos expelled from the womb resembled eggs – one of the observations in favour of *ova* – only because they conformed to the oval shape of the womb.[23] Even Pierre Dionis, demonstrator of anatomy in the Jardin du roi in Paris, hesitated before defending the *ovaristes* in his *Traité général des accouchemens* of 1718. The surgeon man-midwife described the mechanical action by which the first two drops of male semen were conducted to the ovary, penetrating the first egg they touched. The fertile human egg then detached from the ovary, fell into the *trompes* [tubes], and was conducted into the womb. When Dionis insisted the potent drops of semen were akin to a spiritual substance, he presented the female egg as both more material and less active than the male semen that discovered it.[24] Belief in the *ovum* did not necessarily elevate the role of women in reproduction. Nor did it, however, reduce them to passive containers.

In keeping with descriptions of the active role of women in conception, authors of French obstetrical treatises characterized the intimate relationship of pregnant women with their unborn children throughout gestation. Maternal influence varied widely, with women able to have both a positive and negative impact on the fruit in their wombs. Crucial to the child's sustenance, the maternal body provided food in the form of menstrual blood collected to form the 'cake' or afterbirth.[25] Most treatises also included what we would now call a prenatal regimen for women to follow. Authors urged women to eat well, choosing a diet suited to their particular temperament, custom, condition, and quality.[26] Mauriceau advised the pregnant woman to govern herself as if she were sick because of the many inconveniences that could befall her. He argued: 'the mother cannot be inconvenienced without her child feeling the effects of it.'[27] She should, for example, breathe well-tempered air, as cold air could cause her to cough, a sudden downward motion able to induce miscarriage. Of course, such warnings about how to preserve a pregnancy could have provided women with information about what to do if ending it was their goal, encouraging them to take bumpy carriage rides, lift heavy items, and raise their hands above their heads.

Authors of obstetrical treatises also described the ways in which the mother could affect her progeny through her emotions. Maternal anger or fear were judged to impact the child in the womb, placing it in mortal danger.[28] Peu cautioned women against indulging in such unregulated passions, offering as one example the wife of a master button maker who in a fit of anger went to strike her domestic servant, but instead rammed her own pregnant belly against the corner of a nearby table. Peu described how he managed to deliver this suffering woman, noting that her dead child was badly positioned in the womb.[29] Maternal influence was not always, however, so physical in nature. Authors referred less frequently to what literary scholar Hélène Huet has called the 'maternal imagination,' the early modern belief that women could impress their desires and mental images upon an unformed child.[30] Though Mauriceau insisted such influence could impact an unborn child only immediately after its conception, other authors related examples of the extended effects of maternal imagination.[31] In 1671 surgeon man-midwife Cosme Viardel referred to a pregnant woman who had repeatedly gazed at a painting of a moor and had given birth to a black child, while Peu confirmed that one of his client's monstrous children was caused by her observation of grotesque marionettes at the fair S. Laurent.[32]

Women's active role in their pregnancy did not end once labour began. Authors of obstetrical treatises habitually described the womb as a prison from which the unborn figure attempted to escape once its food supply was depleted, it was overwhelmed by its own waste, or the womb could not accommodate its increased size.[33] While it was generally agreed that the child initiated labour, its exit could also be encouraged by the woman's actions. According to physician Laurent Joubert in 1578, frequent sexual intercourse while pregnant 'shook the fruit' and could trigger labour and delivery.[34] But even those births properly instigated by the child were assisted by the parturient woman. Authors insisted that the woman's pains facilitated the child's efforts to enter the light of day. In 1609 surgeon man-midwife Jacques Guillemeau, for example, wrote that in labour 'the child strives and endeavours to exit, and the womb strains itself and contracts to be delivered of its burden.'[35] He and other writers regularly advised practitioners intervening in a difficult case to work with the woman's pains, attempting to revive them if they had ceased. The delivery would inevitably be difficult if the woman was unable to participate because she was weak or unconscious.[36]

According to the written accounts in early modern French obstetrical treatises, women actively contributed to conception, gestation, and birth. They interacted with the children in their wombs – unborn creatures who did not exist independently or propel themselves at will around spacious uterine containers. Yet the engravings that accompany these texts depict unborn figures in large wombs detached from the maternal body. Clearly, such images do not offer inscriptions of concurrent medical beliefs about the nature of the unborn child in the womb. Instead, the visual and written representations of unborn children in the treatises are at odds with each other. This mismatch raises fundamental questions about the status and function of engraved representations of the unborn. It encourages us to rethink not only how they operated as signifiers but also exactly what they signified.

Discovering the Invisible Womb

Interpretations of early modern engravings of the unborn are ultimately based on opinions about *how* the images communicate. Newman's analysis, for example, insists that we can look at the images and draw conclusions about what people in the past thought about the womb and its contents – an unborn figure shown detached from the maternal body demonstrates a belief in fetal autonomy. Without using the term, Newman assumes the representations are iconic, based on the principle of visual resemblance between the image and the thing it portrays. According to Charles Sanders Peirce, an icon can elicit a concept by resembling an object, sharing in or duplicating certain properties of that object.[37] The previous discussion has demonstrated, however, that early modern images of unborn children in contorted postures do not accord with concurrent discussions about the womb and its contents; they do not resemble beliefs about the womb. At least two conclusions follow from this observation: 1) early modern images of the unborn are not iconic signs referring to the womb; 2) these images are iconic signs but refer to something other than the womb.

Historian Barbara Duden supports the first conclusion, arguing that the early modern representation of the figure in the womb:

> remains a symbol rather than a facsimile. It stands for the invisible unborn, not for its appearance. It speaks for the experience of women, not for medical knowledge about an entity or a process in the womb.[38]

Duden contends that the images are based on convention rather than the principle of visual resemblance. Peirce defines a symbol as a sign that 'refers to the Object that it denotes by virtue of a law, usually an association of general ideas, which operates to cause the Symbol to be interpreted as referring to that Object.'[39] According to Duden, the maternal body remained an opaque and mysterious realm throughout the early modern period. The diagnosis of pregnancy, for example, was fraught with uncertainty.[40] Had the woman's menses ceased and was her belly swelling because of a true conception, or did her womb harbour a false conception – perhaps the kind of fleshy mass known as a mole? In the images, this uncertainty is replaced with a certainty (a child) that could only be revealed in the future, after the birth had taken place. According to Duden, these representations symbolically represent the child-to-come. They do not visually inscribe early modern understandings of a pre-human form.

Largely based on eighteenth-century texts written by German physicians, Duden's argument is not entirely borne out in early modern French obstetrical treatises. The authors of French publications insisted they could indeed acquire knowledge of the unborn child in the womb. At the same time, they recognized how difficult it was to diagnose pregnancy, and recommended that fellow surgeon men-midwives exercise caution when attempting to do so.[41] They also admitted to lacking direct visual access to both the interior and exterior of the pregnant female body. As discussed in Chapter 2, for reasons of propriety labouring women were draped with linens that impeded the visual access of male practitioners. Gazing on the body of the parturient woman was an intimate privilege traditionally accorded to female midwives. Surgeon men-midwives nevertheless attempted to turn these potential shortcomings into advantages. They claimed that obstetrical emergencies were the most demanding type of surgical procedure precisely because practitioners could see neither their clients nor what their own hands were doing inside the opaque womb. Dionis went farthest with this argument by claiming that eyes were worthless to a surgeon man-midwife. He pointed to the successful practice of one Faro des Forges, a blind man-midwife, as proof.[42]

Blindness was not always considered a virtue in obstetrical texts. Surgeon man-midwife Mauquest de La Motte worked in Valognes and the surrounding area, a region he described as isolated and bereft of colleagues, forcing him to rely on his own good sense, 'without submitting blindfold to all the rules generally received.'[43] Dionis similarly claimed to avoid 'blindly following the ancients.'[44] And in an earlier publication, Mauriceau compared those 'learned authors' who had never practised childbirth to 'Geographers who describe for us many lands that they have never seen.'[45] It was rather commonplace for surgeon men-midwives to dismiss a strictly theoretical approach to childbirth, linking it with the limited book-learning of physicians as opposed to insight. By invoking a geographical analogy, Mauriceau implied that for those who exclusively read about childbirth, the female body remained an unexplored (and perhaps unconquered) foreign land. In contrast, an extensive first-hand experience with difficult deliveries was associated with both an intimate knowledge of maternity, and observations worthy of publication.

These considerations of blindness send mixed messages: the experienced surgeon man-midwife is portrayed as simultaneously unable to see and possessed of an insightful understanding of the maternal body. The two apparently contradictory ideas are integrated, however, in discussions of male practitioners' hands. Male authors of French obstetrical treatises suggested that the dark and hidden realm of the womb was enlightened by their perceptive hands able to 'see' inside it.[46] Several treatises provided detailed guidelines encouraging surgeons to distinguish between the different parts of the child, which could resemble each other in the womb.[47] Peu, for example, defined the entire surface of the body of the unborn child according to its tactile qualities. The head could be recognized by its round, hard skull, the eyes by their number, the cavity of their sockets, and elevation of the eyeballs, the nose by its eminence between the eyes and above the mouth, and so on.[48] While reporting a marvellous delivery he had undertaken in 1697, the master surgeon le Duc reaffirmed the belief that 'the eyes of the man-midwife are the ends of his fingers.'[49]

These accounts clearly indicate that an image of the unborn child emerged from the physical manipulation of the womb, not from direct visual access to it. None of the men argued, however, that engravings of unborn figures in the womb actually looked like what their hands saw. A few surgeon men-midwives even refused to include such engravings in their treatises, lest inexperienced readers naively equate seeing the images with knowledge of the maternal body. Mauquest de La Motte argued that 'looking upon the representations of the different situations of the child in the uterus, and the various circumstances of the navel string round it, as of no significance, I have omitted giving any.'[50] Dionis also 'estimat[ed] that they could be useless, because it is not the eyes of the man-midwife that teach him how the child is turned in the womb, it is by touching it that he instructs himself about it.'[51] While both men criticized the visual format of these representations, Dionis' complaint was more specific. He implied images of malpresentations could misconstrue the basis of the surgeon man-midwife's knowledge, obscuring the importance of touch. According to Dionis, the act of looking could not replace the more fundamental act of touching.

Why, then, did visual representations of unborn figures in awkward poses appear with such persistence in other French obstetrical treatises? Peu provided an exceptionally detailed account of the engravings in his own publication. He argued that though his plates portrayed only some of the situations of children 'reduced' by twisted umbilical cords, they 'could serve as a principle idea for conceptualizing an infinity of other possible [situations].'[52] Insisting that the engravings provided partial references to his own hands-on practices, Peu distinguished between seeing the images and achieving a perfect understanding of malpresentations. According to him, the engravings were ideas in visual form that could guide the cerebral activity of practitioners asked to intervene in difficult deliveries. He characterized the representations as modes of interpretation able to encourage the production of new knowledge, not depictions of what would be found in the womb.

Peu essentially described the images as diagrams.[53] Diagrams are typically associated with the expression of scientific ideas. By distilling the scientist's observations into a simple formula, they provide a principle that can be tested and developed in subsequent research. According to Peirce, diagrams support creative thinking because 'it is not by a simple mental stare, or strain of mental vision [that thought is developed]. It is by manipulating on paper, or in the fancy, formulae or other diagrams.'[54] Diagrams can be observed and contemplated in order to discover unnoticed relations among the parts of the thing portrayed.[55] Peirce's description of diagrams as thought experiments that reveal invisible relations is not unlike Peu's account of early modern images of the unborn as ideas enabling surgeon men-midwives to imagine malpresentations they had never encountered before.

At least two potential objections arise from this comparison of Peu with Peirce. The early modern images do not look like diagrams; they lack the familiar lines, axes, points, and shapes. Peirce employed the term diagram, however, in a broad sense that denoted any sensuous image presenting an instance of relations analogous to those upon which an argument turns.[56] According to the philosopher, diagrams are a kind of iconic sign 'which represent the relations...of the parts of one thing by analogous relations in their own parts.'[57] This emphasis on iconic resemblance leads to another misgiving because it is clear that images of the unborn were not meant to look like the womb and its contents. Nonetheless Peirce argued that 'many diagrams resemble their objects not at all in looks; it is only in respect to the relations of their parts that their likeness consists."[58] Iconicity includes similarity of abstract relations or structures. Semiotician Umberto Eco cautions against the conflation of icons with visual resemblance, reminding us that the 'concept of icon...concern[s] nonvisual experiences too.'[59]

Peirce regularly defined the diagram as an analogous presentation of the relations of the parts of another thing. This insistence on the arrangement rather than the properties of the parts is difficult to grasp. Philosopher David A. Pharies explains Peirce's conception with reference to one type of diagram:

> The peaks and troughs of an electrocardiogram, for example, share no significant properties with the various modalities of a beating heart. They may, nevertheless, in conjunction with certain conventions, be graphically representative of the relationships among these modalities.[60]

The electrocardiogram does not look, smell, feel, or sound like the heart muscle, its chambers, or pumping blood. Instead, it represents the relations between these things, emphasizing repeated intervals, and changes in intensity. This interpretation is not self-evident but requires previous knowledge to support it, including an understanding of Western medicine and visual conventions.

At first glance it is difficult to see how Pharies' description of the electrocardiogram illuminates the operation of the early modern images in obstetrical treatises. After all, the lines produced by the contemporary medical technology seem more obviously schematic than those in the early modern images. Nevertheless, Pharies' account of the electrocardiogram can be adapted and applied to the engravings, with the following result: the early modern images do not look, smell, feel, or sound like the womb, its contents, or the surgeon man-midwife's encounter with those contents. They represent the exchanges between these things, emphasizing the interrelated location of the parts and their discernability. The actual space of the womb, which was understood to be cramped and confusing, is not portrayed. Instead, the spatial relations are abstracted in a manner recalling a map or plan. According to Peirce: 'the Diagram represents a definite Form of Relation. This Relation is usually one which actually exists, as in a map, or is intended to exist, as in a Plan.'[61] The early modern images are like maps in that they were meant to facilitate surgeon men-midwives' navigation of the womb, and yet they do not portray relations which actually exist. They are more like plans – signs which both precede and generate other signs. The engravings represent a form of relation that is intended to exist, and then be reshaped in the process of mental reconstruction.

In keeping with the electrocardiogram, this interpretation is not self-evident but requires previous knowledge to support it. Such an understanding of the images is unfathomable without a familiarity with the arguments made by early modern medical practitioners. French surgeon men-midwives maintained they could envision the external features of the unborn child in the womb, and use them to perceive new situations. The men thus produced an imaginary and in fact impossible unborn child, one that cooperated with their endeavours. Although such representations might appear to be strictly symbolic – replacing one thing for another – they are not.

According to Peirce, symbols enable us to create abstractions (allowing us to count, for example), but rest on learned habits that do not 'furnish any observation even of themselves.'[62] In contrast, diagrams are not offered as rules to be repeated, but rather as structures promoting thought.

Peu's description of how the images functioned accords with the second conclusion drawn above from the mismatch between visual image and written text in obstetrical treatises: engravings of the unborn are iconic signs, but they refer to something other than the womb. They are diagrams meant to provide support for surgeon men-midwives' haptic acquisition of knowledge of the womb without offering a visual likeness of the womb, which could harbour a multitude of malpresentations. This interpretation goes a long way to explaining why written descriptions of the womb do not match the visual images. If understood to encourage the surgeon man-midwife's skilled encounter with the womb, then the images respond rather than correspond to the texts surrounding them. While written passages stress that in difficult deliveries unborn children are cramped and their limbs muddled, engravings provide the means to guide the surgeon man-midwife's interventions as he remedies the situation. The images thus aid in the production of the surgeon man-midwife's point of view, ultimately referring more to him than to the womb itself.

Shifting Signifiers

The previous analysis has not exhausted the significance of images of the unborn. Though Peu offered an explanation of their use, it is unclear whether or not readers actually followed his advice. There were certainly other ways of understanding the representations, given their complex visual elements. Considering additional interpretations of the engravings does not undermine the appreciation of them as diagrams. Peirce noted there are no absolutely pure icons, indexes, or symbols; these aspects vary in their relative prominence from sign to sign, with conventional codes underpinning all signification.[63] His sophisticated system of signs was not meant to classify visual images into types, determining their final meaning. Instead, the philosopher was primarily interested in providing more precise ways of thinking about the processes of interpretation, recognizing that a sign behaving as an icon in one semiosis could become a symbol in another.[64] Peirce's theories are especially useful for contemplating early modern images of the unborn, as diverse viewers likely tried to make sense of these representations in ways that may or may not have been intended. Authors such as Peu provided directions, but the objectives of the artists commissioned to make the images remain unknown. Unlike author portraits, representations of the unborn were rarely signed by artists and engravers. Nevertheless in each treatise containing such images, stylistic disparities suggest that the artists who produced them were not the same as those who had made the portraits.[65]

In any case, images of the unborn are in dialogue with a host of other representations. The images include references to, among other things, anatomical dissection and angelic cherubs, invoking a broader medical as well as popular culture. According to the theory of intertextuality, this diversity is not unusual. All texts depend on a host of prior conventions, codes, and other texts for their existence. Literary scholar Julia Kristeva argues that 'every text builds itself as a mosaic of quotations, every text is absorption and transformation of another text.'[66] Similar claims can be made about visual representation, as art historians have long known that visual images refer more to other images than to the external world.[67] Any written or visual text therefore contains an unavoidable multiplicity of references, with signifiers referring to other signifiers, and meaning constantly deferred.[68] Reading in terms of intertextuality necessitates abandoning the idea that a final, utterly consistent interpretation of a text is possible. According to Kristeva, 'in the space of a given text, several utterances, taken from other texts, intersect and neutralize one another.'[69] This emphasis on convergence and contradiction challenges analyses that position the author or artist as a stable ground for analysis because multifarious texts do not reflect the intentions of a single creative mind.

Early modern images of the unborn such as those in Peu's treatise bear a visual resemblance to other images of the unborn, not to ideas about the womb. As indicated in Chapter 1, these figures were not invented by surgeon men-midwives but stemmed from Muscio's ninth-century translation of the ancient text by Soranus of Ephesus.[70] When French authors included similar images in their own treatises centuries later, they invoked an established tradition of representation. The images may have signified the authors' familiarity with obstetrical authorities such as Soranus, while providing evidence of the enduring nature of the practice of male midwifery. Attacks on man-midwifery as an unprecedented and shocking development by critics including physician Philippe Hecquet could be undermined with reference to the history of publications on childbirth.[71] Surgeon men-midwives certainly linked themselves with ancient tradition in the written segments of the treatises, particularly their prefaces.[72] At the same time, including conventional images of the unborn placed an author's work within a genre of publication, ensuring it would be recognizable as an obstetrical treatise. Though images of the unborn floating in oversized wombs did not appear in all early modern obstetrical treatises, they were found in many of them, including those of English, German, Italian, and Dutch origin.

Despite eliciting a longstanding tradition of representation, early modern French images of the unborn differ from their ancient forebears. Whereas the images from the translation of Soranus portray figures with adult proportions, the lively children shown in early modern engravings look like pudgy toddlers. Some of the engravings in Guillemeau's publication of 1609 include unborn figures with particularly long arms and legs, but for the most part the figures in French treatises resemble the playful *putti* that populate the broader visual culture of the period. Numerous paintings and drawings produced by Nicolas Poussin during the seventeenth century, for example, depict robust male infants cavorting in mythological scenes of pleasure, while his contemporary Jacques Stella produced a series of images of *putti* at play, called *Les jeux et plaisirs de l'enfance* [The games and pleasures of childhood].[73] Sometimes *putti* appear as mischievous cupids able to transgress the rules of social interaction, or as angelic figures floating above religious scenes in a range of contorted postures.[74] Learning to portray *putti* from diverse angles was a standard part of artistic training during the early modern period, and artists likely drew on this knowledge to produce images of unborn figures. Depictions of *putti* would certainly have been familiar to many viewers at the time, adding another layer of meaning to images of the unborn. These delightful figures alluded to child-like pleasure, innocence, and faith, positive connotations capable of counteracting the association of surgeon men-midwives with danger and sexual deviance.

Early modern images additionally diverge from earlier depictions of the unborn by construing the womb as a fleshy container instead of a transparent vessel. In most French images, the womb consists of layers of viscera that have been surgically breached to reveal the figure inside. The plates in Denis Fournier's obstetrical treatise of 1677, for example, feature jagged flesh that has apparently been ripped open or cut by an instrument (Figure 6.3). In contrast, the books by Mauriceau and Peu contain images that are more peaceful, showing flimsy flaps of skin peeled back with little resistance. All the engravings, however, include indexical references to medical manipulation. Peirce defines an index as:

> a sign which would, at once, lose the character which makes it a sign if its object were removed, but would not lose that character if there were no interpretant. Such, for instance, is a piece of mould with a bullet-hole in it as sign of a shot; for without the shot there would have been no hole; but there is a hole there, whether anybody has the sense to attribute it to a shot or not.[75]

Though Peirce's example draws attention to a real contiguity between the sign (the bullet-hole) and the object (the shot), the connection does not need to be based in reality, but can appear within the image itself.[76] The severed flesh shown in images of the unborn invokes cutting as well as the invasive physical operations required to produce knowledge of the womb. These references potentially reaffirm the arguments of surgeon men-midwives, who insisted that their hands-on manipulations revealed the contents of an otherwise opaque and mysterious womb. Yet the images also emphasize vision in a way that contradicts the men's emphasis on touching the womb rather than looking at it. Dionis was aware of these conflicting messages, fearing that readers could misinterpret the engravings as visions of the womb itself. References to opening the womb and looking inside it furthermore invoke anatomical illustrations, which regularly show flaps of skin pulled back to expose the interior of the human body. Well-known examples include Charles Estienne's anatomical treatise of 1546, in which the abdomen of a standing female figure is stripped of its skin to reveal an unborn child curled in a ball, and Berengario da Carpi's tract of 1521, which shows a male figure peeling back his own skin[77] (Figure 6.6). Conjuring up such imagery could link obstetrical treatises with an esteemed anatomical tradition, reinforcing surgeon men-midwives' affirmations of their thorough understanding of the human body by means of anatomical demonstrations and the autopsies they performed.[78] As indicated in Chapter 5, anatomical knowledge was a recurring issue in early modern debates about the medical hierarchy. While physicians claimed surgeons lacked this crucial knowledge, surgeons argued that female midwives were bereft of it. Yet references to anatomical dissection could also allude to death and dismemberment, medical realities with which surgeon men-midwives did not want to be associated. In their obstetrical treatises, they regularly downplayed their use of surgical instruments, while assuring readers they were not responsible for the deaths of labouring clients and unborn children.[79]

The connotations of danger in the images are nevertheless alleviated by the lively unborn children shown inhabiting the mutilated wombs. Though the unborn creatures are depicted in awkward positions and occasionally ensnared in long umbilical cords, they are also active, with smiles on their plump faces. Sending mixed messages by combining visual references to death with living creatures was a strategy used by anatomical illustrators. The plates from da Carpi's treatise, for example, feature an animated human figure actively inviting viewers to gaze at the interior of his body. According to literary critic Jonathan Sawday, this type of representation was meant to abate social anxieties surrounding the potentially invasive observation of mutilated bodies.[80] He argues that by displaying an ambiguous union of life and death, the images simultaneously revealed and attempted to surmount the contradiction at the heart of anatomical dissection – the practice destroyed the human body in order to construct an elevated understanding of it.[81] Early modern images of the unborn often include similarly discrepant messages, alluding to both danger and health, dismemberment and vitality.

The plates in at least one early modern obstetrical treatise exclude all references to the violent opening of the womb. The 1673 edition of Viardel's book reverts to the earlier convention by showing transparent wombs severed from the maternal body (Figure 6.7). This mode of representation was unusual at the time, and it may be related to Viardel's contention that the surgeon man-midwife should use his hands alone to assist at deliveries, foregoing all instruments.[82] The images in his tract tend to directly refer to the hands-on practices of the male practitioner, portraying strong

CHAP.   XXXVII.

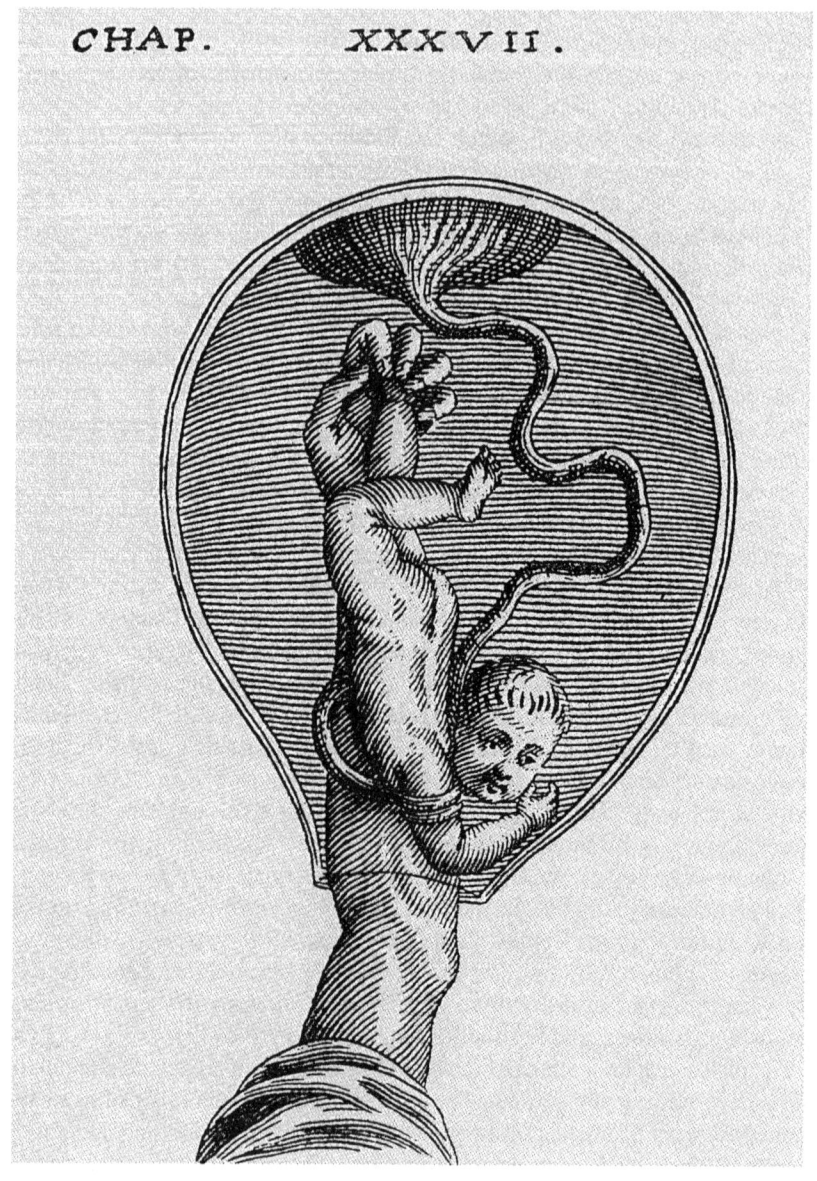

Figure 6.6   Unborn figure, from Cosme Viardel's *Observations sur la pratique des accouchemens naturels, contre nature & monstrueux*, 1673, Paris. Courtesy of the National Library of Medicine, Bethesda, MD

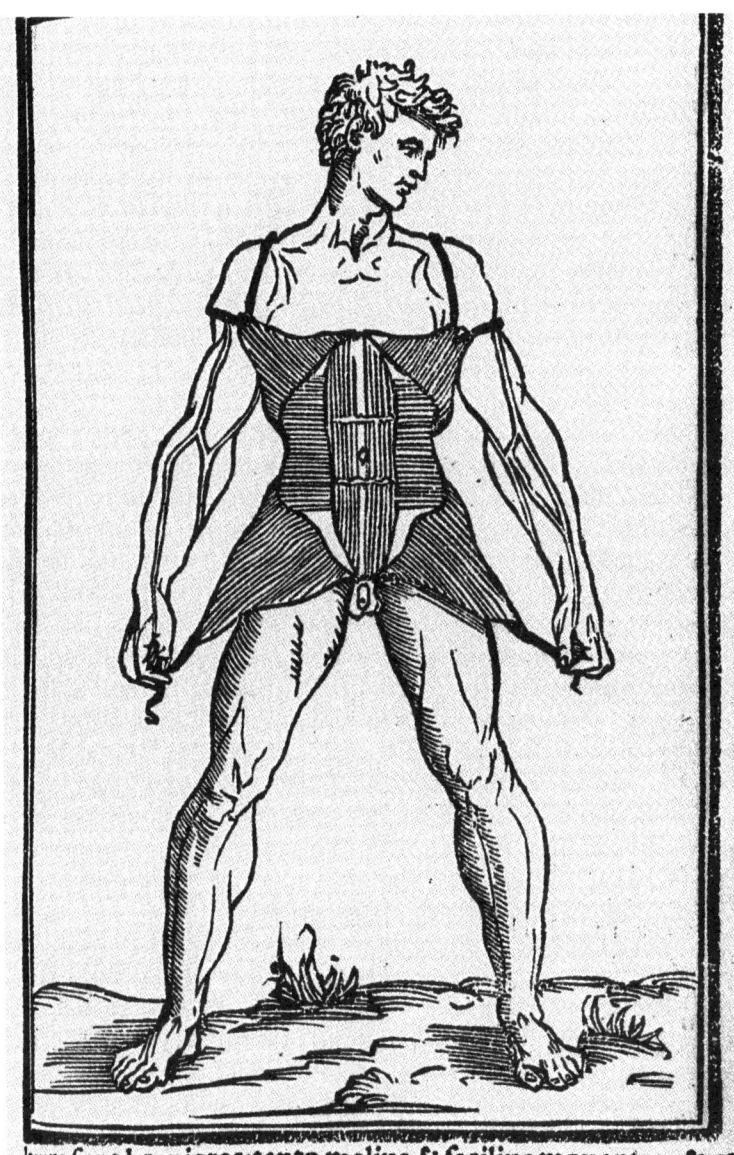

lorum funt breniores:tanto melius & facilius mouentur. & cc

Figure 6.7   Anatomized figure, from Berengario da Carpi's *Commentaria*, 1521,
            Bologna. Courtesy of the National Library of Medicine, Bethesda, MD

male hands and even entire arms entering spacious wombs to manipulate badly positioned unborn children. These fragmentary appendages operate on the principle of synecdoche – a part represents the whole surgeon – but are also indexical signs insisting on the 'real' presence of the surgeon man-midwife and his direct experience of the womb. This message is in keeping with the author portrait of Viardel, which shows him touching the head of a dead child, as discussed in Chapter 4.

Such direct representations of intervening hands do not always represent male practitioners. The engravings in the publication of German midwife Justine Siegemund in 1690 depict slender, feminine arms that labour to remove malpositioned figures from the womb[83] (Figure 6.8). In a similar way, Madame du Coudray's obstetrical treatise of 1769 features slight female hands adorned with white cuffs undertaking medical interventions (Figure 6.9). The images in both publications insist on women's capacity to handle difficult deliveries, while alluding to the authors' anatomical knowledge of the female body. Though the plates in Siegemund's book include the standard flaps of viscera pulled back to reveal the large oval womb, du Coudray's images are significantly different. In her treatise, the maternal body has been reduced to a set of pelvic bones rather than a schematic womb. Noting this distinction, Nina Rattner Gelbart argues that the images in the female midwife's text 'break entirely with all conventions of obstetrical representation used by du Coudray's male predecessors or contemporaries.'[84] This claim is an overstatement, for the plates in the traveling midwife's treatise not only conventionally separate the unborn child from the maternal body, they also resemble the images of the unborn in an earlier treatise by Dutch man-midwife Hendrik van Deventer, which similarly emphasize women's pelvic bones.[85] It is more accurate to say that the images in the treatises of both Siegemund and du Coudray simultaneously absorb and transform the visual conventions typically linked with male knowledge to make gendered statements about women's authority in childbirth. Such cases reveal that early modern images of the unborn were continually reinscribed with signs of knowledge, ability, and identity.

Early modern images of the unborn are complex representations, laden with paradoxical references to both pleasure and danger, looking and touching, and health as well as destruction. Informed by visual conventions in addition to iconic and indexical elements, these images did not have the same meaning for every early modern viewer. Dionis' rejection of the engravings provides one instance of disagreement about their value. Nor did images of the unborn remain the same, for the plates in Viardel's treatise portrayed the hands of the male practitioner, while those in subsequent books by female midwives were recoded to signify the interventions performed by women. Though it is difficult to generalize about early modern images of the unborn, their flexible nature and ability to support multiple meanings helps to explain why such representations continued to appear in obstetrical treatises into the eighteenth century.

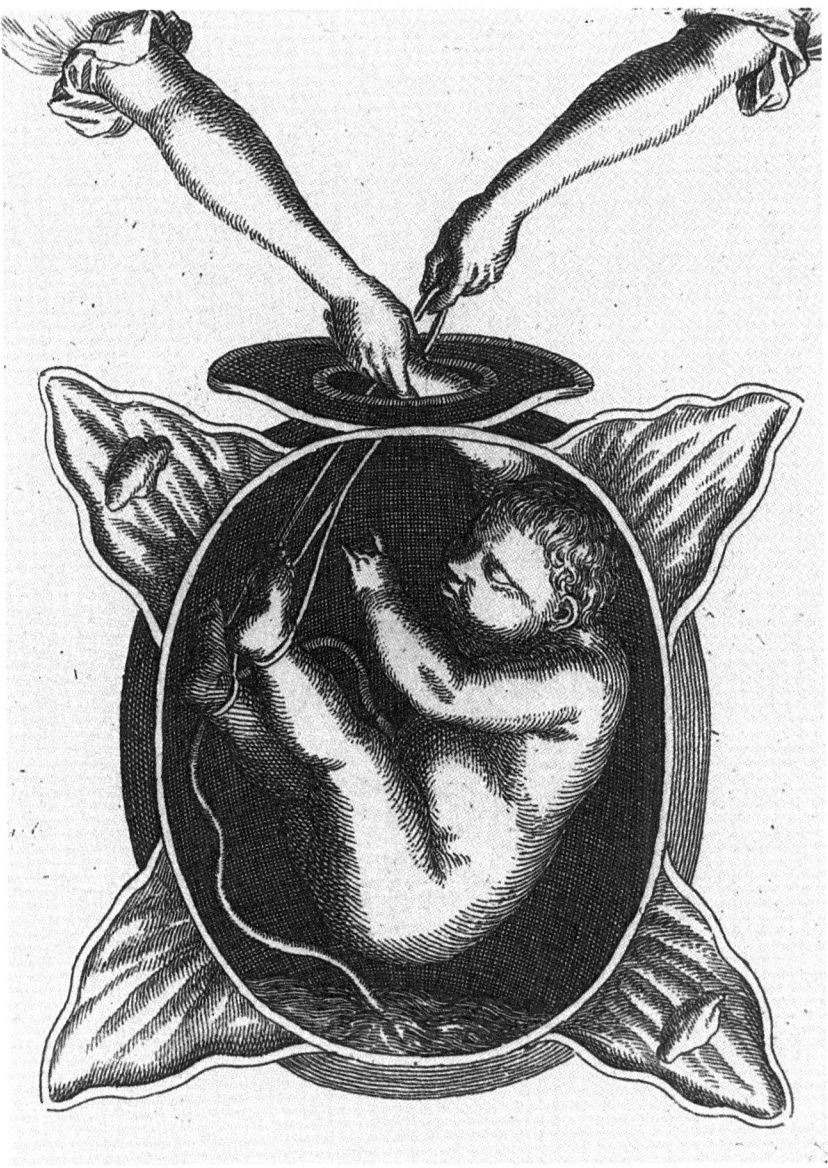

Figure 6.8   Unborn figure, from Justine Siegemund's *Die Chur-Brandenburgische Hoff-Wehe-Mutter*, 1690, Cölln an der Spree. Courtesy of the Edward G. Miner Library, University of Rochester Medical Center, Rochester, NY

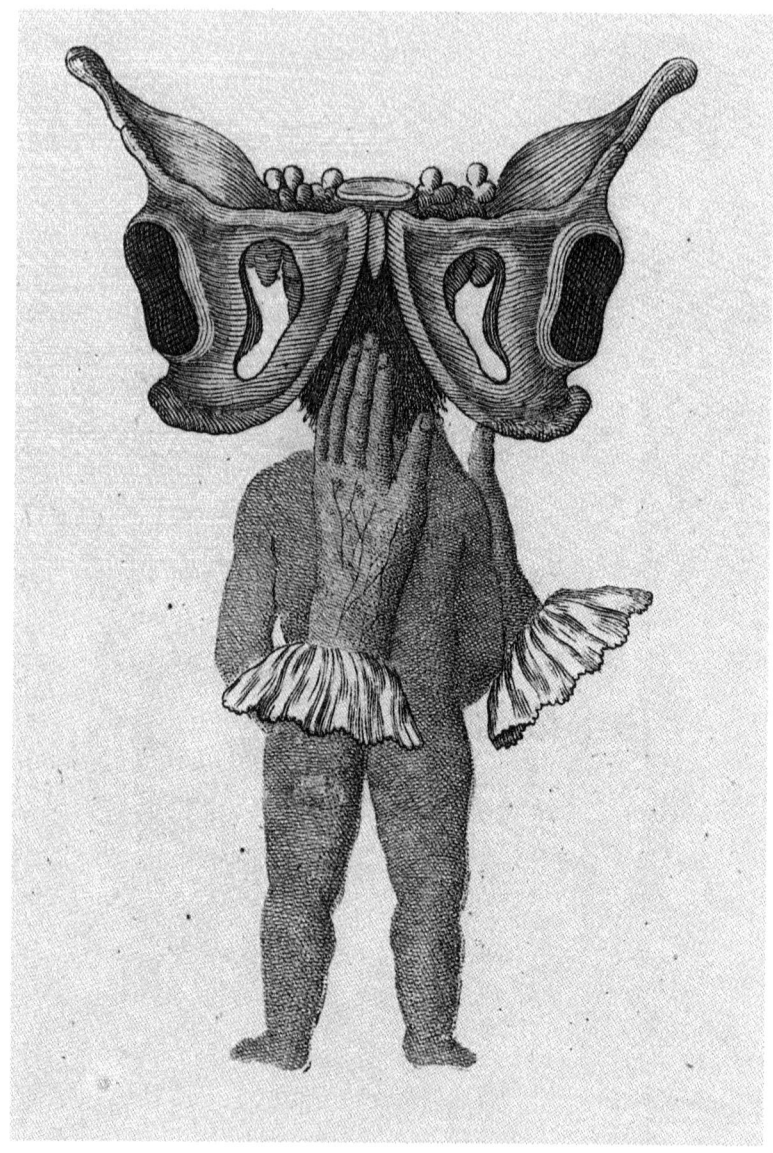

Figure 6.9   Unborn figure, from Angélique Marguerite Le Boursier du Coudray's *Abrégé de l'art des accouchements*, 1777, Paris. Courtesy of the Edward G. Miner Library, University of Rochester Medical Center, Rochester, NY

Unnatural Maternity

The most striking feature of early modern French images of the unborn may well be what is absent from them, namely the maternal body. While the written passages of obstetrical treatises present a pregnant body that actively participates in gestation and birth, in visual images the mother is displaced by the unborn child. Newman contends that this child offers an 'image *par excellence* of rights-bearing Enlightenment Man ferociously rendered in the fabled state of nature.'[86] The unborn figure is indeed always shown as male, considered the ideal product of conception during the early modern period.[87] Yet in obstetrical treatises he is rarely portrayed in what medical writers described as a natural state. According to every author, in natural births the child remained curled in a round ball until it was ready to exit the womb head-first, aided by both its own efforts and those of its mother.[88] Surgeon men-midwives argued that these deliveries could be handled by female midwives if they were patient and simply encouraged the labouring woman, refusing to intervene unnecessarily in the birth.[89] Considered a strictly natural rather than medical event, straightforward births were linked with the agricultural cycle of growth and harvest. The treatise published in 1671 by London midwife Jane Sharp includes an engraving that can be more accurately described as representing the unborn figure in a 'fabled state of nature.' The compact child appears as a ripe fruit or flower produced by its fertile mother[90] (Figure 6.10).

In contrast, obstetrical treatises predominantly display the unborn in positions which early modern authors considered both awkward and dangerous. With legs and arms akimbo, the unborn figures appear to be hopelessly trapped in the womb, a condition sometimes reinforced by the long umbilical cords binding them. Surgeon men-midwives noted that a badly positioned child struggled in vain to exit the womb, while exhausting its mother's attempts to expel it.[91] Such unborn children were separated from both the sustenance of the maternal body and the productivity of the natural order. Their situation was considered utterly unnatural. According to Mauriceau, there were three kinds of troublesome births: laborious, difficult, and unnatural. In both laborious and difficult deliveries the unborn child conformed to a natural posture and was assisted by nature, but its birth was especially painful or delayed.[92] He insisted that in cases of malpresentation, however, nature was absent, leaving the unborn child in a vulnerable state.

Mauriceau and other surgeon men-midwives argued that such unnatural births were hopeless unless a male surgeon was called to intervene. They claimed that malpresentations could never be delivered by the efforts of the mother or the child, while female midwives lacked both the intellectual and manual abilities to accomplish them. Only a man equipped with skilled hands would be able to discern the unborn child's awkward position, and remove it from the womb.[93] Distinguishing themselves from women as well as from nature, surgeon men-midwives linked their

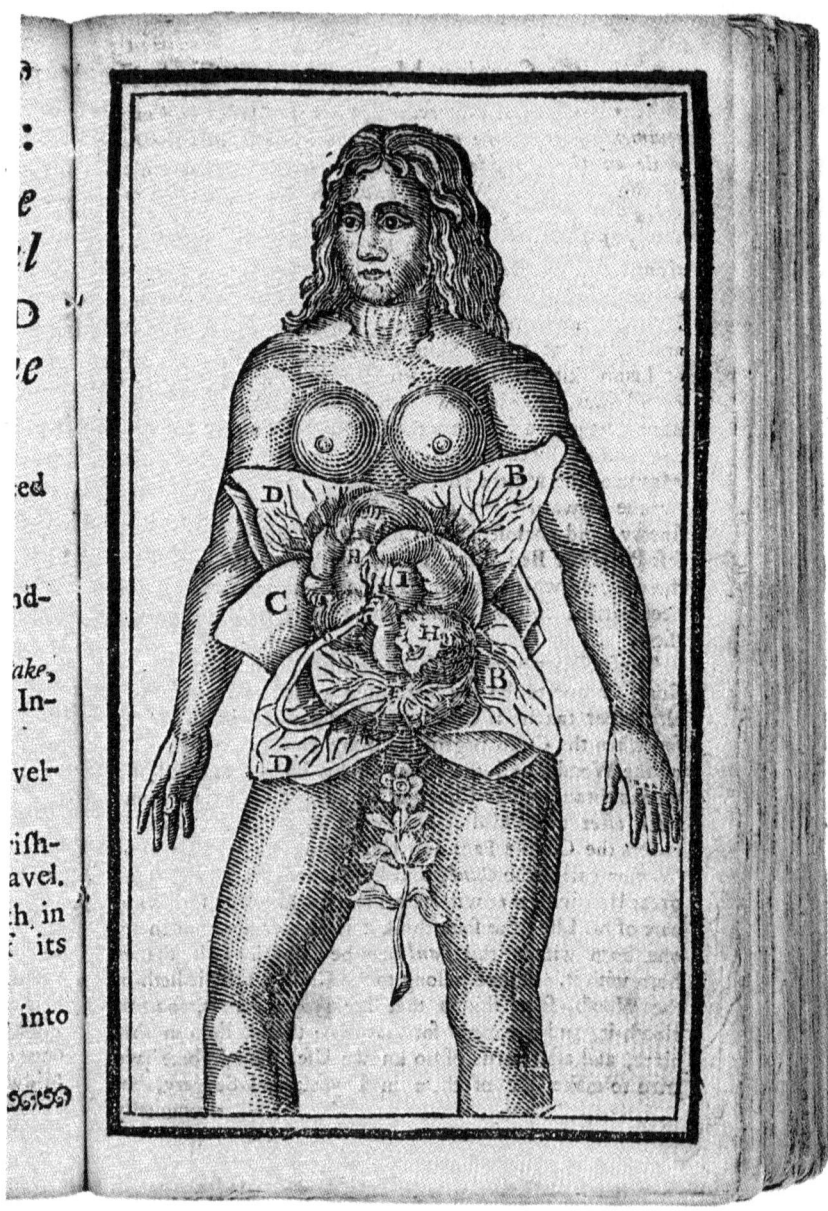

Figure 6.10   Fertile woman, from Jane Sharp's *The Compleat Midwife's Companion*,
1724, London. Courtesy of the Wellcome Library, London

abilities with learned culture. They implied their knowledge and training could supplant nature in its absence. Yet the men also described the physicality of their interventions, explaining how their sensitive and perceptive hands entered the womb to correct malpresentations. They insisted that these endeavours were not easy, but rather required bodily strength and endurance, asserting that repositioning an unborn child regularly left them exhausted or drenched in sweat.[94] As indicated in Chapters 4 and 5, surgeon men-midwives simultaneously distanced themselves from and associated themselves with the corporeality of the maternal body, claiming their own bodily labour could substitute for that of women.

Images of the unborn contribute to arguments about when and how men should perform the maternal role traditionally assigned to women. The absence of the maternal body is shown to coincide with the entry of medical expertise. Representations of endangered unborn children are accompanied by indexical signs of medical presence in the form of physically opened wombs or intervening hands, participating in efforts to associate the hands of medical men with the ability to perceive the invisible womb. This interpretation is not at odds with earlier discussions of both the diagrammatic character of the images and their role in the creation of medical identity. By providing rhetorical rather than strictly intellectual support for surgeon men-midwives' haptic acquisition of knowledge of the womb, images of the unborn demonstrate the necessity and legitimacy of male intervention. They continue to point to the male practitioner and his knowledge instead of reflecting understandings of the womb itself.

Images of the unborn present arguments about obstetrical authority, not representations of dominant beliefs about childbirth. For even as surgeon men-midwives insisted on the superiority of male expertise in their obstetrical treatises, they complained about women's lack of cooperation. The men noted that labouring women and their female midwives often refused to summon male surgeons in difficult cases, relinquishing their maternal privileges to the men.[95] At the same time, women were hardly absent from the lying-in chamber even when men were called. Accounts written by surgeon men-midwives describe female clients who questioned the men's interpretations of their bodies, and doubted that male practitioners would be able to complete the birth.[96] Resistance to the arguments made by male midwives is also found in the treatises produced by female practitioners, including those images of the unborn reshaped to signify women's ability to intervene manually in the womb.

The lack of a maternal body in the images enhances the subjectivity of the medical expert, not the unborn child. Newman mistakenly assumes that the fetus is the object represented, and that it is portrayed as a unique individual endowed with rights. There is neither visual nor written support for her claims in early modern French obstetrical treatises. According to Duden, the concept of a fetus did not even exist until the late eighteenth century.[97] She argues that the earliest disembodied vision of the fetus appeared in the treatise, *Icones Embryonum Humanorum* [Images of human embryos], published by German physician Thomas Soemmerring in 1799. Advocating a drawing technique based on careful architectonic-geometric measurement, Soemmerring produced the first objective fetus. Duden concludes that the fetus is not a natural object, but rather the historical result of mechanically produced records.[98] She criticizes Newman's unhistorical approach to the topic, which presupposes the existence of the fetus as an object that is simply represented in different sources over time.[99] By examining the ways in which the fetus was invented towards the end of the early modern period, Duden undermines the idea that there have been relatively stable inscriptions of it since the ninth century.

There was certainly no stable representation of a 'fetus' in the obstetrical treatises produced by French authors. Those about to be born were almost always referred to as children, not fetuses. Calling the unborn figure a child did not evoke notions of its independence but rather placed it in a familial relationship. Surgeon men-midwives were often summoned to assist at difficult deliveries by family members that could include parents, husbands, and relatives in addition to suffering women and their female midwives.[100] The men operated within the environment of the family, a situation reinforcing the identity of the unborn child in relation to others. According to historian Natalie Zemon Davis, the family was the primary unit from which early modern people took identity.[101] Boundaries between people were not rigid at the time, particularly those separating parents and their children – progeny who were officially subject to parents until the age of consent. Davis nevertheless finds evidence that women and children managed to achieve some forms of self-presentation even within the patriarchal and hierarchical family structure.[102]

An implicit understanding of this hierarchy informs the case studies reported in obstetrical treatises. Both male and female midwives agreed that in difficult cases their primary duty was to save the life of the mother.[103] Few undertook theological discussions about whether or not her life was of greater value than that of the unborn child. They clearly did not comprehend, however, the unborn child as an inviolable figure endowed with rights equal to those of the mother. Mauriceau was not alone when he claimed that a living unborn child could be sacrificed because 'we ought always to prefer the mother's life before that of the child's.'[104] Rival surgeon man-midwife Peu disagreed, defending the use of *crochets* to remove a mutilated child that could be baptised even if it did not survive.[105] He was apparently more concerned with saving the child's soul than with preserving its bodily integrity. Though surgeon men-midwives trumpeted their capacity to remove malpositioned children from the womb, the survival of these children was given less attention than that of the mother. The case studies in obstetrical treatises regularly mentioned her recovery, sometimes noting how quickly she 'got up' from her bed.[106] This situation resulted partly because men were often called to remove dead children from the wombs of women who had laboured in vain for days and were themselves on the verge of death.

Authors of obstetrical treatises did not always refer to the unborn as children. They used the term embryo when providing an overview of the processes of conception, information included in 13 of the books published between 1550 and 1730. Drawing on a Galenic model to describe the sequence of events, writers affirmed that after the early formation of the heart, liver, and brain, all the parts were 'complete' in about five to six weeks, and able to move gently in the womb at three months for males and four for females.[107] Unlike authors of anatomical or embryological publications, those writing obstetrical treatises supplied brief summaries of well-established theories, not extended evaluations of them.[108] In 1573, barber-surgeon Ambroise Paré produced one of the longest discussions of the embryo, arguing that after the seed fermented in the womb, three bubbles formed the rudimentary beginnings of the major organs, and then the bones and interconnecting channels were covered with a protective skin. The embryo was finally endowed with a soul, a change occurring after 40 days for boys, and 45 days for colder girls.[109] His synopsis was echoed with slight changes in subsequent treatises, including that of midwife La Marche in 1677, who similarly noted that the 'three noble parts' were discernible after 26 days of gestation, with all of the parts perfectly formed between 33 and 42 days according to its sex.[110] Yet later writers paid considerably less attention than Paré to the question of ensoulment, mentioning it only in passing if at all.[111] The first volume of Louise Bourgeois' treatise in 1609 provides one exception. She claimed that a woman three and a half months pregnant had produced a tiny child with a visible head, spine, and partially formed limbs. Disparaging those people with little regard for that which had neither life nor a rational soul, the midwife argued against the practice of abortion. Though Paré followed Augustine by asserting that the child received its immortal soul after its parts were formed, Bourgeois invoked the ancient understanding of the tripartite soul by arguing that it was wrong to prevent a child endowed with only a vegetative soul from receiving its sensitive and rational souls.[112] She alluded to the belief that an unborn child was finally infused with a rational soul after about six months of gestation, and then grew stronger during its final months in the womb.[113]

Both Paré and Bourgeois drew on theories of the development of the unborn figure, insisting that it progressed from an unformed to a perfected state. The terms embryo and child are not usually tied, however, to precise or measurable stages in early modern French obstetrical treatises. Though Paré confirmed that until its parts were formed and soul infused, it could not be called child but only 'fetus, embryo, bubbling, beginning, or ripening,' Bourgeois simultaneously referred to the tiny figure she encountered as child and unformed.[114] Later authors would also use the terms embryo and child synonymously, along with the designation fetus, which increased in obstetrical treatises after 1650, perhaps in response to the intensified publication of anatomical and embryological studies.[115] In 1694 Peu referred to unborn figures interchangeably as children and fetuses, while in 1714 surgeon man-midwife Pierre Amand claimed to have examined two fetuses expelled from the womb before 25 days of gestation.[116] Mauquest de La Motte's later treatise did not attach the designation of fetus to a specific object. He insisted that pregnancy could not be verified until the fourth month 'because before that time, what the uterus contains, is so small, that it is impossible to affirm whether it be a fetus, mole, water, wind, or only a suppression of the menses.'[117] In keeping with Duden's arguments about the unpredictable contents of the early modern womb, he insisted that fetus was an uncertain classification, only one possibility among others.

It is impossible to link the terms embryo, fetus, and child with solid definitions in most obstetrical treatises, but some patterns of their use can be discerned. Authors primarily reserved the labels embryo and fetus for the early rather than later stages of pregnancy, though in 1693 physician Théodore Turquet de Mayerne uniquely and without explanation called even fully developed children about to be born 'fetuses.'[118] At the same time, authors used such terms almost exclusively in theoretical discussions of the conception and growth of the unborn figure. Peu, for example, referred to fetuses only in his summaries of the formation of the placenta and purpose of the umbilical cord.[119] Authors typically employed the words embryo and fetus in anatomical descriptions of early development in general, not in specific case studies which mentioned individual pregnant women and their families. This limited usage suggests the references linked authors with anatomical and embryological theories, displaying the breadth of their medical knowledge rather than pointing to specific objects enclosed in the womb.

Discussions of theories of conception and the development of the embryo are remarkably consistent in early modern French obstetrical treatises, avoiding innovative beliefs in the *ova* and preformation until well into the eighteenth century. Yet some changes in the publications occurred during the second half of the seventeenth century. At that point, several surgeon men-midwives began to include descriptions of the dissections they had performed on minuscule creatures simultaneously referred to as fetuses, embryos, and children. While this blurring of categories was not unusual, a few authors found signs of the formed child in even the tiniest unborn figures. In his treatise of 1685, for example, surgeon man-midwife Paul Portal recounted how he had dissected a hard blood clot excreted by an ill woman, discovering the early formation of a child in 'an embryo or child of the size and length of a fly, or a clove.'[120] Noting the woman was three months pregnant, Portal reasoned the undersized embryo must have been deprived of food at the beginning of its generation. Mauriceau also drew on his own experiences with tiny figures expelled from the womb, arguing that in 1679 he had seen a five-week-old fetus that was no bigger than a fingernail and yet had all the parts of its body as perfectly formed as those of a nine-month-old child. This encounter confirmed his opinion that the fetus was entirely formed and endowed with life from the first days of conception, though its parts were difficult to see because of their infinitesimal size and softness.[121] Unlike early writers such as Paré, both Mauriceau and Portal recognized the formation of a child very soon after conception.

The surgeon men-midwives invoked what literary scholar Eve Keller has called the metamorphic embryo, a mechanistic approach to conception not necessarily at odds with the established two seed theory. In contrast to descriptions of the sequential development of the embryo, metamorphosis held that all aspects of the child were formed simultaneously after fecundation, even if they were not immediately visible.[122] Analysing embryological scholarship during the second half of the seventeenth century, Keller argues that the theory of the metamorphic embryo insisted on the immediate evidence of human identity in response to mechanical accounts of reproduction that threatened to remove human agency from the process. She concludes that 'the more mechanistic the theory, the earlier the attribution of identity' to the unborn figure.[123] Extending her arguments to visual representation, Keller contends that when seen in the light of new embryological theories, longstanding images of children about to be born potentially invoked the prospect of fetal and even embryonic personhood.

Keller is correct to point out that changing historical understandings of conception could alter interpretations of images of the unborn. It does not follow, however, that unborn figures were considered rights-bearing individuals because some authors saw signs of humanity in tiny figures discharged from the womb. Unborn creatures were certainly not treated as persons. Obstetrical treatises uniformly describe them as objects of medical manipulation. Those about to be born were handled by surgeon men-midwives, while those expelled before their time were subject to dissection. These creatures were also squashed underfoot when dropped on the floor, cast into the fire, and preserved as marvelous specimens in medical collections.[124] Portal reported saving his minuscule embryo in water, and though Mauriceau argued against inducing abortion while making special efforts to baptize the tiny children, he too displayed them in flasks filled with alcohol as part of his personal collection.[125] Amand likewise placed his 'perfectly formed' 25-day-old embryos in vials of alcohol for display in his home.[126] The curiosities were furthermore likened to a host of non-human items, including seeds, honey bees, and peas. According to Jacques Duval in 1612, a one-month-old unborn child was the size of a large ant, whereas Portal equated an embryo with a hazelnut, and Mauquest de La Motte described it with reference to a grain of wheat.[127] Such comparisons were not unusual, given that embryologists often based their arguments about conception and the formation of the child on analogies with the rest of nature.[128] Although insisting that the unborn bore unmistakably human characteristics distinguishing them from other creatures, the continuing use of analogy simultaneously related them to their inhuman counterparts.

Neither the visual nor the written contents of early modern French obstetrical treatises characterize the unborn as beings able to exist apart from others. Images show imperiled unborn figures requiring medical assistance, while the shifting classifications of embryo, fetus, and unborn child do not point to objects with fixed meanings. Instead, the terms always assume significance in relation to other concepts. Though associated with pregnant women and their families, in discussions of conception the categories were linked with various products of nature, including fruit, insects, and grains. According to at least one surgeon man-midwife, while in the womb the uncertain fetus could scarcely be distinguished from wind or retained menstrual blood. When separated from the maternal body and its productivity, the unborn were related to medical experts, especially surgeon men-midwives. In these cases, embryos, fetuses, and unborn children were produced by the perceptive hands of these men, or endowed with significance within their marvelous collections. Representations of the unborn provided modes of interpretation and sites for the production of medical identity; they did not portray the unborn as unique individuals endowed with rights.

Conclusions

Early modern French images of the unborn do not represent a modern fetus. Nor do they depict beliefs about the physiology of the womb. These complex images primarily combine iconic and indexical signs to make arguments about the haptic knowledge and gendered medical identity of the practitioner who intervenes in difficult deliveries, substituting for the maternal body. But even this conclusion is reductive. For early modern images of the unborn in treatises penned by both male and female midwives are riddled with contradictions, referring to anatomical expertise, delightful male *putti*, and an exhausted maternal body, among other things. By recognizing this diversity, modern scholars can avoid mistaking both the purpose and meaning of these images. At the same time, they can think more complexly about early modern representation in general, refusing to assume that images are exclusively based on the principle of visual resemblance, reflecting social, cultural, or medical beliefs.

My interpretation applies only to early modern French images of the unborn. It cannot simply be transferred to other malpresenting birth figures, such as those found in concurrent English treatises, no matter how similar they appear to be. Part of my argument is that different images have different meanings. I have nevertheless suggested a way to approach other images of the unborn. Each representation requires its own careful visual analysis, one that pays as much attention to how the image signifies as to what it signifies. This analysis should move beyond the image proper, considering the publication in which it was reproduced as well as the social site of its enunciation, including obstetrical discourses and debates at the time. Attending to intertextuality ought to reveal how each particular image both transforms and incorporates a broader system of signs related to obstetrical authority, medical identity, anatomical knowledge, and other arenas not considered here. At the same time, scholars should be prepared to find contradictory messages that refuse to gel into a tidy conclusion.

Modern scholars who see fetal persons when they look at early modern images of the unborn have not simply made an unhistorical error. Their interpretations are based on the continuing effects of intertextuality. Although earlier texts are transformed in later ones, the opposite is also true. Subsequent transformations affect the entire system of signs, reshaping their predecessors. In other words, early modern birth figures look different now. They appear to be undeniably endowed with subjectivity because of the meanings currently attached to fetal imagery. This interpretation reveals the success of the anti-abortion insistence that fetal images are signifiers linked with only one signified – fetal personhood. Concluding that early modern images of the unborn represent independent persons is not simply wrong, it is reductive. Such readings do little justice to the layered, flexible, and paradoxical images, replacing their ambiguities with a static interpretation.

Notes

1.   Barbara Duden, 'The Fetus as an Object of Our Time,' *Res* 25 (Spring 1994), 132–5, E. Ann Kaplan, 'Look Who's Talking, Indeed: Fetal Images in Recent North American Visual Culture,' Evelyn Nakano Glenn, Grace Chang, and Linda Rennie Forcey, eds, *Mothering: Ideology, Experience, and Agency* (New York: Routledge, 1994), 121–37, Janelle S. Taylor, 'The Public Fetus and the Family Car: From Abortion Politics to a Volvo Advertisement,' *Public Culture* 4, 2 (1992), 67–80, and Bruce Mink, 'American Cancer Society's "Smoking Fetus,"' *American Cinematographer* 66 (August 1985), 77–80.

2.   Susan Squier, 'Fetal Subjects and Maternal Objects: Reproductive Technology and the New Fetal/Maternal Relation,' *Journal of Medicine and Philosophy* 21 (October 1996), 515–35, Jessie Givner, 'Reproducing Reproductive Discourse: Optical Technologies in *The Silent Scream* and *Eclipse of Reason*,' *Journal of Popular Culture* 28 (Winter 1994), 229–44, Lauren Berlant, 'America, "Fat," the Fetus,' *Boundary* 21 (Fall 1994), 145–95, Valerie Hartouni, 'Fetal Exposures: Abortion Politics and the Optics of Allusion,' *Camera Obscura* 29 (May 1992), 130–149, and Sarah Franklin, 'Fetal Fascinations: New Dimensions to the Medical-Scientific Construction of Fetal Personhood,' Sarah Franklin, Celia Lury, and Jackie Stacey, eds, *Off-Centre: Feminism and Cultural Studies* (London: Harper Collins, 1991), 190–205.

3.   Carol A. Stabile, 'The Traffic in Fetuses,' Lynn M. Morgan and Meredith W. Michaels, eds, *Fetal Subjects, Feminist Positions* (Philadelphia: University of Pennsylvania Press, 1999), 133–58, Barbara Duden, *Disembodying Women: Perspectives on Pregnancy and the Unborn*, Lee Hoinacki, trans. (Cambridge, MA:

Harvard University Press, 1993), 99–106, and Rosalind Pollack Petchesky, 'Foetal Images: The Power of Visual Culture in the Politics of Reproduction,' Michelle Stanworth, ed., *Reproductive Technologies: Gender, Motherhood and Medicine* (Minneapolis: University of Minnesota Press, 1987), 57–80.

4.   Karen Newman, *Fetal Positions: Individualism, Science, Visuality* (Stanford: Stanford University Press, 1996), 26.

5.   *Ibid.*, 67.

6.   François Mauriceau, *Des maladies des femmes grosses et accouchées* (Paris, 1668), 285–90.

7.   *Ibid.*, 300–33.

8.   Paul Portal, *La pratique des accouchemens* (Paris, 1685), 44. On 204 Portal insisted that distinguishing by touch between the child's mouth, ear, and anus, was not easy. Jacques Bury, *Le propagatif de l'homme* (Paris, 1623), 93–4, argued that the unborn child's body parts were easy to confuse in stomach presentations.

9.   Mauriceau, *Des maladies des femmes grosses et accouchées*, 209–20, Cosme Viardel, *Observations sur la pratique des accouchemens naturels, contre nature & monstrueux* (Paris, 1671), 6, and Pierre Dionis, *Traité général des accouchemens* (Paris, 1718), 100–106.

10. Dionis, *Traité général des accouchemens*, 248.

11. For an account of how quickening, the first perceptible movement of the unborn child, was linked with its religious and legal status see Duden, *Disembodying Women*, 59–60, 79–82, and 94–6.

12. Viardel, *Observations sur la pratique des accouchemens naturels, contre nature & monstrueux*, 15–16, Mauriceau, *Des maladies des femmes grosses et accouchées*, 232–3, and Guillaume Mauquest de La Motte, *Traité complet des accouchemens* (Paris, 1729; orig. 1721), 93.

13. Mauquest de La Motte, *Traité complet des accouchemens*, 97.

14. See, for example, François Mauriceau, *Observations sur la grossesse et l'accouchement des femmes* (Paris, 1695), 30 and 48, and Philippe Peu, *La pratique des accouchemens* (Paris, 1694), 377 and 390.

15. Newman, *Fetal Positions*, 33.

16. Marguerite de La Marche [du Tertre], *Instruction familière et très utile aux sages-femmes pour bien pratiquer les accouchemens* (Paris, 1710; orig. 1677), 22: 'Conception est une vivification des semences procurée par le pouvoir de la matrice.'

17. Charles de Saint-Germain, *L'eschole méthodique et parfaite des sages-femmes* (Paris, 1650), 49.

18. Helen King, *Hippocrates' Woman: Reading the Female Body in Ancient Greece* (London: Routledge, 1998), 9, discusses the 'sliding scale' of gendered distinctions in the Hippocratic corpus, with various men and women producing seed of differing quality.

19. D. M. Balme, 'Ανθρωπος 'ανθρωπον γεννᾷ: Human is Generated by Human,' G. R. Dunstan, ed., *The Human Embryo: Aristotle and the Arabic and European Traditions* (Exeter: University of Exeter Press, 1990), 20–31.

20. William Harvey, *Exercitationes de generatione animalium* (London, 1651).

21. Jacques Roger, *The Life Sciences in Eighteenth-Century French Thought*, Robert Ellrich, trans. (Stanford: Stanford University Press, 1997), 215. See also 206–35 for differing theories about where the egg was produced.

22. Pierre Amand, *Nouvelles observations sur la pratique des accouchemens* (Paris, 1714), 58.

23. Mauquest de La Motte, *Traité complet des accouchemens*, 22. For the standard comparison of the miscarried embryo to an egg see Roger, *The Life Sciences in Eighteenth-Century French Thought*, 206.

24. Dionis, *Traité général des accouchemens*, 88–9. Pierre Dionis, *Dissertation sur la génération de l'homme* (Paris, 1698), 56–7, had already noted that the two semen theory was not generally accepted by anatomists.

25. For a few examples of this commonplace see Louise Bourgeois, *Observations diverses sur la stérilité, perte de fruict, foecondité, accouchements et maladies des femmes et enfants nouveaux naiz*, Françoise Olive, ed. (Paris: Côté-Femmes, 1992; orig. 1652), 60, and Dionis, *Traité général des accouchemens*, 93–8.

26. Almost every treatise includes advice for pregnant women, but see for example, Mauriceau, *Des maladies des femmes grosses et accouchées*, 105–17, Bury, *Le propagatif de l'homme*, 47–51, and Dionis, *Traité général des accouchemens* 137–43.

27. Mauriceau, *Des maladies des femmes grosses et accouchées*, 105: 'la mere ne peut pas estre incommodée, sans que son enfant ne s'en ressente.'

28. Bourgeois, *Observations diverses*, 51, 168, advised women to avoid anger, while Peu, *La pratique des accouchemens*, 64–86, devoted an entire chapter to the negative effects of pregnant women's uncontrolled passions.

29. Peu, *La pratique des accouchemens*, 71–2.

30. Marie-Hélène Huet, *Monstrous Imagination* (Cambridge, MA: Harvard University Press, 1993).

31. Mauriceau, *Des maladies des femmes grosses et accouchées*, 59–60.

32. Viardel, *Observations sur la pratique des accouchemens naturels, contre nature & monstrueux*, 49, and Peu, *La pratique des accouchemens*, 463.

33. See Mauquest de La Motte, *Traité complet des accouchemens*, 122, for a description of the child initiating delivery. For the womb as a prison see Viardel, *Observations sur la pratique des accouchemens naturels, contre nature & monstrueux*, 16, and Peu, *La pratique des accouchemens*, 477.

34. Laurent Joubert, *Popular Errors*, Gregory David de Rocher, trans. (Tuscaloosa: University of Alabama Press, 1989), 142–3.

35. Jacques Guillemeau, *De l'heureux accouchement des femmes* (Paris, 1609), 168: 'l'enfant s'efforce & roidist pour sortir dehors, & que la matrice se bande & reserre pour estre delivree de ce fardeau.' See also Mauquest de La Motte, *Traité complet des accouchemens*, 679, for an account of the uterus assisting the child with its pains. According to de La Marche [du Tertre], *Instruction familière et très utile aux sages-femmes pour bien pratiquer les accouchemens*, 54, both mother and child participated in the birth.

36. Peu, *La pratique des accouchemens*, 159–65, for example, advised surgeons to work with the woman's pains and attempt to conserve her strength. See also the anatomical treatise by André Du Laurens, *Toutes les oeuvres de Me André Du Laurens* (Rouen,

1621), 437, for unnatural childbirth resulting when the efforts of either the mother or the child were lacking.

37.   Charles Sanders Peirce, 'Prolegomena to an Apology for Pragmaticism,' James Hoopes, ed., *Peirce on Signs: Writings on Semiotics by Charles Sanders Peirce* (Chapel Hill: University of North Carolina Press, 1991), 251–2. Charles Sanders Peirce, *Collected Papers*, vol. 1–6, Charles Hartshorne and Paul Weiss, eds (Cambridge, MA: Belknap Press of Harvard University Press, 1931–1935), characterized the icon as 'a sign which stands for something merely because it resembles it' (vol. 3, 211), as 'partaking in the characters of the object' (vol. 4, 414), or as a sign whose 'qualities resemble those of that object, and excite analogous sensations in the mind for which it is a likeness' (vol. 2, 168).

38.   Duden, *Disembodying Women*, 36.

39.   Peirce, *Collected Papers*, 2, 143–4. See also Kaja Silverman, *The Subject of Semiotics* (New York: Oxford University Press, 1983), 14–25.

40.   Barbara Duden, 'The Fetus on the "Farther Shore": Toward a History of the Unborn,' Lynn M. Morgan and Meredith W. Michaels, eds, *Fetal Subjects, Feminist Positions*, 16–18.

41.   Almost every treatise includes advice about how to determine a 'true' pregnancy. See, for example, Viardel, *Observations sur la pratique des accouchemens naturels, contre nature & monstrueux*, 8–12, Mauriceau, *Des maladies des femmes grosses et accouchées*, 76–80, Peu, *La pratique des accouchemens*, 10–21, Dionis, *Traité général des accouchemens*, 122–8.

42.   Dionis, *Traité général des accouchemens*, 247.

43.   Guillaume Mauquest de La Motte, *A General Treatise of Midwifry*, Thomas Tomkyns, trans. (London, 1746), ix.

44.   Dionis, *Traité général des accouchemens*, vij: 'à n'avoir pas une soumission aveugle pour tout ce que nos Anciens.'

45.   Mauriceau, *Des maladies des femmes grosses et accouchées*, unpaginated preface: 'De quantité de sçavans Auteurs...n'ayant jamais pratiqué l'Art qu'il nous ont voulu enseigner, ressemblent (à mon avis) à ces Geographes, qui nous font la description de plusieurs terres qu'ils n'ont jamais veuës.'

46.   Mauquest de La Motte, *Traité complet des accouchemens*, 192, conflated touching with seeing, or verifying the truth. Peu, *La pratique des accouchemens*, 408, wrote: 'Je la glissai le long du corps pour découvrir l'épine & le ventre, & reconnoître ensuite lequel des deux pieds.' Peu, 450, lamented he was not able to use his hand to enlighten himself in a particularly difficult case: 'Je ne pouvois pas introduire la main pour m'en éclaircir.' Portal, *La pratique des accouchemens*, 2, 5, 79, linked touching with recognizing, examining and observing. Portal, 53, also wrote: 'Pour en avoir cependant une connoissance plus certaine, je glissay mes doigts plus avant.'

47.   Portal, *La pratique des accouchemens*, 27, advised the surgeon man-midwife: 'examiner doucement avec le doigt, si on sent la bouche, le nez, les yeux, le front, & le menton de l'Enfant. En ayant observé & reconnu que c'est la face.'

48.   Peu, *La pratique des accouchements*, 54.

49.   The report by le Duc, 'Observation d'une flâme sortie du ventre d'une femme en couche,' appeared in Claude Brunet's *Le Progrès de la médecine* (Paris, 1709), 73–8.

According to Brunet, le Duc described how a hot, violet flame was expelled from the vagina of his newly-delivered client. The master surgeon concluded that because the womb was always dark and shrouded in obscurity (forcing the man-midwife to see with his fingers), the flame must have come from without – most likely, a candle ignited the vapours being discharged from the woman's body.

50. Mauquest de La Motte, *Traité complet des accouchemens*, xii.

51. Dionis, *Traité général des accouchemens*, xj–xij: 'estimant qu'elles seroient inutiles, parce que ce ne sont point les yeux de l'Accoucheur qui lui apprennent comment l'enfant est tourné dans la matrice, c'est en la touchant qui'l [sic] s'en instruit.'

52. Peu, *La pratique des accouchemens*, 441: 'qui peuvent servir comme d'idée principale pour s'en réprésenter une infinité d'autres possibles.'

53. I thank Steven Turner for suggesting this interpretation to me.

54. Peirce, *Collected Papers*, vol. 4, 87. See also Hugh Joswick, 'The Object of Semeiotic,' Vincent M. Colapietro and Thomas M. Olshewsky, eds, *Peirce's Doctrine of Signs: Theory, Applications, and Connections* (Berlin: Mouton de Gruyter, 1996), 100.

55. Roland Daube-Schackat, 'Peirce and Hermeneutics,' Colapietro and Olshewsky, eds, *Peirce's Doctrine of Signs*, 389. See also David Savan, *An Introduction to C.S. Peirce's Semiotics*, vol. 1 (Toronto: Toronto Semiotic Circle, 1976), 44.

56. Daube-Schackat, 'Peirce and Hermeneutics,' 386.

57. Peirce, *Collected Papers*, vol. 2, 157.

58. *Ibid.*, vol. 2, 159. Algebraic formulas, for example, only 'exhibit, by means of the algebraic signs (which are not themselves icons), the relations of the quantities concerned.' For an excellent explanation of Peirce's conception of the iconic sign see Thomas A. Sebeok, 'Iconicity,' *MLN* 91, 6 (December 1976), 1427–56.

59. Umberto Eco, *Kant and the Platypus: Essays on Language and Cognition*, Alastair McEwen, trans. (San Diego: Harcourt, 1999), 340.

60. David A. Pharies, *Charles S. Peirce and the Linguistic Sign* (Amsterdam: John Benjamins Publishing, 1985), 36.

61. Charles Sanders Peirce, *The New Elements of Mathematics*, Carolyn Eisele, ed. (The Hague: Mouton, 1976), 315–16, note 1. For Peirce's discussion of existential graphs as the graphic representation of thought and the thought process see Don D. Roberts, *The Existential Graphs of Charles S. Peirce* (The Hague: Mouton, 1973).

62. Peirce, 'Prolegomena to an Apology for Pragmaticism,' 251.

63. Eco, *Kant and the Platypus*, 343, argues that Peirce never denied the broadly conventional content of the icon.

64. Gérard Deledalle, *Charles S. Peirce's Philosophy of Signs: Essays in Comparative Semiotics* (Bloomington: Indiana University Press, 2000), 20, argues that 'nothing is in itself icon, index, or symbol. ... It is the analysis of a given semiosis (and not the formal analysis of the semiotic triad) which will tell us the "nature" of its constituents.' Sebeok, 'Iconicity,' 1433, note 2, claims 'it is inane to ask whether any given object "is," or is represented by, an icon, an index, or a symbol, for all signs are situated in a complex network of syntagmatic and paradigmatic contrasts and oppositions. ... It is their position at a particular moment that will determine the predominance of the aspect in focus.'

65. Mauriceau, *Des maladies des femmes grosses et accouchées*, provides an exception because many of the engravings are signed. While Antoine Paillet and Guillaume Vallet produced his author portrait, the anatomical plates were designed by Pierre Lombard and engraved by Paul Androuet de Cerceau, and Karl Audran drew the unborn figures. Though Mauriceau's treatise indicates that an array of artists were commissioned to make the images, both Portal's portrait and some of the figures inside his treatise were produced by the same artists, Gabriel Revel and Matthieu Lefebvre.

66. Cited in Jeanine Parisier Plottel, 'Introduction,' Jeanine Parisier Plottel and Hanna Charney, eds, *Inter-textuality: New Perspectives in Criticism* (New York: New York Literary Forum, 1978), xiv.

67. A belief in the conventional nature of visual art underpins, for example, the practice of iconographical analysis. See Erwin Panofsky, *Studies in Iconology: Humanistic Themes in the Art of the Renaissance* (New York: Harper and Row, 1962).

68. Jacques Derrida, 'Différance,' Hazard Adams and Leroy Searle, eds, *Critical Theory Since 1965* (Tallahassee: Florida State University Press, 1986), 120–36. See also Graham Allen, *Intertextuality* (London: Routledge, 2000), 64–5.

69. Julia Kristeva, *Desire in Language: A Semiotic Approach to Literature and Art* (New York: Columbia University Press, 1980), 36.

70. E. Ingerslev, 'Rösslin's "Rosegarten": Its Relation to the Past (the Muscio Manuscripts and Soranos), particularly with regard to Podalic Version,' *The Journal of Obstetrics and Gynaecology of the British Empire* 15, 1 (1909), 1–25.

71. Philippe Hecquet, *De l'indécence aux hommes d'accoucher les femmes* (Paris, 1708).

72. See, for example, Guillemeau, *De l'heureux accouchement des femmes*, unpaginated preface, Viardel, *Observations sur la pratique des accouchemens naturels, contre nature & monstrueux*, unpaginated preface, and Dionis, *Traité général des accouchemens*, unpaginated preface.

73. See, for example, Poussin's *Putti Fighting on Goats*, of the 1630s, his *Echo and Narcissus* of 1627, and engravings after the works by Stella in Anthony Blunt, *Nicolas Poussin* (London: Pallas Athene, 1995), 111, colour plate III, and 324.

74. For angelic *putti* see Poussin's *The Rest on the Flight into Egypt*, and *The Assumption of the Virgin*, both early works though not firmly dated, in Blunt, *Nicolas Poussin*, 428–9.

75. Charles Sanders Peirce, 'Sign,' James Hoopes, ed., *Peirce on Signs*, 239–40.

76. Mieke Bal and Norman Bryson, 'Semiotics and Art History,' *Art Bulletin* 73, 2 (June 1991), 190.

77. Charles Estienne, *La dissection des parties du corps humain* (Paris, 1546), and Berengario da Carpi, *Commentaria* (Bologna, 1521).

78. See Chapter 2, notes 45–8. Though the opened wombs might also seem to refer to the caesarean operation, postmortem caesareans were rarely performed, and early modern medical images of the caesarean operation show a tidy crescent-shaped incision, not a gaping wound.

79. See Chapter 2, notes 63–5 and 71–5.

80. Jonathan Sawday, *The Body Emblazoned: Dissection and the Human Body in Renaissance Culture* (London: Routledge, 1995), 110–29.

81.   For an excellent analysis of this paradox in both early modern and contemporary anatomies see Catherine Waldby, *The Visible Human Project* (New York: Routledge, 2000). For the gendered connotations of early modern anatomical images see Valerie Traub, 'Gendering Mortality in Early Modern Anatomies,' Valerie Traub, M. Lindsay Kaplan and Dympna Callaghan, eds, *Feminist Readings of Early Modern Culture: Emerging Subjects* (Cambridge: Cambridge University Press, 1996), 44–92.

82.   Viardel, *Observations sur la pratique des accouchemens naturels, contre nature & monstrueux*, 222–30.

83.   For Siegemund see Lynne Tatlock, 'Speculum Feminarum: Gendered Perspectives on Obstetrics and Gynecology in Early Modern Germany,' *Signs* 17, 4 (1992), 725–60.

84.   Nina Rattner Gelbart, *The King's Midwife: A History and Mystery of Madame du Coudray* (Berkeley: University of California Press, 1998), 130–31.

85.   See Hendrik van Deventer, *The Art of Midwifery Improv'd*, 3rd edn (London, 1728).

86.   Newman, *Fetal Positions*, 67.

87.   For this commonplace see, for example, Saint-Germain, *L'eschole méthodique et parfaite des sages-femmes*, 49. In keeping with ancient tradition, the physician argued that stronger semen formed boys who developed more quickly than more feeble girls. Boys were also linked with the increased health of the pregnant woman. See Guillemeau, *De l'heureux accouchement des femmes*, 14–17, for male children produced by hotter and younger women, who consequently had good complexions and bright eyes while pregnant.

88.   See, for example, Mauriceau, *Des maladies des femmes grosses et accouchées*, 194–5, and 209, as well as Portal, *La pratique des accouchemens*, 7.

89.   See, for example, Guillemeau, *De l'heureux accouchement des femmes*, 167–9, Peu, *La pratique des accouchemens*, 145–6, and Amand, *Nouvelles observations sur la pratique des accouchemens*, 54.

90.   Jane Sharp, *The Midwives' Book* (London, 1671). See also Jacques Gélis, *L'arbre et le fruit: la naissance dans l'Occident moderne, XVIe–XIXe siècle* (Paris: Fayard, 1984).

91.   Bury, *Le propagatif de l'homme*, 78–82, and Peu, *La pratique des accouchemens*, 257–8.

92.   Mauriceau, *Des maladies des femmes grosses et accouchées*, 256–7.

93.   See, for example, Mauriceau, *Des maladies des femmes grosses et accouchées*, 256, and Amand, *Nouvelles observations sur la pratique des accouchemens*, 15, and 228.

94.   See Chapter 5, notes 90–93.

95.   Mauriceau, *Des maladies des femmes grosses et accouchées*, 243, Portal, *La pratique des accouchemens*, 9, and Dionis, *Traité général des accouchemens*, 218, recounted cases when the surgeon was called too late to be of assistance. For women's resistance to men see also Chapter 2, notes 14–17.

96.   Both Dionis, *Traité général des accouchemens*, 133, and Amand, *Nouvelles observations sur la pratique des accouchemens*, 193, described female clients who refused to believe the men's diagnoses of pregnancy. Mauriceau, *Des maladies des femmes grosses et accouchées*, 193, provided advice about how to convince women to submit to the surgeon man-midwife's operations, using gentle words to convince them they could not give birth without his help.

97.   Duden, 'The Fetus on the "Farther Shore",' 13.

98. *Ibid.*, 22–23.

99. *Ibid.*, 21.

100. Though Portal, *La pratique des accouchemens*, regularly indicated he was sent for by female midwives, he also noted, 251, that a labouring woman requested his assistance. Viardel, *Observations sur la pratique des accouchemens naturels, contre nature & monstrueux*, 120, argued that a woman's husband sent for him. According to David Harley, 'Provincial Midwives in England: Lancashire and Cheshire, 1660–1760,' Hilary Marland, ed., *The Art of Midwifery: Early Modern Midwives in Europe* (London: Routledge, 1993), 43, by the mid-eighteenth century husbands may have increasingly selected the man-midwife.

101. Natalie Zemon Davis, 'Boundaries and the Sense of Self in Sixteenth-Century France,' Thomas C. Heller, Morton Sosna, and David E. Wellbery, eds, *Reconstructing Individualism: Autonomy, Individuality, and the Self in Western Thought* (Stanford: Stanford University Press, 1986), 53–63.

102. *Ibid.*, 62–3.

103. See, for example, Denis Fournier, *L'accoucheur méthodique* (Paris, 1677), 108, and 346–8. He argued that it was not permissible to put a woman in danger or cause her death in order to save her child.

104. Mauriceau, *Des maladies des femmes grosses et accouchées*, 299: 'nous devons toûjours préferer la vie de la mere à celle de l'enfant.' Citing both the anatomist Jean Riolan and Tertulien, Mauriceau argued that the child should be sacrificed only in extreme cases, following its baptism.

105. Peu, *La pratique des accouchemens*, 351, argued that the goal of using the *crochet* was to save the life of the mother and ensure the eternal salvation of the child.

106. Portal, *La pratique des accouchemens*, 203, and 217, drew attention to the health of his female clients, but at the end of one case study, 142, he added: 'I forgot to say that the child was dead.' Mauquest de La Motte, *A General Treatise of Midwifry*, 304, 323, noted how quickly his female clients recovered.

107. See, for example, Fournier, *L'accoucheur méthodique*, 44, and Viardel, *Observations sur la pratique des accouchemens naturels, contre nature & monstrueux*, 5–8.

108. A few surgeon men-midwives nevertheless wrote separate treatises on conception and generation. See Dionis, *Dissertation sur la génération de l'homme*, and Guillaume Mauquest de La Motte, *Dissertation sur la génération, sur la superfétation et la réponse au livre intitulé: De l'Indécence aux hommes d'accoucher les femmes* (Paris, 1718).

109. Ambroise Paré, *Deux livres de chirurgie, de la génération de l'homme* (Paris, 1573), 37–48. See also Helen King, 'Making a Man: Becoming Human in Early Greek Medicine,' Dunstan, ed., *The Human Embryo*, 10–19.

110. La Marche [du Tertre], *Instruction familière et très utile aux sages-femmes pour bien pratiquer les accouchemens*, 32–3. For a similar description see Saint-Germain, *L'eschole méthodique et parfaite des sages-femmes*, 119–21.

111. Jacques Duval, *Traité des hermaphrodits, parties génitales, accouchemens des femmes* (Rouen, 1612), 128, accorded with Paré, but Dionis, *Traité général des accouchemens*, 98, argued that the point at which an unborn child possessed a soul was entirely unknown.

112. Bourgeois, *Observations diverses*, 48.
113. For early modern understandings of the soul see Vivian Nutton, 'The Anatomy of the Soul in Early Renaissance Medicine,' Dunstan, ed., *The Human Embryo*, 136–57.
114. Paré, *Deux livres de chirurgie, de la génération de l'homme*, 36: 'lequel ne doibt encores estre appelé enfant, tant que toutes ses parties soient bien formees & figurees, & que l'ame y soit introduicte: mais seulement sera appelé Foetus, ou Embrion, ou pululant, ou naissant, ou meurissant.'
115. Fournier, *L'accoucheur méthodique*, 8, 37, 43, and Mauriceau, *Des maladies des femmes grosses et accouchées*, 37, 41, 176, 187, 195, and 210–17.
116. Peu, *La pratique des accouchemens*, 24–33, and Amand, *Nouvelles observations sur la pratique des accouchemens*, 10.
117. Mauquest de La Motte, *Traité complet des accouchemens*, 49.
118. Théodore Turquet de Mayerne, *La pratique de médecine...avec le régime des femmes grosses* (Lyon, 1693), 429–30, 495, and 498–9.
119. Peu, *La pratique des accouchemens*, 38–40.
120. Portal, *La pratique des accouchemens*, 365: 'un Embrion ou Enfant de la grosseur & longueur d'une mouche, ou d'un clou de girofle.'
121. Mauriceau, *Observations sur la grossesse et l'accouchement des femmes*, 142–3.
122. Eve Keller, 'Embryonic Individuals: The Rhetoric of Seventeenth-Century Embryology and the Construction of Early-Modern Identity,' *Eighteenth-Century Studies* 33, 3 (2000), 321–48.
123. *Ibid.*, 323.
124. Mauquest de La Motte, *Traité complet des accouchemens*, 201, and 213.
125. Portal, *La pratique des accouchemens*, 367, and Mauriceau, *Observations sur la grossesse et l'accouchement des femmes*, 142.
126. Amand, *Nouvelles observations sur la pratique des accouchemens*, 10.
127. Duval, *Traité des hermaphrodits, parties génitales, accouchemens des femmes*, 128, Portal, *La pratique des accouchemens*, 365, Mauquest de La Motte, *Traité complet des accouchemens*, 245. Mauriceau, *Observations sur la grossesse et l'accouchement des femmes*, 63–4, and 135, compared the fetus to a honey bee, pea, and grain of millet.
128. Roger, *The Life Sciences in Eighteenth-Century French Thought*, 148–9, and 191–2, argues that a seventeenth-century interest in the fascinating complexity of insects reshaped understandings of nature. The contemporary vogue for microscopy also helps to explain comparisons of tiny embryos and fetuses with insects, especially Robert Hooke's *Micrographia* of 1665, which included detailed illustrations of plants, insects, and inanimate objects.

Conclusions

I began this book with a question: how did men ever appear to be qualified birthing assistants when women were naturally associated with childbirth? According to the visual and written contents of obstetrical treatises published in France between 1550 and 1730, men struggled to be recognized as authorities in the lying-in chamber. Though men criticized female midwives in their books, these sources do not document the medicalization of women's maternal role. Asserting that male medical practitioners wrested control of childbirth from women during the early modern period both overestimates male prestige in the birthing room and underrates women's continuing ability to limit male practice, or refuse it altogether. When examined carefully, obstetrical treatises reveal anxious male practitioners who attempted to reassure women with gentle words and a pleasing appearance, as well as domineering ones who boasted they could intervene to remedy difficult deliveries when women and female midwives failed to do so. Overall, obstetrical treatises suggest that men's entry into the lying-in chamber was a complex negotiation involving their adaptation to the demands of women.

Obstetrical authority remained tied to bodily experience during the seventeenth and early eighteenth centuries. The treatises written by surgeon men-midwives do not exclusively espouse the value of theoretical learning. Male authors strove to associate themselves with a corporeal perception of pregnancy, invoking the bodily experiences of female relatives as well as their own physical exertions in the lying-in chamber. Though in some ways the men appropriated women's labour, they also conveyed a continuing respect for women's embodied experience. Their publications indicate that traditional maternal values were not suddenly discredited during the early modern period, even by those male midwives wishing to be called more promptly to assist at unnatural labours.

The birthing chamber emerges from obstetrical treatises as a highly visual realm in which women regarded men to determine their abilities and demeanour, in keeping with prevailing physiognomical doctrines. Though male practitioners described looking at those parturient women subject to autopsy, they were regularly prevented from seeing the bodies of female clients. Compensating for their inability to gaze at the bodies of women and unborn children, surgeon men-midwives affirmed that touching the female body was more meaningful than looking at it. Their arguments suggest that modern scholars may have overestimated the powerful looking undertaken by male medical practitioners in the lying-in chamber, while neglecting to consider representations of men's embodied experiences as husbands, brothers, sons, and birth attendants. These men were themselves on display, endeavouring to present an appealing spectacle for the largely female audience in the birthing room. Female midwives were similarly subject to scrutiny, required to exhibit their abilities instead of being automatically associated with obstetrical authority. Though Louise Bourgeois insisted her midwifery skills were visibly evident in her person, she also made efforts to demonstrate her masculine anatomical knowledge and propensity for self-control.

Attending to the visual display of expertise in childbirth reveals a more flexible system of gender than has previously been realized. Obstetrical treatises do not simply pit men against women, but rather delineate surgeon men-midwives who adopt feminine qualities such as tenderness and charity, as well as female midwives who espouse medical theory and a masculine character. The images of male and female midwives emerging from treatises written by both men and women are unstable, shifting between gendered roles instead of solidifying them. Distinctions of gender were clearly important, placing women at a disadvantage in relation to the official medical hierarchy and rendering them more vulnerable to medical criticism. Yet gender was not the only factor used to distinguish between practitioners. The age, social status, and physical appearance of birthing attendants of both sexes were also considered crucial to their successful performance at deliveries. Furthermore, the relative importance of these elements could change depending on the circumstances. Bourgeois emphasized her youth when asserting her superiority to the older midwife Madame Dupuis, but stressed her controlled courtly body when describing her role at the first labour of Queen Marie de Médicis.

Obstetrical treatises were sites for the display of identity, producing and contesting understandings of obstetrical authority. Both male and female authors drew on an established genre of visual and written representation to defend as well as legitimate their practices. Though my study ostensibly ends around 1730, the texts did not abruptly change after that date. After all, my discussion included Angélique Marguerite Le Boursier du Coudray's publication of 1759, a treatise attesting to the endurance of visual and written conventions. Male authors also revisited similar themes in later publications. Surgeon man-midwife Jacques Mesnard, for example, continued to describe the manipulation of malpresenting unborn children in the womb in his *Le guide des accoucheurs* [Guide for men-midwives] of 1743. And though Jean Astruc's *L'art d'accoucher réduit à ses principes* [Art of delivery reduced to its principles] of 1766 pays less attention to unnatural deliveries, it is largely a synthesis of the earlier publications on childbirth produced by his fellow physicians.

There are, however, noticeable changes in other obstetrical treatises published during the eighteenth century. André Levret's *L'art des accouchemens* [Art of childbirth] of 1753, emphasizes difficult birth presentations, but does so without reference to embodied experience or personal case studies. Instead, the surgeon man-midwife described the mechanical nature of childbirth, providing measurements of the female pelvis and advocating the use of forceps. The plates in his book do not feature the usual unborn children in the womb, but rather map the stages of growth in normal labours and plot the pelvic structure of women. Presenting childbirth as a knowable activity that can be discussed abstractly, this treatise differs significantly from earlier ones instead of providing a culmination of their goals. Yet texts such as Levret's should not be interpreted as signs that medicalization had actually occurred, with both men and women increasingly viewing childbirth as a standardized event that required professional management. In keeping with earlier obstetrical treatises, texts advocating the mechanical nature of childbirth were persuasive, participating in promoting a new kind of medical expert. This alternative version of obstetrical authority was not uncontested, given that more traditional treatises continued to be published throughout the eighteenth century. Though a new conception of the maternal body was being produced, it was not yet dominant.

My study extended beyond rethinking the function of obstetrical treatises. It also demonstrated that visual images participated in the creation of knowledge during the early modern period without being subordinate to written texts. Insisting on the careful analysis of individual images, I encouraged an interdisciplinary approach to the study of early modern culture, drawing on sources from art history, literary studies, sociology, anthropology, women's studies, history, film studies, and gender studies. At the same time, my research shed light on the display culture permeating early modern France by exploring the visual aspects of gender, identity, and professional reputation. Even as the lying-in chamber was in some ways a distinctive realm where traditional hierarchies could be both reshaped and temporarily overturned, it remained imbricated in broader social structures. Investigating the visual politics of childbirth offered a concentrated look at the way in which bodies, appearances, gestures, clothing, and facial expressions conveyed meaning. This book showed that childbirth was part of the visual culture of early modern France, a period when authority was largely determined by the precarious act of putting onself on display.

Selected Bibliography

French Obstetrical Treatises (1550–1730)

Amand, Pierre. *Nouvelles observations sur la pratique des accouchements* (Paris, 1714).

Baudoin, M., 'Lettre sur les accouchements,' Paul-Émile Le Maguet, ed. *Le monde médical parisien sous le Grand Roi, suivi du portefeuille de Vallant* (Paris: Maloine, 1899; orig. 1671), 314–40.

Bourgeois, Louise. *Observations diverses sur la stérilité, perte de fruict, foecondité, accouchements et maladies des femmes et enfants nouveaux naiz* (Paris, 1626).

Bury, Jacques. *Le propagatif de l'homme* (Paris, 1623).

Dionis, Pierre. *Traité général des accouchemens* (Paris, 1718).

Duval, Jacques. *Traité des hermaphrodits, parties génitales, accouchemens des femmes* (Rouen, 1612).

Fontaine, Jacques. *Deux paradoxes, appartenant à la chirurgie, le premier contient la façon de tirer les enfans du ventre de leur mère par la violence extraordinaire* (Paris, 1611).

Fournier, Denis. *L'accoucheur méthodique* (Paris, 1677).

Franco, Pierre. *Traité des hernies contenant une ample déclaration de toutes leurs espèces, et autres excellentes parties de la chirurgie* (Paris, 1561).

Guillemeau, Jacques. *De l'heureux accouchement des femmes* (Paris, 1609).

Joubert, Laurent. *Erreurs populaires* (Bordeaux, 1578).

La Marche, Marguerite [du Tertre]. *Instruction familière et très utile aux sages-femmes pour bien pratiquer les accouchemens* (Paris, 1710; orig. 1677).

Mauquest de la Motte, Guillaume. *Traité complet des accouchemens* (Paris, 1729; orig. 1721).

Mauriceau, François. *Des maladies des femmes grosses et accouchées* (Paris, 1668).

———. *Observations sur la grossesse et l'accouchement des femmes et sur leurs maladies* (Paris, 1695).

Paré, Ambroise, 'La manière de extraire les enfans tant mors que vivans hors le ventre de la mère,' *Briefve collection de l'administration anatomique* (Paris, 1550), 88–96.

———. *Deux livres de chirurgie, de la génération de l'homme* (Paris, 1573).

Peu, Philippe. *La pratique des accouchemens* (Paris, 1694).

Portal, Paul. *La pratique des accouchemens* (Paris, 1685).

Rousset, François. *Traitté nouveau de l'hysterotomotokie, ou enfantement caesarien* (Paris, 1581).

Ruleau, Jean. *Traité de l'opération cesarienne, et des accouchemens difficiles & laborieux* (Paris, 1704).

Saint-Germain, Charles de. *L'eschole méthodique et parfaite des sages-femmes* (Paris, 1650).

———. *Traité des fausses couches* (Paris, 1655).

Viardel, Cosme. *Observations sur la pratique des accouchemens naturels, contre nature & monstrueux* (Paris, 1671).

Other Primary Literature

Arrêt de la cour de parlement concernant la réception et prestation de serment des sages-femmes (Paris, 1726).

Arrêt de la cour du parlement rendu en faveur des jurées sages femmes en titre d'office et leurs aspirantes, contre les prévots gardes et communauté des maîtres chirurgiens de Saint Cosme et tous démonstrateurs anatomiques (Paris, 1732).

Arrêt de parlement portant nouveau réglement pour les apprentissages et réceptions des sages-femmes (Paris, 1675).

The Compleat Midwife's Practice Enlarged, 3rd edn (London, 1663).

Déclaration...portant défenses à ceux de la religion prétendüe réformée de faire les fonctions de sages-femmes (Saint-Germain-en-Laye, 1680).

Mémoire signifié pour les prévôts et communauté des chirurgiens-jurez à Saint-Côme de la ville de Paris, demandeurs, contre Louise Blanchon femme Jaunet et Lamare, jurées-sages-femmes en titre d'office au Châtelet de Paris, defenderesses (Paris, 1737).

Monomachie ou response d'un compagnon chirurgien nouvelement arrivé de Montpellier, aux calomnieuses invectives de la Gigantomachie de Riolan, docteur la en [sic] faculté d'ignorance, contre l'honneur du College des chirurgiens de Paris (n.l., n.d.).

Rapport de l'ouverture du corps de feu Madame (1627), François Rouget and Colette H. Winn, eds. *Récit véritable de la naissance de messeigneurs et dames les enfans de France* (Geneva: Droz, 2000), 108–9.

Récit exact d'une grossesse extraordinaire á l'Hôtel-Dieu de Paris (n.l., n.d.).

Sentence du prevôt de Paris concernant les sages-femmes (Paris, 1678).

Sentence rendue par le lieutenant criminel contre plusieurs sages-femmes qui n'ont point prêté serment au Châtelet (Paris, 1730).

Statuts et reiglemens ordonnez pour toutes les Matronnes ou Saiges femmes de la ville (n.l., 1587).

Statuts et reiglemens ordonnez pour toutes les matronnes, ou saiges femmes de la ville, faulxbourgs, prevosté, et vicomté de Paris (Paris, n.d.).

Statuts pour la communauté des maistres chirurgiens jurez de Paris (Paris, 1699 and 1701).

Arons, Wendy. trans. and intro. *Eucharius Rösslin: When Midwifery Became the Male Physician's Province* (Jefferson: McFarland, 1994).

Astruc, Jean. *L'art d'accoucher réduit à ses principes* (Paris, 1766).

Bartholin, Caspar Thomesen. *De ovariis mulierum et generationis historia epistola anatomica* (Rome, 1677).

Bayle, François. *Histoire anatomique d'une grossesse de 25 ans* (Toulouse, 1678).

Bernier, Jean. *Histoire chronologique de la médecine, et des médecins* (Paris, 1695).

Bourgeois, Louise. *Observations diverses sur la stérilité, perte de fruict, foecondité, accouchements et maladies des femmes et enfants nouveaux naiz*, Françoise Olive, ed. (Paris: Côté-Femmes, 1992; orig. 1652).

————. *Récit véritable de la naissance de messeigneurs et dames les enfans de France* (1617), François Rouget and Colette H. Winn, eds. *Récit véritable de la naissance de messeigneurs et dames les enfans de France* (Geneva: Droz, 2000), 57-96.

————. *Fidelle relation de l'accouchement, maladie et ouverture du corps de feu Madame* (1627), François Rouget and Colette H. Winn, eds. *Récit véritable de la naissance de messeigneurs et dames les enfans de France* (Geneva: Droz, 2000), 99-107.

Brunet, Claude, ed. *Le progrès de la médecine* (Paris, 1697).

————, 'D'une grossesse d'home [sic],' *Le progrès de la médecine*, (Paris, 1697), 62–5.

————. *Traité raisonné sur la structure des organes des deux sexes destinez à la génération* (Paris, 1696).

Bulwer, John. *Chirologia: Or the Naturall Language of the Hand* (London, 1644).

Carpi, Berengario da. *Commentaria* (Bologna, 1521).

Chamberlen, Hugh, trans. *The Accomplisht Midwife, Treating of the Diseases of Women with Child, and in Child-bed* (London, 1673).

Chéreau, Achille, ed. and intro. *Les six couches de Marie de Médicis* (Paris: Léon Willem and Paul Daffis, 1875).

Cureau de La Chambre, Marin. *The art how to know men*, John Davies, trans. (London, 1665).

Deventer, Hendrik van. *The Art of Midwifery Improv'd*, 3rd edn (London, 1728).

Dionis, Pierre. *Histoire anatomique d'une matrice extraordinaire* (Paris, 1683).

Dubois, Jacques [Jacobus Silvius]. *De mensibus mulierum, et hominis generatione* (Paris, 1555).

Du Laurens, André. *Toutes les oeuvres de Me André Du Laurens* (Rouen, 1621).

Estienne, Charles. *La dissection des parties du corps humain* (Paris, 1546).

Faret, Nicolas. *L'honneste homme ou l'art de plaire à la court*, M. Magendie, ed. (Paris: Les presses universitaires de France, 1925).

Foisil, Madeleine, ed. *Journal de Jean Héroard*, vol. 1 (Paris: Fayard, 1989).

Fournier, Édouard. *Les caquets de l'accouchée* (Paris: Jannet, 1855).

Franco, Pierre. *Chirurgie*, E. Nicaise, intro. (Geneva: Slatkine Reprints, 1972).

Green, Monica H., ed. and trans. *The Trotula: A Medieval Compendium of Women's Medicine* (Philadelphia: University of Pennsylvania Press, 2001).

Guillemeau, Charles, attr. *Remonstrance à Madame Bourcier, touchant son apologie* (1627), François Rouget and Colette H. Winn, eds. *Récit véritable de la naissance de messeigneurs et dames les enfans de France* (Geneva: Droz, 2000), 111–20.

————, attr. *Discours apologétique touchant la verité des geants. Contre la Gigantomachie d'un soy disant escollier en Medecine* (Paris, 1615).

Habicot, Nicolas. *Antigigantologie, ou contrediscours de la grandeur des géans* (Paris, 1618).

————. *Gigantostéologie, ou discours des os d'un géant* (Paris, 1613).

Harvey, William. *Exercitationes de generatione animalium* (London, 1651).

Hecquet, Philippe. *De l'indécence aux hommes d'accoucher les femmes* (Paris, 1708).

Joubert, Laurent. *Popular Errors*, Gregory David de Rocher, trans. (Tuscaloosa: University of Alabama Press, 1989).

Le Duc, M., 'Observation d'une flâme sortie du ventre d'une femme en couche,' Claude Brunet, ed. *Le progrès de la médecine* (Paris, 1709), 73–8.

L'Honoré, Germain. *Description d'un monstre dont une femme de la ville de Rouen accoucha le mois d'octobre 1672* (Rouen, 1673).

Liébault, Jean. *Thrésor des remèdes secrets pour les maladies des femmes* (Paris, 1582).

Le Brun, Charles. *Conférence de M. Le Brun sur l'expression générale et particulière* (Paris, 1698).

Levret, André. *L'art des accouchemens* (Paris, 1753).

Maillard, Claude. *Le bon mariage, ou le moyen d'estre heureux et faire son salut en estat de mariage* (Douay, 1643).

Marinelli, Giovanni. *Le medicine partenenti alle infermità delle donne* (Venice, 1574).

Matthieu, Pierre. *Histoire de France soubs les règnes de François I. Henry II. François II. Charles IX. Henry III. Henri IV*, vol. 2 (Paris, 1631).

Maubray, John. *The Female Physician* (London, 1724).

Mauquest de La Motte, Guillaume. *A General Treatise of Midwifry*, Thomas Tomkyns, trans. (London, 1746).

————. *Dissertation sur la génération, sur la superfétation et la réponse au livre intitulé: De l'Indécence aux hommes d'accoucher les femmes* (Paris, 1718).

Mauriceau, François. *Aphorismes touchant la grossesse, l'accouchement, les maladies, et autres dispositions des femmes* (Paris, 1694).

Mayerne, Théodore Turquet de. *La pratique de médecine...avec le régime des femmes grosses* (Lyon, 1693).

Mercurio, Girolamo. *La commare o riccoglitrice* (Venice, 1601).

Mesnard, Jacques. *Le guide des accoucheurs* (Paris, 1743).

Nihell, Elizabeth. *A Treatise on the Art of Midwifery* (London, 1760).

Paré, Ambroise. *Des monstres et prodiges*, Jean Céard, ed. (Geneva: Droz, 1971).

————. *Oeuvres complètes d'Ambroise Paré*, 3 vol., J.-F. Malgaigne, ed. (Paris: Baillière, 1840–41).

————. *Les oeuvres de M. Paré* (Paris, 1575).

————. *Responce de M. Ambroise Paré, premier chirurgien du Roy, aux calomnies d'aucuns médecins, et chirurgiens, touchant ses oeuvres* (n.l., n.d.).

Peu, Philippe. *Réponse de M. Peu aux observations particulières de M. Mauriceau sur la grossesse et l'accouchement des femmes* (n.l., n.d.).

————. *Réponse à l'avertissement* (n.l., n.d.)

Portal, Paul. *The Compleat Practice of Men and Women Midwives* (London, 1705).

Refuge, Eustache de. *The accomplish'd courtier*, H. W. Gent, trans. (London, 1660).

Riolan, Jean, fils, attr. *Gigantomachie, pour respondre à la Gigantostologie* (n.l., 1613).

————, attr. *L'imposture descouverte des os humains supposés et faussement attribués au roy Theutobochus* (Paris, 1614).

————. *Gigantologie. Discours sur la grandeur des geants. Où il est demonstré, que de toute ancienneté les plus grands hommes, & geants, n'ont esté plus hauts que ceux de ce temps* (Paris, 1618).

Ripa, Caesar. *Iconologia*, P. Tempest, trans. (London, 1709).

Risko, Agnes, '*"Gott Zu Ehren, Dem Neben=Christen Zu Nutz..."*': Anna Elisabeth Horenburg's Manual for Midwives' (Ph.D. Diss., Ohio State University, 1998).

Saviard, Barthélemy. *Nouveau recueil d'observations chirurgicales* (Paris, 1702).

————. *Réponse de M. Saviard,...à la critique de l'extrait de sa lettre* (Paris, 1698).

Sermon, William. *The Ladies Companion, or the English Midwife* (London, 1671).

Serres, Louys de. *Discours de la nature, causes, signes et curation des empeschemens de la conception, et de la stérilité des femmes* (Lyon, 1625).

Sharp, Jane. *The Midwives Book* (London, 1671).

Simon, M. *Factum ou lettre écrite par Mr. Simon à Mr. Peu sur la falsification d'un fait qui se trouve à la fin du premier livre de sa Pratique des accouchemens* (n.l., n.d.).

Soranus. *Gynecology*, Owsei Temkin, trans. and intro. (Baltimore: The Johns Hopkins University Press, 1956).

Spieghel, Adriaan van den. *De humani corporis fabrica* (Venice, 1627).

Stone, Sarah. *A Complete Practice of Midwifery* (London, 1737).

Tousche, Gervais de la. *La Tres haute et tres souveraine science de l'art et industrie naturelle d'enfanter, contre la maudicte et perverse impericie des femmes que l'on appelle saiges femmes ou belles meres, lesquelles par leur ignorance font journellement perir une infinité de femmes et d'enfans à l'enfantement* (Paris, 1587).

Venette, Nicholas. *De la génération de l'homme ou tableau de l'amour conjugal* (Cologne, 1702).

Willughby, Percival. *Observations on Midwifery*, Henry Blenkinsop, ed. (Wakefield: S. R. Publishers, 1972; orig. manuscript 1863).

Secondary Literature

Ackerknecht, Erwin H., 'Midwives as Experts in Court,' *Bulletin of the New York Academy of Medicine* 52 (1976), 1224–8.

Adams, Ann Jensen, 'The Three-Quarter Length Life-Sized Portrait in Seventeenth-Century Holland: The Cultural Functions of *Tranquillitas*,' Wayne Franits, ed. *Looking at Seventeenth-Century Dutch Art: Realism Reconsidered* (Cambridge: Cambridge University Press, 1997), 158–74.

Allen, Graham. *Intertextuality* (London: Routledge, 2000).

Ang, Ien. *Watching Dallas: Soap Opera and the Melodramatic Imagination* (London: Methuen, 1985).

Apostolidès, Jean-Marie. *Le Roi-machine: spectacle et politique au temps de Louis XIV* (Paris: Minuit, 1981).

Arms, Suzanne. *Immaculate Deception: A New Look at Women and Childbirth in America* (Boston: Houghton Mifflin, 1975).

Bal, Mieke, 'Visual Essentialism and the Object of Visual Culture,' *Journal of Visual Culture* 2, 1 (2003), 5–32.

————, 'Intention,' *Travelling Concepts in the Humanities: A Rough Guide* (Toronto: University of Toronto Press, 2002), 253–85.

Bal, Mieke and Bryson, Norman, 'Semiotics and Art History,' *Art Bulletin* 73, 2 (1991), 174–208.

Balme, D. M., 'Άνθρωπος 'ανθρωπον γεννᾷ: Human is Generated by Human,' G. R. Dunstan, ed. *The Human Embryo: Aristotle and the Arabic and European Traditions* (Exeter: University of Exeter Press, 1990), 20–31.

Baskins, Cristelle L. *Cassone Painting, Humanism, and Gender in Early Modern Italy* (Cambridge: Cambridge University Press, 1998).

Bellier de la Chavignerie, Émile. *Dictionnaire général des artistes de l'école française* (Paris: Renouard, 1885).

Bénézit, Emmanuel. *Dictionnaire critique et documentaire des peintres, sculpteurs, dessinateurs et graveurs* (Paris: Gründ, 1966).

Berger, Harry, Jr. *Fictions of the Pose: Rembrandt Against the Italian Renaissance* (Stanford: Stanford University Press, 2000).

Berlant, Lauren, 'America, "Fat," the Fetus,' *Boundary* 21 (Fall 1994), 145–95.

Berriot-Salvadore, Evelyne. *Les femmes dans la société française de la renaissance* (Geneva: Droz, 1990).

Bertrand, Pierre, 'L'Univers de la naissance en France dans la peinture et la gravure (1550–1700): La poétique de l'image face à la rhétorique médicale' (Mémoire de D.E.A. en histoire de l'art, Paris I, 1990).

————, 'Graver la naissance au XVIIe siècle,' *Ethnologie française* 26, 2 (1996), 329–39.

————, 'Le portrait de Gabrielle d'Estrées au Musée Condé de Chantilly ou la gloire de la maternité,' *Gazette des beaux-arts* 6, 122 (1993), 73–82.

Bicks, Caroline. *Midwiving Subjects in Shakespeare's England* (Aldershot: Ashgate, 2003).

Bideau, Alain, 'Accouchement "naturel" et accouchement à "haut risque",' *Annales de demographie historique* (1981), 4–66.

Blumenfeld-Kosinski, Renate. *Not of Woman Born: Representations of Caesarean Birth in Medieval and Renaissance Culture* (Ithaca: Cornell University Press, 1990).

Blunt, Anthony. *Nicolas Poussin* (London: Pallas Athene, 1995).

Boss, Berenice and Boss, Jeffrey, 'Ignorant Midwives – a Further Rejoinder,' *Society for the Social History of Medicine Bulletin* 33 (1983), 71.

Bourdieu, Pierre, 'Some Properties of Fields,' *Sociology in Question*, Richard Nice, trans. (London: Sage, 1993), 72–7.

————. *The Logic of Practice*, Richard Nice, trans. (Stanford: Stanford University Press, 1990).

Breitenberg, Mark. *Anxious Masculinity in Early Modern England* (Cambridge: Cambridge University Press, 1996).

Brockliss, Laurence and Jones, Colin. *The Medical World of Early Modern France* (Oxford: Clarendon Press, 1997).

Brockliss, Laurence, 'The Embryological Revolution in the France of Louis XIV: The Dominance of Ideology,' G. R. Dunstan, ed. *The Human Embryo: Aristotle and the Arabic and European Traditions* (Exeter: University of Exeter Press, 1990), 158–86.

————, 'The Medico-Religious Universe of an Early Eighteenth-Century Parisian Doctor: The Case of Philippe Hecquet,' Roger French and Andrew Wear, eds. *The Medical Revolution of the Seventeenth Century* (Cambridge: Cambridge University Press, 1989), 191–221.

Bronfen, Elisabeth. *Over Her Dead Body: Death, Femininity, and the Aesthetic* (New York: Routledge, 1992).

Broomhall, Susan. *Women's Medical Work in Early Modern France* (Manchester: Manchester University Press, 2004).

————, '"Women's Little Secrets": Defining the Boundaries of Reproductive Knowledge in Sixteenth-Century France,' *Social History of Medicine* 15, 1 (2002), 1–15.

————. *Women and the Book Trade in Sixteenth-Century France* (Aldershot: Ashgate, 2002).

Brun, Robert. *Le livre français* (Paris: Larousse, 1948).

Bryson, Norman, 'The Legible Body: LeBrun,' *Word and Image: French Painting of the Ancien Régime* (Cambridge: Cambridge University Press, 1981), 29–57.

Burke, Peter. *Eyewitnessing: The Uses of Images as Historical Evidence* (Ithaca: Cornell University Press, 2001).

————. *The Fabrication of King Louis XIV* (New Haven: Yale University Press, 1992).

Bury, Emmanuel, 'Civiliser la "personne" ou instituer le "personnage"? Les deux versants de la politesse selon les théoriciens français du XVIIe siècle,' Alain Montandon, ed. *Etiquette et politesse* (Clermont-Ferrand: Association des publications de la Faculté des lettres et sciences humaines de Clermont-Ferrand, 1992), 125–38.

Butler, Judith. *Gender Trouble: Feminism and the Subversion of Identity* (New York: Routledge, 1990).

————, 'Imitation and Gender Insubordination,' Diana Fuss, ed. *Inside/Out: Lesbian Theories, Gay Theories* (New York: Routledge, 1991), 13–31.

Carlino, Andrea. *Books of the Body: Anatomical Ritual and Renaissance Learning* (Chicago: University of Chicago Press, 1999).

Carrier, Henriette. *Origines de la Maternité de Paris. Les maîtresses sages-femmes et l'office des accouchées de l'ancien Hôtel Dieu (1378–1796)* (Paris: Steinheil, 1888).

Chartier, Roger. *The Order of Books: Readers, Authors, and Libraries in Europe between the Fourteenth and Eighteenth Centuries*, Lydia G. Cochrane, trans. (Stanford: Stanford University Press, 1994).

————, 'The Practical Impact of Writing,' Roger Chartier, ed. *A History of Private Life, vol. 3, Passions of the Renaissance*, Arthur Goldhammer, trans. (Cambridge, MA: Harvard University Press, 1989), 111–59.

————. *The Cultural Uses of Print in Early Modern France*, Lydia G. Cochrane, trans. (Princeton: Princeton University Press, 1987).

Cianfrani, Theodore. *A Short History of Obstetrics and Gynecology* (Springfield: Thomas, 1960).

Cody, Lisa Forman, 'The Birth of the Nation: Man-Midwifery and the Conception of Eighteenth-Century Britain' (unpublished manuscript, forthcoming from Oxford University Press).

————, 'The Politics of Reproduction: From Midwives' Alternative Public Sphere to the Public Spectacle of Man-Midwifery,' *Eighteenth-Century Studies* 32, 4 (1999), 477–95.

Coe, Richard, Lingard, Lorelei and Tatiana Teslenko, eds. *The Rhetoric and Ideology of Genre* (Cresskill: Hampton, 2002).

Cohen, Michele. *Fashioning Masculinity: National Identity and Language in the Eighteenth Century* (London: Routledge, 1996).

Cohen, Sarah R. *Art, Dance, and the Body in French Culture of the Ancien Régime* (Cambridge: Cambridge University Press, 2000).

Collins, Harry M. *Changing Order: Replication and Induction in Scientific Practice* (London: Sage, 1985).

Colwill, Elizabeth, 'Sex, Savagery, and Slavery in the Shaping of the French Body Politic,' Sara E. Melzer and Kathryn Norberg, eds. *From the Royal to the Republican Body: Incorporating the Political in Seventeenth- and Eighteenth-Century France* (Berkeley: University of California Press, 1998), 198–223.

Coquery, Emmanuel, 'Le portrait vu du Grand Siècle,' *Visages du Grand Siècle: Le portrait français sous le règne de Louis XIV, 1660–1715* (Paris: Somogny, 1997), 21–31.

Courtine, Jean-Jacques and Haroche, Claudine. *Histoire du visage: exprimer et taire ses émotions XVIe–début XIXe siècle* (Paris: Rivages, 1988).

Crary, Jonathan, 'Modernity and the Problem of the Observer,' *Techniques of the Observer: On Vision and Modernity in the Nineteenth Century* (Cambridge, MA: MIT Press, 1998), 1–24.

Crawford, Patricia, 'Sexual Knowledge in England, 1500–1750,' Roy Porter and Mikuláš Teich, eds. *Sexual Knowledge, Sexual Science: The History of Attitudes to Sexuality* (Cambridge: Cambridge University Press,1994), 82–106.

Cressy, David. *Birth, Marriage, and Death: Ritual, Religion, and the Life-Cycle in Tudor and Stuart England* (Oxford: Oxford University Press, 1997).

————, 'Books as Totems in Seventeenth-Century England and New England,' *Journal of Library History* 21 (1986), 92–106.

Cunningham, Andrew. *The Anatomical Renaissance: The Resurrection of the Anatomical Projects of the Ancients* (Aldershot: Ashgate, 1997).

Cutter, Irving Samuel and Viets, Henry R. *A Short History of Midwifery* (Philadelphia: Saunders, 1964).

Darmon, Pierre. *Le tribunal de l'impuissance: Virilité et défaillances conjugales dans l'ancienne France* (Paris: Seuil, 1979).

Darnton, Robert, 'Reading, Writing, and Publishing in Eighteenth-Century France: A Case Study in the Sociology of Literature,' *Daedalus* (Winter 1971), 214–56.

Daube-Schackat, Roland, 'Peirce and Hermeneutics,' Vincent M. Colapietro and Thomas M. Olshewsky, eds. *Peirce's Doctrine of Signs: Theory, Applications, and Connections* (Berlin: Mouton de Gruyter, 1996), 381–90.

Davidson, Jane P., 'The Myth of the Persecuted Female Healer,' *Journal of the Rocky Mountain Medieval and Renaissance Association* 14 (1993), 115–29.

Davis, Natalie Zemon, 'Boundaries and the Sense of Self in Sixteenth-Century France,' Thomas C. Heller, Morton Sosna, and David E. Wellbery, eds. *Reconstructing Individualism: Autonomy, Individuality, and the Self in Western Thought* (Stanford: Stanford University Press, 1986), 53–63.

————, 'Women on Top: Symbolic Sexual Inversion and Political Disorder in Early Modern Europe,' Barbara A. Babcock, ed. *The Reversible World: Symbolic Inversion in Art and Society* (Ithaca: Cornell University Press, 1978), 147–90.

————, 'Printing and the People,' *Society and Culture in Early Modern France* (Stanford: Stanford University Press, 1975), 189–225.

————, 'Proverbial Wisdom and Popular Errors,' *Society and Culture in Early Modern France* (Stanford: Stanford University Press, 1975), 227–67.

Dawson, Warren R. *The Custom of Couvade* (Manchester: Manchester University Press, 1929).

Dechambre, Amédée, ed. *Dictionnaire encylopédique des sciences médicales* (Paris: Masson, 1879).

Declercq, Eugene, DeVries, Raymond, Kirsi Viisainen, Helga B. Salvesen, and Sirpa Wrede, 'Where to Give Birth? Politics and the Place of Birth,' Raymond DeVries, Cecilia Benoit, Edwin R. van Teijlingen, and Sirpa Wrede, eds. *Birth by Design: Pregnancy, Maternity Care, and Midwifery in North America and Europe* (New York: Routledge, 2001), 7–27.

Delacoux, A. *Biographie des sages-femmes célèbres, anciennes, modernes, contemporaines* (Paris: Trinquart, 1833).

Deledalle, Gérard. *Charles S. Peirce's Philosophy of Signs: Essays in Comparative Semiotics* (Bloomington: Indiana University Press, 2000).

Derrida, Jacques, 'Différance,' Hazard Adams and Leroy Searle, eds. *Critical Theory Since 1965* (Tallahassee: Florida State University Press, 1986), 120–36.

DiPiero, Thomas. *Dangerous Truths and Criminal Passions: The Evolution of the French Novel, 1569–1791* (Stanford: Stanford University Press, 1992).

Dobbie, B. M. Willmott, 'An Attempt to Estimate the True Rate of Maternal Mortality, Sixteenth to Eighteenth Centuries,' *Medical History* 26 (1982), 79–90.

Donnison, Jean. *Midwives and Medical Men* (New York: Schocken Books, 1977).

Duchatel, François, 'Paul Portal (1630?–1er juillet 1703): Un accoucheur méconnue du XVIIe siècle,' *Histoire des sciences médicales* 14, 4 (1980), 407–18.

Duden, Barbara, 'The Fetus on the "Farther Shore": Toward a History of the Unborn,' Lynn M. Morgan and Meredith W. Michaels, eds. *Fetal Subjects, Feminist Positions* (Philadelphia: University of Pennsylvania Press, 1999), 13–25.

————, 'The Fetus as an Object of Our Time,' *Res* 25 (Spring 1994), 132–5.

————. *Disembodying Women: Perspectives on Pregnancy and the Unborn*, Lee Hoinacki, trans. (Cambridge, MA: Harvard University Press, 1993).

Duff, David, 'Introduction,' David Duff, ed. *Modern Genre Theory* (Harlow: Pearson Education Limited, 2000), 1–24.

Dumaitre, Paule. *Ambroise Paré: chirurgien de quatre rois de France* (Paris: Librairie Académique Perrin Fondation Singer-Polignac, 1986).

————, 'Autour d'Ambroise Paré, ses élèves, ses amis,' *Histoire des sciences médicales* 30, 3 (1996), 351–7.

Dumont, Martial, 'Histoire et petite histoire du forceps,' *Journal de gynécologie, obstétrique, et biologie* 13, 7 (1984), 743–57.

Dunn, Peter M., 'The Chamberlen Family (1560–1728) and Obstetric Forceps,' *Archives of Disease in Childhood* 81, 3 (1999), 232–5.

Eccles, Audrey. *Obstetrics and Gynaecology in Tudor and Stuart England* (London: Croom Helm, 1982).

Eco, Umberto. *Kant and the Platypus: Essays on Language and Cognition*, Alastair McEwen, trans. (San Diego: Harcourt, 1999).

Ehrenreich, Barbara and English, Deirdre. *Witches, Midwives, and Nurses: A History of Women Healers* (New York: The Feminist Press, 1973).

Eisenstein, Elizabeth. *The Printing Press as an Agent of Change*, vol. 1 (Cambridge: Cambridge University Press, 1979).

Elias, Norbert. *The Court Society*, Edmund Jephcott, trans. (Oxford: Blackwell, 1983).

————. *The Civilizing Process, vol. 1, The History of Manners*, Edmund Jephcott, trans. (New York: Urizen Books, 1978).

Éloy, Nicolas-François-Joseph. *Dictionnaire historique de la médecine ancienne et moderne* (Mons: H. Hoyois, 1778).

Erickson, Robert A., '"The Books of Generation": Some Observations on the Style of the British Midwife Books, 1671–1764,' Paul-Gabriel Boucé, ed. *Sexuality in Eighteenth-Century Britain* (Manchester: Manchester University Press, 1982), 74–94.

Evenden, Doreen. *The Midwives of Seventeenth-Century London* (Cambridge: Cambridge University Press, 2000).

Febvre, Lucien and Martin, Henri-Jean. *The Coming of the Book*, David Gerard, trans. (London: Verso, 1976).

Ficheux, D., 'François Mauriceau, accoucheur sous le Roi Soleil' (Thèse pour le doctorat en médecine, Université d'Amiens, 1985).

Filippini, Nadia Maria, 'The Church, the State and Childbirth: The Midwife in Italy During the Eighteenth Century,' Hilary Marland, ed. *The Art of Midwifery: Early Modern Midwives in Europe* (London: Routledge, 1993), 152–75.

Finucci, Valeria and Brownlee, Kevin, eds. *Generation and Degeneration: Tropes of Reproduction in Literature and History from Antiquity to Early Modern Europe* (Durham: Duke University Press, 2001).

Finucci, Valeria, 'Maternal Imagination and Monstrous Birth: Tasso's *Gerusalemme liberata*,' Valeria Finucci and Kevin Brownlee, eds. *Generation and Degeneration: Tropes of Reproduction in Literature and History from Antiquity to Early Modern Europe* (Durham: Duke University Press, 2001), 41–77.

Fisher, Will, 'The Renaissance Beard: Masculinity in Early Modern England,' *Renaissance Quarterly* 54 (2001), 155–87.

Fissell, Mary E., 'Readers, Texts, and Contexts: Vernacular Medical Works in Early Modern England,' Roy Porter, ed. *The Popularization of Medicine 1650–1850* (London: Routledge, 1992), 72–96.

ffolliott, Sheila, 'Catherine de' Medici as Artemesia: Figuring the Powerful Widow,' Margaret W. Ferguson, Maureen Quilligan, and Nancy J. Vickers, eds. *Rewriting the Renaissance: The Discourses of Sexual Difference in Early Modern Europe* (Chicago: University of Chicago Press, 1986), 227–41.

Forbes, Thomas Rogers. *The Midwife and the Witch* (New Haven: Yale University Press, 1966).

Fosseyeux, Marcel, 'Sages-femmes et nourrices à Paris au XVIIIe siècle,' *Revue de Paris* 19 (October 1921), 535–54.

Foucault, Michel, 'What is an Author?' Donald Bouchard and Sherry Simon, trans. and Josué V. Harari, ed. *Textual Strategies: Perspectives in Post-Structuralist Criticism* (Ithaca: Cornell University Press, 1979), 141–60.

————. *The Birth of the Clinic: An Archaeology of Medical Perception*, A. M. Sheridan Smith, trans. (New York: Vintage, 1975).

Franklin, Sarah, 'Fetal Fascinations: New Dimensions to the Medical-Scientific Construction of Fetal Personhood,' Sarah Franklin, Celia Lury, and Jackie Stacey, eds. *Off-Centre: Feminism and Cultural Studies* (London: Harper Collins, 1991), 190–205.

Freccero, Carla, 'Politics and Aesthetics in Castiglione's *Il Cortegiano*: Book III and the Discourse on Women,' David Quint et al., eds. *Creative Imitation: New Essays on Renaissance Literature in Honor of Thomas M. Greene* (Binghamton: Medieval and Renaissance Texts and Studies, 1992), 259–79.

Gardiner, Judith Kegan, ed. *Masculinity Studies and Feminist Theory* (New York: Columbia University Press, 2002).

Gelbart, Nina Rattner. *The King's Midwife: A History and Mystery of Madame du Coudray* (Berkeley: University of California Press, 1998).

Gelfand, Toby. *Professionalizing Modern Medicine: Paris Surgeons and Medical Science and Institutions in the 18th Century* (Westport: Greenwood, 1980).

Gélis, Jacques. *Accoucheur de campagne sous le Roi-Soleil: Le traité des accouchements de G. Mauquest de La Motte* (Paris: Imago, 1989).

————. *La sage-femme ou le médecin: une nouvelle conception de la vie* (Paris: Fayard, 1988).

————. *L'arbre et le fruit: la naissance dans l'Occident moderne, XVIe–XIXe siècle* (Paris: Fayard, 1984).

Gélis, Jacques, Laget, Mireille, and Marie-France Morel, *Entrer dans la vie – Naissances et enfances dans la France traditionelle* (Paris: Gallimard, 1978).

Givner, Jessie, 'Reproducing Reproductive Discourse: Optical Technologies in *The Silent Scream* and *Eclipse of Reason*,' *Journal of Popular Culture* 28 (Winter 1994), 229–44.

Gledhill, Christine, 'History of Genre Criticism,' Pam Cook, ed. *The Cinema Book* (London: British Film Institute, 1985), 58–64.

Grieco, Sara F. Matthews. *Ange ou diablesse: La représentation de la femme au XVIe siècle* (Paris: Flammarion, 1991).

Grundy, Isobel, 'Sarah Stone: Enlightenment Midwife,' *Clio Medica* 29 (1995), 128–44.

Hahn, André, Dumaitre, Paule, and Janine Samion-Content. *Histoire de la médecine et du livre médical* (Paris: Olivier Perrin, 1962).

Halberstam, Judith. *Female Masculinity* (Durham: Duke University Press, 1998).

Hall, Nor and Dawson, Warren R. *Broodmales: A Psychological Essay on Men in Childbirth* (Dallas: Spring Publications, 1989).

Hall, Stuart, 'Encoding, Decoding,' Simon During, ed. *The Cultural Studies Reader* (London: Routledge, 1993), 90–103.

Hamby, Wallace B. *Ambroise Paré: Surgeon of the Renaissance* (St. Louis: Warren H. Green, 1967).

Hanley, Sarah, 'Engendering the State: Family Formation and State Building in Early Modern France,' *French Historical Studies* 16 (1989), 4–27.

Harth, Erica. *Ideology and Culture in Seventeenth-Century France* (Ithaca: Cornell University Press, 1983).

Harley, David, 'Review of Jonathan Sawday, *The Body Emblazoned*,' *Medical History* 40 (1996), 253–4.

————, 'Provincial Midwives in England: Lancashire and Cheshire, 1660–1760,' Hilary Marland, ed. *The Art of Midwifery: Early Modern Midwives in Europe* (London: Routledge, 1993), 27–48.

————, 'Historians as Demonologists: The Myth of the Midwife-witch,' *Journal of the Society for the Social History of Medicine* 3, 1 (1990), 1–26.

————, 'Ignorant Midwives – A Persistent Stereotype,' *Society for the Social History of Medicine Bulletin* 28 (1981), 6–9.

Harrison, Peter, 'Reading the Passions: The Fall, the Passions, and Dominion Over Nature,' Stephen Gaukroger, ed. *The Soft Underbelly of Reason: The Passions in the Seventeenth Century* (London: Routledge, 1998), 49–78.

Hartouni, Valerie, 'Fetal Exposures: Abortion Politics and the Optics of Allusion,' *Camera Obscura* 29 (May 1992), 130–49.

Harvey, Elizabeth D., 'Matrix as Metaphor: Midwifery and the Conception of the Voice,' *Ventriloquized Voices: Feminist Theory and English Renaissance Texts* (London: Routledge, 1992), 76–115.

Heinich, Nathalie. *Du peintre à l'artiste: Artisans et académiciens à l'âge classique* (Paris: Minuit, 1993).

Herrle-Fanning, Jeanette, 'Figuring the Reproductive Woman: The Construction of Medical Identity in Eighteenth-Century British Midwifery Texts,' Mary M. Lay, et al., eds. *Body Talk: Rhetoric, Technology, Reproduction* (Madison: University of Wisconsin Press, 2000), 29–48.

Hofer, Philip. *Baroque Book Illustration: A Short Survey from the Collection in the Department of Graphic Arts, Harvard College Library* (Cambridge, MA: Harvard University Press, 1951).

Hoopes, James, ed. *Peirce on Signs: Writings on Semiotic by Charles Sanders Peirce* (Chapel Hill: University of North Carolina Press, 1991).

Huard, Pierre and Drazen Grmek, Mirko. *La chirurgie moderne. Ses débuts en occident XVIe–XVIIe–XVIIIe siècles* (Paris: Dacosta, 1968).

Huet, Marie-Hélène. *Monstrous Imagination* (Cambridge, MA: Harvard University Press, 1993).

Hults, Linda C. *The Print in the Western World: An Introductory History* (Madison: University of Wisconsin Press, 1996).

Ingerslev, E., 'Rösslin's "Rosegarten": Its Relation to the Past (the Muscio Manuscripts and Soranos), particularly with regard to Podalic Version,' *The Journal of Obstetrics and Gynaecology of the British Empire* 15, 1 (1909), 1–25.

Jameson, Edwin A. *Gynecology and Obstetrics* (New York: Hoeber, 1936).

Johns, Adrian. *The Nature of the Book: Print and Knowledge in the Making* (Chicago: University of Chicago Press, 1998).

Johnson, W. McAllister. *French Royal Academy of Painting and Sculpture Engraved Reception Pieces: 1672–1798* (Kingston: Agnes Etherington Art Centre, Queen's University, 1982).

Jordan, Brigitte, 'Authoritative Knowledge and Its Construction,' Robbie E. Davis-Floyd and Carolyn F. Sargent, eds. *Childbirth and Authoritative Knowledge: Cross-Cultural Perspectives* (Berkeley: University of California Press, 1997), 55–79.

————. *Birth in Four Cultures: A Cross-Cultural Investigation of Childbirth in Yucatan, Holland, Sweden and the United States* (Prospect Heights: Waveland Press, 1993).

Jordanova, Ludmilla. *Nature Displayed: Gender, Science and Medicine 1760–1820* (London: Longman, 1999).

————, 'Medical Men 1780–1820,' Joanna Woodall, ed. *Portraiture: Facing the Subject* (Manchester: Manchester University Press, 1997), 101–15.

————. *Sexual Visions: Images of Gender in Science and Medicine between the Eighteenth and Twentieth Centuries* (New York: Harvester Wheatsheaf, 1989).

————, 'Gender, Generation and Science: William Hunter's Obstetrical Atlas,' W.F. Bynum and Roy Porter, eds. *William Hunter and the Eighteenth-Century Medical World* (Cambridge: Cambridge University Press, 1985), 385–412.

Joswick, Hugh, 'The Object of Semeiotic,' Vincent M. Colapietro and Thomas M. Olshewsky, eds. *Peirce's Doctrine of Signs: Theory, Applications, and Connections* (Berlin: Mouton de Gruyter, 1996), 93–102.

Jouan, Andrée, 'Thomas de Leu et le portrait français de la fin du XVIe siècle,' *Gazette des beaux-arts* 58 (1961), 203–22.

Kalisch, Philip A., Scobey, Margaret, and Beatrice J. Kalisch, 'Louyse Bourgeois and the Emergence of Modern Midwifery,' *Journal of Nurse-Midwifery* 26, 4 (1981), 3–17.

Kaplan, E. Ann, 'Look Who's Talking, Indeed: Fetal Images in Recent North American Visual Culture,' Evelyn Nakano Glenn, Grace Chang, and Linda Rennie Forcey, eds. *Mothering: Ideology, Experience, and Agency* (New York: Routledge, 1994), 121–37.

Kapsalis, Terri. *Public Privates: Performing Gynecology from Both Ends of the Speculum* (Durham: Duke University Press, 1997).

Keller, Eve, 'The Subject of Touch: Medical Authority in Early Modern Midwifery,' Elizabeth D. Harvey, ed. *Sensible Flesh: On Touch in Early Modern Culture* (Philadelphia: University of Pennsylvania Press, 2003), 62–80.

————, 'Embryonic Individuals: The Rhetoric of Seventeenth-Century Embryology and the Construction of Early-Modern Identity,' *Eighteenth-Century Studies* 33, 3 (2000), 321–48.

Kelly, Joan, 'Early Feminist Theory and the *Querelle des Femmes*, 1400–1789,' *Signs* 8, 1 (1982), 4–28.

King, Helen. *Hippocrates' Woman: Reading the Female Body in Ancient Greece* (London: Routledge, 1998).

————, '"As if None Understood the Art that Cannot Understand Greek": The Education of Midwives in Seventeenth-Century England,' Vivian Nutton and Roy Porter, eds. *The History of Medical Education in Britain* (Amsterdam: Rodopi, 1995), 184–98.

————, 'Making a Man: Becoming Human in Early Greek Medicine,' G. R. Dunstan, ed. *The Human Embryo: Aristotle and the Arabic and European Traditions* (Exeter: University of Exeter Press, 1990), 10–19.

————. 'Agnodike and the Profession of Medicine,' *Proceedings of the Cambridge Philological Society* 32 (1986), 53–77.

Kloosterman, G. J., 'Some Obstetric Remarks on Vrouw Schrader's Notebook and Memoirs,' Hilary Marland, trans. *'Mother and Child Were Saved'. The Memoirs (1693–1740) of the Frisian Midwife Catharina Schrader* (Amsterdam: Rodopi, 1987), 29–41.

Kristeva, Julia. *Desire in Language: A Semiotic Approach to Literature and Art* (New York: Columbia University Press, 1980).

Kuchta, David. *The Three-Piece Suit and Modern Masculinity: England, 1550–1850* (Berkeley: University of California Press, 2002).

Laget, Mireille. *Naissances: L'accouchement avant l'âge de la clinique* (Paris: Seuil, 1982).

————, 'Childbirth in Seventeenth- and Eighteenth-Century France: Obstetrical Practices and Collective Attitudes,' Robert Forster and Orest Ranum, eds. *Medicine and Society in France: Selections from the Annales Economies, Sociétés, Civilizations*, vol. 6 (Baltimore: Johns Hopkins Press, 1980), 137–76.

————, 'La césarienne ou la tentation de l'impossible: XVIIe et XVIIIe siècle,' *Annales de bretagne et des pays de l'ouest* 86 (1979), 177–89.

Laqueur, Thomas, 'Sex in the Flesh,' *Isis* 94 (2003), 300–306.

————. *Making Sex: Body and Gender from the Greeks to Freud* (Cambridge, MA: Harvard University Press, 1990).

Lawrence, Christopher, 'Incommunicable Knowledge: Science, Technology and the Clinical Art in Britain 1850–1914,' *Journal of Contemporary History* 20 (1985), 503–20.

Lazard, Madeleine, 'Femmes, littérature, culture au XVIe siècle en France,' Danielle Haase-Dubosc and Eliane Viennot, eds. *Femmes et pouvoirs sous l'Ancien Régime* (Paris: Rivages, 1991), 101–19.

————. *Images littéraires de la femme à la Renaissance* (Paris: Presses universitaires de France, 1985).

————, 'Médecins contre matrones au 16e siècle: La difficile naissance de l'obstétrique,' Marc Bertrand, ed. *Popular Tradition and Learned Culture in France* (Saratoga: Anma Libri, 1985), 25–41.

Lehoux, Françoise. *Le cadre de vie des médecins parisiens aux XVIe et XVIIe siècles* (Paris: Picard, 1976).

Lévy-Valensi, Joseph. *La médecine et les médecins français au XVIIe siècle* (Paris: Baillière, 1933).

Lindemann, Mary. *Medicine and Society in Early Modern Europe* (Cambridge: Cambridge University Press, 1999).

————, 'Professionals? Sisters? Rivals? Midwives in Braunschweig, 1750–1800,' Hilary Marland, ed. *The Art of Midwifery: Early Modern Midwives in Europe* (London: Routledge, 1993), 176–91.

Lingo, Alison Klairmont, 'Print's Role in the Politics of Women's Health Care in Early Modern France,' Barbara B. Diefendorf and Carla Hesse, eds. *Culture and Identity in Early Modern Europe (1500–1800): Essays in Honor of Natalie Zemon Davis* (Ann Arbor: The University of Michigan Press, 1993), 203–21.

————, 'Empirics and Charlatans in Early Modern France: The Genesis of the Classification of the "Other" in Medical Practice,' *Journal of Social History* 19 (1986), 583–604.

Long, Kathleen P., ed. *High Anxiety: Masculinity in Crisis in Early Modern France* (Kirksville: Truman State University Press, 2002).

————, 'Jacques Duval on Hermaphrodites,' Kathleen Long, ed. *High Anxiety: Masculinity in Crisis in Early Modern France* (Kirksville: Truman State University, 2002), 107–38.

Loudon, Irvine. *Death in Childbirth: An International Study of Maternal Care and Maternal Mortality 1800–1950* (Oxford: Clarendon, 1992).

————, 'Deaths in Childbed from the Eighteenth Century to 1935,' *Medical History* 30 (1986), 1–41.

Maclean, Ian. *Woman Triumphant: Feminism in French Literature 1610–1652* (Oxford: Clarendon, 1977).

Marin, Louis. *Portrait of the King*, Martha M. Houle, trans. (Minneapolis: University of Minnesota Press, 1988).

Marland, Hilary, '"Stately and Dignified, Kindly and God-fearing": Midwives, Age and Status in the Netherlands in the Eighteenth Century,' Hilary Marland and Margaret Pelling, eds. *The Task of Healing: Medicine, Religion and Gender in England and the Netherlands 1450–1800* (Rotterdam: Erasmus Publishing, 1996), 271–305.

————, 'The *"burgerlijke"* Midwife: The *stadsvroedvrouw* of Eighteenth-Century Holland,' Hilary Marland, ed. *The Art of Midwifery: Early Modern Midwives in Europe* (London: Routledge, 1993), 192–213.

————, trans. and ed. *'Mother and Child Were Saved'. The Memoirs (1693–1740) of the Frisian Midwife Catharina Schrader* (Amsterdam: Rodopi, 1987).

Martin, Henri-Jean. *The History and Power of Writing*, Lydia G. Cochrane, trans. (Chicago: University of Chicago Press, 1994).

————. *Print, Power, and People in 17th-Century France*, David Gerard, trans. (Metuchen: Scarecrow, 1993).

————. *Le livre français sous l'Ancien Régime* (Paris: Promodis, 1987).

————. *Livre, pouvoirs et société à Paris au XVIIe siècle (1598–1701)*, vol. 1 (Geneva: Droz, 1969).

Martin, Henri-Jean, Chartier, Roger and Jean-Pierre Vivet. *Histoire de l'édition française* (Paris: Promodis, 1982).

Maruitte, Émile-Jules-Alfred. *Paul Portal. Sa vie. Son oeuvre* (Paris: Steinheil, 1900).

McCartney, Elizabeth, 'The King's Mother and Royal Prerogative in Early-Sixteenth-Century France,' John Carmi Parsons, ed. *Medieval Queenship* (New York: St. Martin's Press, 1993), 117–41.

McClive, Cathy, 'The Hidden Truths of the Belly: The Uncertainties of Pregnancy in Early Modern Europe,' *Social History of Medicine* 15, 2 (2002), 209–27.

McGrath, Roberta. *Seeing Her Sex: Medical Archives and the Female Body* (Manchester: Manchester University Press, 2002).

McLaren, Angus. *A History of Contraception: From Antiquity to the Present Day* (Oxford: Blackwell, 1990).

McTavish, Lianne, 'On Display: Portraits of Seventeenth-Century French Men-Midwives,' *Social History of Medicine* 14.3 (December 2001), 389–415.

————, 'Figuring the Hand: Portraits of Artists and Surgeons in Seventeenth-Century France'(unpublished paper presented at the Portraiture and Scientific Identity conference, National Portrait Gallery, London, 2000).

Melot, Michel, Griffiths, Antony, Richard S. Field, and André Béguin, *Prints: History of an Art* (New York: Rizzoli, 1981).

Melzer, Sara E. and Norberg, Kathryn, eds. *From the Royal to the Republican Body: Incorporating the Political in Seventeenth- and Eighteenth-Century France* (Berkeley: University of California Press, 1998).

Middelkoop, Norbert E., '"Large and Magnificent Paintings, all Pertaining to the Chirurgeon's Art". The Art Collection of the Amsterdam Surgeons' Guild,' Ben Broos et al., eds. *Rembrandt Under the Scalpel: The Anatomy Lesson of Dr Nicolaes Tulp Dissected* (Mauritshuis, The Hague: Six Art Promotion, 1998), 9–38.

Millepierres, François. *La vie quotidienne des médecins au temps du Molière* (Paris: Hachette, 1964).

Miller, Naomi J. and Yavneh, Naomi, eds. *Maternal Measures: Figuring Caregiving in the Early Modern Period* (Aldershot: Ashgate, 2000).

Mink, Bruce, 'American Cancer Society's "Smoking Fetus,"' *American Cinematographer* 66 (August 1985), 77–80.

Moi, Toril, 'Appropriating Bourdieu: Feminist Theory and Pierre Bourdieu's Sociology of Culture,' *New Literary History* 22 (1991), 1017–49.

Montagu, Jennifer. *The Expression of the Passions: The Origin and Influence of Charles Le Brun's 'Conférence sur l'expression générale et particulière'* (New Haven: Yale University Press, 1994).

Mortimer, Ruth. *A Portrait of the Author in Sixteenth-Century France* (Chapel Hill: University of North Carolina Press, 1980).

Nance, Brian. *Turquet de Mayerne as Baroque Physician: The Art of Medical Portraiture* (Amsterdam: Rodopi, 2001).

Neale, Stephen, 'Genre and Cinema,' Tony Bennett et al., eds. *Popular Television and Film* (London: British Film Institute/Open University Press, 1981), 6–25.

Newman, Karen. *Fetal Positions: Individualism, Science, Visuality* (Stanford: Stanford University Press, 1996).

Nutton, Vivian, 'Beyond the Hippocratic Oath,' Andrew Wear et al., eds. *Doctors and Ethics: The Earlier Historical Setting of Professional Ethics* (Amsterdam: Rodopi, 1993), 10–37.

————, 'The Anatomy of the Soul in Early Renaissance Medicine,' G. R. Dunstan, ed. *The Human Embryo: Aristotle and the Arabic and European Traditions* (Exeter: University of Exeter Press, 1990), 136–57.

Oakley, Ann, 'Wisewoman and Medicine Man: Changes in the Management of Childbirth,' Juliet Mitchell and Ann Oakley, eds. *The Rights and Wrongs of Women* (Harmondsworth: Penguin, 1976), 17–58.

Olivier, Louis, '"Curieux", Amateurs and Connoisseurs: Laymen and the Fine Arts in the Ancien Régime' (Ph.D. Diss., The Johns Hopkins University, 1976).

Olson, Todd P. *Poussin and France: Painting, Humanism, and the Politics of Style* (New Haven: Yale University Press, 2002).

Orr, Clarissa Campbell, ed. *Queenship in Britain, 1660–1837* (Manchester: Manchester University Press, 2002).

Panel, G. *Jacques Mesnard, chirurgien et accoucheur (1685–1746) et ses oeuvres* (Rouen: Lestringant, 1889).

Panofsky, Erwin. *Studies in Iconology: Humanistic Themes in the Art of the Renaissance* (New York: Harper and Row, 1962).

Park, Katharine and Nye, Robert A., 'Destiny is Anatomy,' *The New Republic* (February 18, 1991), 53–7.

Pears, Iain. *The Discovery of Painting: The Growth of Interest in the Arts in England, 1680–1768* (New Haven: Yale University Press, 1988).

Peirce, Charles Sanders, 'Prolegomena to an Apology for Pragmaticism,' James Hoopes, ed. *Peirce on Signs: Writings on Semiotics by Charles Sanders Peirce* (Chapel Hill: University of North Carolina Press, 1991), 249–52.

————. *Collected Papers*, vol. 1–6, Charles Hartshorne and Paul Weiss, eds (Cambridge, MA: Belknap Press of Harvard University Press, 1931–1935).

————. *The New Elements of Mathematics*, Carolyn Eisele, ed. (The Hague: Mouton, 1976).

Perkins, Wendy. *Midwifery and Medicine in Early Modern France: Louise Bourgeois* (Exeter: University of Exeter Press, 1996).

————, 'Midwives versus Doctors: The Case of Louise Bourgeois,' *Seventeenth Century* 3 (1988), 135–57.

Petchesky, Rosalind Pollack, 'Foetal Images: The Power of Visual Culture in the Politics of Reproduction,' Michelle Stanworth, ed. *Reproductive Technologies: Gender, Motherhood and Medicine* (Minneapolis: University of Minnesota Press, 1987), 57–80.

Petrelli, Richard L., 'The Regulation of French Midwifery during the *Ancien Régime*,' *Journal of the History of Medicine* 27 (1971), 276–92.

Pharies, David A. *Charles S. Peirce and the Linguistic Sign* (Amsterdam: John Benjamins Publishing, 1985).

Placet, Émile. *L'obstétrique aux XVIIe et XVIIIe siècles. Viardel, Portal, et Mauquest de La Motte* (Paris: Baillière, 1892).

Plottel, Jeanine Parisier and Charney, Hanna, eds. *Inter-textuality: New Perspectives in Criticism* (New York: New York Literary Forum, 1978).

Pointon, Marcia. *Hanging the Head: Portraiture and Social Formation in Eighteenth-Century England* (New Haven: Yale University Press, 1993).

Pollock, Griselda. *Vision and Difference: Femininity, Feminism and Histories of Art* (London: Routledge, 1988).

Pomata, Gianna, 'Menstruating Men: Similarity and Difference of the Sexes in Early Modern Medicine,' Valeria Finucci and Kevin Brownlee, eds. *Generation and Degeneration: Tropes of Reproduction in Literature and History from Antiquity to Early Modern Europe* (Durham: Duke University Press, 2001), 109–52.

Porter, Roy. *Bodies Politic: Disease, Death, and Doctors in Britain, 1650–1900* (London: Reaktion Books, 2001).

————. *Quacks: Fakers and Charlatans in English Medicine* (Stroud, Gloucestershire: Tempus, 2000).

————. *Medicine: A History of Healing* (New York: Marlowe, 1997).

————, 'A Touch of Danger: The Man-Midwife as Sexual Predator,' G. S. Rousseau and Roy Porter, eds. *Sexual Underworlds of the Enlightenment* (Chapel Hill: University of North Carolina Press, 1988), 206–32.

Posner, Donald, 'Concerning the "Mechanical" Parts of Painting and the Artistic Culture of Seventeenth-Century France,' *Art Bulletin* 75 (1993), 583–98.

Pouchelle, Marie-Christine. *The Body and Surgery in the Middle Ages*, Rosemary Morris, trans. (New Brunswick: Rutgers University Press, 1990).

Poulain, François. *La vie et l'oeuvre de deux chirurgiens: Jacques Guillemeau (1550–1613) et Charles Guillemeau (1588–1656)* (Université de Montpellier I, Faculté de Médecine, 1993).

Préaud, Maxime. *Inventaire du fonds français: graveurs du XVIIe siècle*, vol. 10 (Paris: Bibliothèque nationale, 1989).

Radcliffe, Walter. *Milestones in Midwifery* (Bristol: Wright & Sons, 1967).

Ramsey, Matthew, 'The Popularization of Medicine in France, 1650–1900,' Roy Porter, ed. *The Popularization of Medicine, 1650–1850* (New York: Routledge, 1992), 97–133.

Ravel, Jeffrey, 'Le Derrière du cocher: une soirée interrompue au XVIIIe siècle' (unpublished communication presented at the École normale supérieure, Paris in 2003).

Read, Kirk, 'Mother's Milk from Father's Breast: Maternity without Women in Male French Renaissance Lyric,' Kathleen P. Long, ed. *High Anxiety: Masculinity in Crisis in Early Modern France* (Kirksville: Truman State University Press, 2002), 71–92.

Ricci, James V. *The Genealogy of Gynaecology: History of the Development of Gynaecology throughout the Ages, 2000 B.C.–1800 A.D.* (Philadelphia: Blakiston, 1943).

Riddle, John M. *Eve's Herbs: A History of Contraception and Abortion in the West* (Cambridge, MA: Harvard University Press, 1997).

————. *Contraception and Abortion from the Ancient World to the Renaissance* (Cambridge, MA: Harvard University Press, 1992).

Rigal, Jeanne. *La communauté des maîtres-chirurgiens jurés de Paris au XVIIe et au XVIIIe siècle* (Paris: Vigot Frères, 1936).

Roach, Joseph, 'Body of Law: The Sun King and the Code Noir,' Melzer, Sara E. and Norberg, Kathryn, eds. *From the Royal to the Republican Body: Incorporating the Political in Seventeenth- and Eighteenth-Century France* (Berkeley: University of California Press, 1998), 113–30.

Roberts, Don D. *The Existential Graphs of Charles S. Peirce* (The Hague: Mouton, 1973).

Roberts, K. B. and Tomlinson, J. D. W. *The Fabric of the Body: European Traditions of Anatomical Illustrations* (Oxford: Clarendon, 1992).

Roger, Jacques. *The Life Sciences in Eighteenth-Century French Thought*, Robert Ellrich, trans. (Stanford: Stanford University Press, 1997).

Roodenburg, Herman, 'How to Sit, Stand, and Walk: Toward a Historical Anthropology of Dutch Paintings and Prints,' Wayne Franits, ed. *Looking at Seventeenth-Century Dutch Art: Realism Reconsidered* (Cambridge: Cambridge University Press, 1997), 175–86.

————, 'The Maternal Imagination: The Fears of Pregnant Women in Seventeenth-Century Holland,' *Journal of Social History* 21, 4 (1988), 701–16.

Rose, Gillian. *Visual Methodologies* (London: Sage, 2001).

Rosso, Jeannette Geffriaud. *Études sur la féminité aux XVIIe et XVIIe siècles* (Pisa: Libreria Goliardica, 1984).

Rouget, François, 'De la sage-femme à la femme sage: réflexion et réflexivité dans les *Observations* de Louise Boursier,' *Papers on French Seventeenth-Century Literature* 25, 49 (1998), 483–96.

Rowland, Beryl. *Medieval Woman's Guide to Health: The First English Gynecological Handbook* (Kent: Kent State University Press, 1981).

Savan, David. *An Introduction to C.S. Peirce's Semiotics*, vol. 1 (Toronto: Toronto Semiotic Circle, 1976).

Sawday, Jonathan. *The Body Emblazoned: Dissection and the Human Body in Renaissance Culture* (London: Routledge, 1995).

Schofield, Roger, 'Did the Mothers Really Die? Three Centuries of Maternal Mortality in "The World We Have Lost",' Lloyd Bonfield et al., eds. *The World We Have Gained* (Oxford: Blackwell, 1986), 231–60.

Scott, Joan Wallach. *Gender and the Politics of History* (New York: Columbia University Press, 1999).

Scott, Katie and Warwick, Genevieve, eds. *Commemorating Poussin: Reception and Interpretation of the Artist* (Cambridge: Cambridge University Press, 1999).

Sebeok, Thomas A., 'Iconicity,' *MLN* 91, 6 (December 1976), 1427–56.

Sedgwick, Eve Kosofsky, 'Gosh, Boy George, You Must be Awfully Secure in your Masculinity!' Maurice Berger, Brian Wallis, and Simon Watson, eds. *Constructing Masculinity* (New York: Routledge, 1995), 11–20.

————. *Epistemology of the Closet* (Berkeley: University of California Press, 1990).

Sheridan, Bridgette, 'At Birth: The Modern State, Modern Medicine, and the Royal Midwife Louise Bourgeois in Seventeenth-Century France,' *Dynamis* 19 (1999), 145–66.

Sheriff, Mary D. *The Exceptional Woman: Elisabeth Vigée-Lebrun and the Cultural Politics of Art* (Chicago: University of Chicago Press, 1996).

Siebold, Eduard Kaspar Jakob von. *Essai d'une histoire de l'obstétricie*, vol. 2 (Paris: Steinheil, 1891–1892).

Silverman, Kaja. *The Subject of Semiotics* (New York: Oxford University Press, 1983).

Silverman, Lisa. *Tortured Subjects: Pain, Truth, and the Body in Early Modern France* (Chicago: University of Chicago Press, 2001).

Siraisi, Nancy G. *Medieval and Early Renaissance Medicine: An Introduction to Knowledge and Practice* (Chicago: University of Chicago Press, 1990).

Smith, Hilda, 'Gynecology and Ideology in Seventeenth-Century England,' Berenice A. Carroll, ed. *Liberating Women's History: Theoretical and Critical Essays* (Urbana: University of Illinois Press, 1976), 97–114.

Solomon-Godeau, Abigail, 'Male Trouble,' Maurice Berger, Brian Wallis, and Simon Watson, eds. *Constructing Masculinity* (New York: Routledge, 1995), 68–76.

Speert, Harold. *Obstetric and Gynecologic Milestones Illustrated* (New York: Parthenon, 1996).

Spicer, Joaneath, 'The Renaissance Elbow,' Jan Bremmer and Herman Roodenburg, eds. *A Cultural History of Gesture* (Ithaca: Cornell University Press, 1991), 84–128.

Squier, Susan, 'Fetal Subjects and Maternal Objects: Reproductive Technology and the New Fetal/Maternal Relation,' *Journal of Medicine and Philosophy* 21 (October 1996), 515–35.

Stabile, Carol A., 'The Traffic in Fetuses,' Lynn M. Morgan and Meredith W. Michaels, eds. *Fetal Subjects, Feminist Positions* (Philadelphia: University of Pennsylvania Press, 1999), 133–58.

Stafford, Barbara Maria. *Body Criticism: Imaging the Unseen in Enlightenment Art and Medicine* (Cambridge, MA: MIT Press, 1991).

Stam, Robert. *Film Theory: An Introduction* (Oxford: Blackwell, 2000).

Stanton, Domna C., 'Recuperating Women and the Man Behind the Screen,' James Grantham Turner, ed. *Sexuality and Gender in Early Modern Europe: Institutions, Texts, Images* (Cambridge: Cambridge University Press, 1993), 247–65.

Stofft, Henri, 'Ambroise Paré, accoucheur,' *Histoire des sciences médicales* 32, 4 (1998), 399–407.

Stolberg, Michael, 'A Woman Down to Her Bones: The Anatomy of Sexual Difference in the Sixteenth and Early Seventeenth Centuries,' *Isis* 94 (2003), 274–99.

Swales, John M. *Genre Analysis* (Cambridge: Cambridge University Press, 1990).

Tatlock, Lynne, 'Speculum Feminarum: Gendered Perspectives on Obstetrics and Gynecology in Early Modern Germany,' *Signs* 17, 4 (1992), 725–60.

Talvacchia, Bette, 'Mythology, Sexuality, and Science in Charles Estienne's Manual of Anatomy,' *Taking Positions: On the Erotic in Renaissance Culture* (Princeton: Princeton University Press, 1999), 161–87.

Taylor, Janelle S., 'The Public Fetus and the Family Car: From Abortion Politics to a Volvo Advertisement,' *Public Culture* 4, 2 (1992), 67–80.

Thomas, T H. *French Portrait Engraving of the XVIIth and XVIIIth Centuries* (London: G. Bell, 1910).

Thuillier, Jacques, 'Académie et classicisme en France: Les débuts de l'Académie royale de peinture et de sculpture (1648–63),' S. Bottari, ed. *Il Mito del Classicismo nel Seicento* (Messina/Florence: G. d'Anna, 1964), 181–209.

Trafton, Dain A., 'Politics and the Praise of Women: Political Doctrine in the *Courtier*'s Third Book,' Robert W. Hanning and David Rosand, eds. *Castiglione: The Ideal and the Real in Renaissance Culture* (New Haven: Yale University Press, 1983), 29–44.

Traub, Valerie, Kaplan, M. Lindsay and Dympna Callaghan, eds. *Feminist Readings of Early Modern Culture: Emerging Subjects* (Cambridge: Cambridge University Press, 1996).

Traub, Valerie, 'Gendering Mortality in Early Modern Anatomies,' Valerie Traub, M. Lindsay Kaplan and Dympna Callaghan, eds. *Feminist Readings of Early Modern Culture: Emerging Subjects* (Cambridge: Cambridge University Press, 1996), 44–92.

Tucker, Holly. *Pregnant Fictions: Childbirth and the Fairy Tale in Early-Modern France* (Detroit: Wayne State University Press, 2003).

Vigarello, Georges, 'The Upward Training of the Body from the Age of Chivalry to Courtly Civility,' Michel Feher, ed. *Zone: Fragments for a History of the Human Body*, vol. 2 (New York: Urzone, 1989), 149–99.

———. *Concepts of Cleanliness: Changing Attitudes in France since the Middle Ages*, Jean Birrell, trans. (Cambridge: Cambridge University Press, 1988).

Waldby, Catherine. *The Visible Human Project* (New York: Routledge, 2000).

Weiden, R. M. F. van der and Hoogsteder, W. J., 'A New Light Upon Hendrik van Deventer (1651–1724): Identification and Recovery of a Portrait,' *Journal of the Royal Society of Medicine* 90 (October 1997), 567–9.

Weigert, Roger-Armand. *Inventaire du fonds français: graveurs du XVIIe siècle*, vol. 3 (Paris: Bibliothèque nationale, 1954).

Welch, Evelyn. *Art and Society in Italy 1350–1500* (Oxford: Oxford University Press, 1997).

Wells, Robin Headlam. *Shakespeare on Masculinity* (Cambridge: Cambridge University Press, 2000).

Wiesner, Merry E. *Women and Gender in Early Modern Europe* (Cambridge: Cambridge University Press, 1993).

———, 'Early Modern Midwifery: A Case Study,' *International Journal of Women's Studies* 6, 1 (1983), 26–43.

Wilson, Adrian. *The Making of Man-Midwifery: Childbirth in England 1660–1770* (London: UCL Press, 1995).

———, 'The Perils of Early Modern Procreation: Childbirth With or Without Fear?' *British Journal for Eighteenth-Century Studies* 16 (Spring 1993), 1–19.

————, 'The Ceremony of Childbirth and its Interpretation,' Valerie Fildes, ed. *Women as Mothers in Pre-Industrial England* (London: Routledge, 1990), 68–107.

————, 'Ignorant Midwives – a Rejoinder,' *Society for the Social History of Medicine Bulletin* 32 (1983), 46–9.

Wind, Barry. *'A Foul and Pestilent Congregation': Images of 'Freaks' in Baroque Art* (Aldershot: Ashgate, 1998).

Winn, Colette H., 'De sage (-) femme à sage (-) fille: Louise Boursier, *Instructions à ma Fille* [1626],' *Papers on French Seventeenth-Century Literature* 24, 46 (1997), 61–83.

Wolfe, Michael, ed. *Changing Identities in Early Modern France* (Durham: Duke University Press, 1996).

Zanger, Abby. *Scenes from the Marriage of Louis XIV: Nuptial Fictions and the Making of Absolutist Power* (Stanford: Stanford University Press, 1997).

Zapperi, Roberto. *The Pregnant Man* (Chur, Switzerland: Harwood Academic Publishers, 1991).

Index

Index

251